FOCUS Psychiatry Review:
Volume 2

AMERICAN PSYCHIATRIC ASSOCIATION

FOCUS Psychiatry Review: Volume 2

A workbook with questions covering the
ABPN outline of topics for recertification:

Anxiety Disorders
Child and Adolescent Psychiatry
Disorders of Sleep, Eating, and Sex
Ethics and Professionalism
Genetics and Genomics
Geriatric Psychiatry
Mood Disorders
Obsessive-Compulsive Disorder
Personality and Temperament
Posttraumatic Stress Disorder and Disaster Psychiatry
Psychopharmacology
Psychosomatic Medicine
Psychotherapy
Schizophrenia
Substance Abuse

Editors

Deborah J. Hales, M.D.

Mark Hyman Rapaport, M.D.

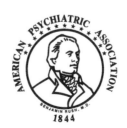

American Psychiatric Association
1000 Wilson Boulevard
Arlington, VA 22209-3901
www.psych.org

ISBN-13: 978-0-89042-346-2

Contents

Introduction

In today's world it is hard to keep up with the explosive growth in knowledge. Psychiatric practice is rapidly improving thanks to developments in evidence-based practice and advances in neuroscience research. The editors of *FOCUS* developed the *FOCUS Psychiatry Review* as an aid for psychiatrists in lifelong learning in the field. This workbook contains 400 board-type multiple-choice questions from *FOCUS*'s annual Self-Assessment Examinations that can help psychiatrists prepare for examinations and identify areas for further study. The questions, developed by the *FOCUS* self-assessment board, are consistent in form and process with the questions used by high-stakes examinations. They cover important clinical areas of psychiatric practice and closely follow the American Board of Psychiatry and Neurology (ABPN) outline of topics for the recertification examination in psychiatry.

The *FOCUS Psychiatry Review* is designed to test current knowledge and its clinical application. The workbook is flexible in format, allowing readers to use the educational approach that works best for them. Readers can review resource materials prior to answering questions, or they can use the workbook to review the references listed in the critiques after scoring test sections.

The workbook will be useful for anyone committed to lifelong learning in the field—psychiatric residents, practicing psychiatrists, and psychiatrists preparing for examinations.

- The *FOCUS Psychiatry Review* contains 400 clinical questions that can be used to identify areas of strength and weakness.
- It provides up-to-date critiques and current references to facilitate further study.
- It is a complementary component to a larger overall program of lifelong learning for the psychiatrist who wants to keep current in the field.

This volume covers the following topics:

Anxiety Disorders

Child and Adolescent Psychiatry

Disorders of Sleep, Eating, and Sex

Ethics and Professionalism

Genetics and Genomics

Geriatric Psychiatry

Mood Disorders

Obsessive-Compulsive Disorder

Personality and Temperament

Posttraumatic Stress Disorder and Disaster Psychiatry

Psychopharmacology

Psychosomatic Medicine

Psychotherapy

Schizophrenia

Substance Abuse

The *FOCUS Psychiatry Review* provides up to 50 hours of Continuing Medical Education Credit.

APA is accredited by ACCME to provide continuing medical education for physicians.
APA designates this educational activity for a maximum of 50 AMA PRA Category 1 Credits.™ Physicians should claim only the credit commensurate with the extent of their participation in the activity.

Educational Objectives

At the completion of the activity, participants will
1) have an increased understanding of new developments in psychiatric diagnosis and treatment;
2) be aware of resources available for learning more about these developments; and
3) recognize areas of strength and areas where more study is needed.

FOCUS Self-Assessment Editors and Editorial Board
Disclosure of Financial Interests or Other Affiliations With Commercial Organizations

Annette M. Matthews, M.D.
Psychiatrist, Portland Veterans Affairs Medical Center, Portland, Oregon, Assistant Professor of Psychiatry, Oregon Health and Science University, Portland, Oregon
No financial affiliations with commercial organizations

David W. Preven, M.D.
Clinical Professor in the Department of Behavioral Sciences and Psychiatry, Albert Einstein College of Medicine, Montefiore Medical Center, Bronx, New York
Speaker: Pfizer, Forest

Rima Styra, M.D.
Toronto General Hospital, University Health Network, Department of Psychiatry, Toronto, Ontario, Canada
No financial affiliations with commercial organizations

Lowell D. Tong, M.D.
Associate Chair of Education, Department of Psychiatry, University of California San Francisco School of Medicine
No financial affiliations with commercial organizations

Marcia L. Verduin, M.D.
Associate Professor of Psychiatry, Assistant Dean for Students, University of Central Florida College of Medicine, Orlando, Florida
Grant/Research Support: Robert Wood Johnson Foundation

Eric R. Williams, M.D.
Assistant Professor of Child and Adolescent Psychiatry, University of South Carolina School of Medicine, Charleston, South Carolina
No financial affiliations with commercial organizations

Isaac K. Wood, M.D.
Associate Professor of Psychiatry and Pediatrics, Associate Dean of Student Activities, Director of Medical Student Education in Psychiatry, Virginia Commonwealth University School of Medicine, Richmond, Virginia
No financial affiliations with commercial organizations

Joel Yager, M.D.
Professor, Department of Psychiatry, School of Medicine, University of Colorado; Emeritus Professor, Department of Psychiatry at the University of New Mexico School of Medicine and Department of Psychiatry and Biobehavioral Sciences at the the David Geffen School of Medicine at UCLA
No financial affiliations with commercial organizations

Disclosure of Unapproved or Investigational Use of a Product

FOCUS examination questions may contain information on off-label uses of particular medications. Off-label use of medications by individual physicians is permitted and common. Decisions about off-label use can be guided by the evidence provided in the scientific literature and by clinical experience.

To obtain Continuing Medical Education Credit, complete and send this page to:

American Psychiatric Association
Department of CME
1000 Wilson Blvd., Suite 1825
Arlington, VA 22209
Fax: 703-907-7849
educme@psych.org

Begin date: February 2011
End date: February 2014

AMERICAN PSYCHIATRIC ASSOCIATION
FOCUS Psychiatry Review: Volume 2

I have participated for _____ hours (up to 50) in completion of this CME activity.

Name (please print): _____

Address: _____

Address: _____

City/State/Zip: _____

E-mail _____ Fax _____

Please send my certificate by: Mail _____ Fax _____ E-mail _____

1. The quality of the *FOCUS Psychiatry Review* workbook was excellent.
   Strongly agree   Agree   Disagree   Strongly disagree

2. The *FOCUS Psychiatry Review* workbook was useful to me in preparing for examinations.
   Strongly agree   Agree   Disagree   Strongly disagree

3. The workbook was useful in helping me understand my areas of strength and weakness.
   Strongly agree   Agree   Disagree   Strongly disagree

4. The workbook will be helpful to me in my clinical practice.
   Strongly agree   Agree   Disagree   Strongly disagree

5. The material in the *FOCUS Psychiatry Review* was presented without bias.
   Strongly agree   Agree   Disagree   Strongly disagree

6. The questions were: too hard ____, just right ____, too easy ____.

Comments:

_____

_____

_____

Section 1: Self-Assessment Questions

1

An 18-year-old woman is brought to the emergency department after collapsing at a party. She appears delirious and confused, with a temperature of 104°F. The friends who brought her to the emergency room say that she might have taken some pills. She was talking about feeling blissful and dancing a lot until she collapsed. Which of the following is the most likely drug ingested?

(A) Methylenedioxymethamphetamine (MDMA)
(B) Ketamine
(C) Flunitrazepam
(D) Gamma-hydroxybutyrate (GHB)

2

Which one of these terms defines the most common form of genetic variation observed in the genome?

(A) Short tandem repeat
(B) Single nucleotide polymorphism
(C) Haplotype
(D) Allele
(E) Variable number of tandem repeat

3

In adults, which of the following anxiety disorders is diagnosed in equal numbers in men and women?

(A) Generalized anxiety disorder
(B) Panic disorder
(C) Specific phobia
(D) Obsessive-compulsive disorder (OCD)
(E) Obsessive-compulsive personality disorder

4

Which of the following SSRIs is most likely to be "self-tapering," thereby decreasing the chances of withdrawal effects?

(A) Citalopram
(B) Escitalopram
(C) Fluoxetine
(D) Paroxetine
(E) Sertraline

5

Dialectical behavior therapy (DBT) was developed specifically for the treatment symptoms associated with which one of the following personality disorders?

(A) Antisocial
(B) Borderline
(C) Avoidant
(D) Obsessive-compulsive
(E) Histrionic

6

The most common cause of treatment failure in HIV/AIDS patients on antiretroviral medications is that most patients:

(A) have infections that are resistant to most available medications.
(B) fail to maintain the required adherence to the medication regime.
(C) do not start treatment until the infection is in the terminal stages.
(D) refuse to participate in medical treatment and take medications.
(E) have such severe side effects that medications cannot be used.

7

Advanced paternal age is a well established risk factor for which of the following psychiatric illnesses?

(A) Schizophrenia
(B) Substance dependence
(C) Major depressive disorder
(D) Generalized anxiety disorder

8

A 21-year-old woman presents with questions about her risk of developing schizophrenia. She is worried because her 18-year-old brother has recently been diagnosed with schizophrenia and required hospitalization for psychosis. There are no other family members who have a history of schizophrenia. Having a sibling with schizophrenia increases a person's risk of developing schizophrenia by approximately what amount?

(A) the sibling is no more likely to develop schizophrenia
(B) the risk of developing schizophrenia for a sibling is 50%
(C) the risk of developing schizophrenia for a sibling is 10 fold
(D) the risk of developing schizophrenia is 30 fold
(E) it is almost certain the sibling will develop schizophrenia

9

An 18-year-old female has high scores on scales of the personality traits of Harm Avoidance and Reward Dependence. Based on these personality traits, she is at HIGHEST risk for developing which one of the following disorders?

(A) Anorexia nervosa
(B) Major depressive disorder
(C) Obsessive-compulsive disorder
(D) Schizophrenia
(E) Social anxiety disorder

10

A 40-year-old man with a 20-year history of heroin dependence and high tolerance is admitted to the hospital for IV antibiotic treatment of bacterial endocarditis. To prevent opioid withdrawal, considering his opioid tolerance, he is prescribed a moderately high dose of buprenorphine. He is just beginning to experience withdrawal symptoms before the first buprenorphine dose, but shortly thereafter, his anxiety, muscle aches and rhinorrhea worsen. At this point the best option would be to:

(A) increase the dose of buprenorphine.
(B) decrease the dose of buprenorphine.
(C) change to methadone.
(D) add a benzodiazepine.
(E) add naltrexone.

11

A 35-year-old man with obsessive-compulsive disorder presents for treatment. He would prefer not using medication due to possible side effects. Which of the following psychotherapies would be the treatment of choice for his disorder?

(A) Supportive psychotherapy
(B) Exposure with response prevention
(C) Hypnotherapy
(D) Interpersonal therapy
(E) Psychodynamic psychotherapy

12

An adolescent with mild mental retardation continues to be significantly depressed despite actively participating in psychotherapy for several months. Which of the following is the best clinical option?

(A) Start treatment with an atypical antipsychotic
(B) Start treatment with an SSRI
(C) Change psychotherapeutic approaches
(D) Implement intense behavioral management

13

Personalities characterized by the traits of persistence, perfectionism, and decreased flexibility in "set shifting," i.e. the ability to move back and forth between tasks, operations or mental sets, are associated with which of the following disorders?

(A) Alcohol dependence in full-sustained remission
(B) Delusional disorder
(C) Anorexia nervosa
(D) Early Alzheimer's disease
(E) Traumatic brain injury

14

Which of the following treatments is considered the best approach to managing a patient with panic disorder, unresponsive to initial treatments with an SSRI and a benzodiazepine?

(A) SNRI
(B) Buspirone
(C) Atypical antipsychotic
(D) Another SSRI
(E) CBT

15

A 27-year-old man has borderline personality disorder, primarily manifested by an inability to control his urges to hurt himself. As a result, when frustrated, he will frequently superficially cut his wrists. Which of the following medications has been found to be most helpful in curbing this behavior?

(A) Olanzapine
(B) Fluoxetine
(C) Clonazepam
(D) Divalproex
(E) Naloxone

16

A visibly pregnant 29-year-old woman presents seeking treatment for oxycodone dependence. Because of her pregnancy, she wants to stop using all drugs and does not want to take any medications. She went through untreated opiate withdrawal in the past when she couldn't get any pills, and while it was very uncomfortable, she thinks she could do it again with intensive social support and counseling. At this point the best treatment recommendation would be to initiate:

(A) methadone maintenance.
(B) methadone-assisted withdrawal.
(C) clonidine-naltrexone assisted withdrawal.
(D) buprenorphine maintenance.
(E) daily clinic visits to provide support.

17

A 38-year-old female patient with schizophrenia has been treated with haloperidol and risperidone at different times in the past. Currently, she exhibits a non-rhythmical hyperkinetic movement disorder of the lips and jaw. The movement disorder most likely consistent with this finding is:

(A) akathisia (motor restlessness).
(B) Parkinsonian's tremor.
(C) tardive dyskinesia.
(D) tardive dystonia.

18

Which one of the following dimensions assessed on the Temperament and Character Inventory (TCI) is MOST likely to increase with age?

(A) Cooperativeness
(B) Harm avoidance
(C) Persistence
(D) Reward dependence
(E) Self-transcendence

19

A 74-year-old man presents with a history of rapidly progressive cognitive decline with ataxia, multifocal myoclonic jerks and visual field cut. MRI reveals increased T2 and FLAIR signal intensity in the basal ganglia. Which of the following is the most likely diagnosis?

(A) Alzheimer's dementia
(B) Huntington's chorea
(C) Creutzfeldt-Jakob disease
(D) Vascular dementia
(E) Lewy body disease

20

Recent genome-wide association studies (GWAS) have implicated regions of which chromosome in autism spectrum disorders (ASD)?

(A) Chromosome 1
(B) Chromosome 5
(C) Chromosome 8
(D) Chromosome 22

21

A 16-year-old woman presents with fatigue and dehydration. On physical examination she is noted to have swollen salivary glands and calluses on her knuckles. She is also hypokalemic. These findings are most consistent with which of the following diagnoses?

(A) Chronic fatigue syndrome
(B) Bulimia nervosa
(C) Obsessive-compulsive disorder
(D) Anorexia nervosa
(E) Rumination disorder

22

A 21-year old college student is seen in the University counseling center because of relationship problems. He has had one serious relationship with a woman that lasted about six months. He terminated the relationship because he discovered that the woman was seeing someone else. Although he wants to engage in a new relationship, he is extremely reluctant stating: "Women just can't be trusted." Which of the following BEST describes this thinking error?

(A) Arbitrary inference
(B) Dichotomous thinking
(C) Magnification
(D) Overgeneralization
(E) Selective abstraction

23

A 40-year-old patient is diagnosed with Alzheimer's disease. Which of the following genes is associated with this very early form of Alzheimer's disease?

(A) Presenilin 1
(B) Presenilin 2
(C) Apo E2
(D) Apo E3
(E) Apo E4

24

During an interview of a patient with a substance abuse disorder, the therapist asks the patient about the pros and cons of specific behaviors, explores the patient's goals and associated ambivalence about reaching those goals, and listens reflectively to the patient's response. This treatment approach is most consistent with:

(A) cognitive-behavioral therapy.
(B) contingency management.
(C) interpersonal therapy.
(D) motivational enhancement therapy.
(E) psychodynamic psychotherapy.

25

Which of the following antidepressants has the greatest body of evidence for efficacy in treating major depressive disorder in children and adolescents?

(A) Citalopram
(B) Fluoxetine
(C) Fluvoxamine
(D) Sertraline
(E) Paroxetine

26

A city is attacked by terrorists intermittently over a three-week period. There is no indication that the attacks will stop. Which of the following interventions is most likely to be effective in lowering the risk of developing PTSD in the months following exposure?

(A) Educating the public about symptoms of PTSD
(B) Evacuating the most vulnerable population
(C) Limiting exposure to media coverage of the attacks
(D) Providing psychological debriefing to survivors
(E) Reestablishing a relative sense of safety

27

Defining high-risk situations, covert antecedents, and stimulus control techniques are a focus of which of the following therapeutic modalities?

(A) Brief psychodynamic psychotherapy
(B) Cognitive behavioral therapy
(C) Supportive therapy
(D) Interpersonal therapy
(E) Relapse prevention therapy

28

A 42-year-old patient with schizophrenia presents to the emergency department with confusion and agitation following an overdose of antipsychotic medication. The patient has a temperature of 101.7°F, blood pressure of 140/80 mm Hg, and pulse of 112. Physical examination reveals hot, dry skin, dilated pupils, and decreased bowel sounds. This patient's symptoms are most likely caused by medication effects at which of the following receptors?

(A) Muscarinic cholinergic
(B) Nicotinic cholinergic
(C) α1-adrenergic
(D) Histaminergic
(E) Dopaminergic

29

Which of the following therapies for borderline personality disorder incorporates psychoeducation about the illness, emotional management skills training, and behavior skills training?

(A) Mentalization based therapy
(B) Schema-focused therapy
(C) Trauma-focused cognitive-behavior therapy
(D) Eye movement desensitization and reprocessing
(E) Systems Training for Emotional Predictability and Problem Solving

30

When managing a chronically suicidal patient, respecting the patient's preference to remain at home and not be admitted to the psychiatric unit for additional care reflects which of the following ethical principles?

(A) Autonomy
(B) Beneficience
(C) Non-Maleficence
(D) Egalitarianism

31

A 12-year-old boy is hospitalized after a serious suicide attempt. His parents report that they noticed a difference in his behavior about a year ago. He became increasingly withdrawn; was preoccupied with mythical creatures; his academic performance declined significantly, he had difficulty sleeping and a decreased appetite. Over the past two months, he has seemed progressively worse. He has demonstrated both persecutory and somatic delusions; has reported he hears voices telling him to "beware–they are watching you–you're a naughty little boy." Today he heard a voice telling him that he was "rotting inside" and in response, he attempted to hang himself. On examination he denies a mood disturbance. His thinking is illogical and non-linear. What is the most likely diagnosis?

(A) Bipolar disorder
(B) Attention-deficit/hyperactivity disorder
(C) Schizophrenia
(D) Major depressive disorder
(E) Asperger's syndrome

32

Individuals with two copies of which one of the following genes develop Alzheimer's disease eight times more frequently than those without it?

(A) Apo E1
(B) Apo E2
(C) Apo E3
(D) Apo E4
(E) Apo E5

33

In addition to the neuroticism, extraversion, openness, and conscientious facets of personality, the fifth facet of personality being considered as an alternative or complement to the classification for personality disorders in the revision of the Diagnostic and Statistical Manual of Mental Disorders (DSM) is which ONE of the following?

(A) Agreeableness
(B) Brightness
(C) Happiness
(D) Humor
(E) Optimism

34

A 32-year-old man with a history of bipolar I disorder has been off all medication for over six months. He currently presents with symptoms consistent with a moderately severe major depressive episode. Which of the following has the best evidence as a pharmacologic treatment for him?

(A) Clonazepam and lithium
(B) Olanzapine and fluoxetine
(C) Lithium and paroxetine
(D) Valproate and fluoxetine
(E) Bupropion alone

35

Which of the following psychiatric disorders confers the highest genetic relative risk for first degree relatives?

(A) Panic disorder
(B) Alcoholism
(C) Major depression
(D) Bipolar disorder
(E) Schizophrenia

36

A 35-year-old woman began taking citalopram, 20 mg, daily about three months ago when she presented with symptoms consistent with panic disorder. On the current regimen, her symptoms are under control. Until her recent episode of illness she has had no other history of psychiatric symptoms and there is no family history of psychiatric illness. How long should she continue this medication?

(A) Four weeks
(B) Three months
(C) One year
(D) Three years
(E) Indefinitely

37

Based upon the results of the National Institute of Mental Health funded multi-site Multimodal Treatment Study of Children with Attention Deficit-Hyperactivity Disorder (MTA), which of the following interventions was proven to be the MOST effective in treating the majority of children with ADHD?

(A) Medication alone
(B) Medication with an intensive summer treatment program
(C) Medication with community referral
(D) Medication with parent training
(E) Medication with school consultation

38

Which of the following personality disorders is most common in the biological relatives of patients with schizophrenia?

(A) Schizoid
(B) Paranoid
(C) Schizotypal
(D) Histrionic
(E) Antisocial

39

Which of the following symptoms is a diagnostic feature of atypical depression?

(A) Insomnia
(B) Weight loss
(C) Suicidal ideation
(D) Mood reactivity
(E) Inappropriate guilt

40

A 33-year-old man whose bipolar I disorder has been well controlled on medication, presents to the emergency department with severe left upper quadrant pain radiating to his back, nausea and vomiting. Which medication is most likely contributing to these symptoms?

(A) Lamotrigine
(B) Lithium
(C) Olanzapine
(D) Valproate
(E) Ziprasidone

41

A sniper attacks a city hall building, killing 13 individuals and significantly injuring another 12 before he takes his own life. Therapists from the local mental health clinic are dispatched to the scene to provide psychological debriefing to prevent PTSD symptoms. Using an evidence-based framework, what is the most likely impact of this intervention on direct survivors?

(A) It will be ineffective or harmful to the direct survivors.
(B) It will decrease the probability of developing PTSD symptoms.
(C) It will decrease the severity of PTSD symptoms.
(D) It will decrease the time period for recovery from PTSD symptoms.
(E) It will delay the onset of PTSD symptoms.

42

You are asked to write 22 questions for a board-type examination in less than four weeks. Your first thought is, "I will never be able to get all those questions written in such a short time!" You ignore the fact that you seem to have been able to be successful at this several times before. From a cognitive therapy perspective, what is the best description of this type of thinking?

(A) Magnification
(B) Minimization
(C) Personalization
(D) Selective abstraction
(E) Catastrophic thinking

43

A patient with four or more mood disturbances within a single year that meet both the duration and symptom criteria for major depressive, mixed, manic and/or hypomanic episodes demarcated by remission or switch to opposite polarity, meets the DSM-IV criteria for which of the following disorders?

(A) Bipolar disorder with rapid cycling specifier
(B) Bipolar disorder, Not Otherwise Specified
(C) Cyclothymic disorder
(D) Schizoaffective disorder (bipolar type)

44

Which of the following disorders has been shown to have the greatest degree of heritability?

(A) Schizophrenia
(B) Autism
(C) Bipolar disorder
(D) Alcoholism
(E) Attention-deficit/hyperactivity disorder (ADHD)

45

A 42-year-old man presents to a psychiatrist 6 months after a motor vehicle accident. He has difficulty sleeping because he has frequent nightmares about the accident. He has not been able to drive since the accident, and his wife usually drives for him. Even then, he finds it very difficult to be in a car, often panicking if another car is near them on the road. Which of the following medications would be the most appropriate for this man?

(A) Propranolol
(B) Nortriptyline
(C) Clonazepam
(D) Olanzapine
(E) Sertraline

46

A patient presents with involuntary frowning, blinking, grimacing, and choreoathetoid movements of the upper extremities after several years of antipsychotic medication treatment. Which one of the following is the most likely diagnosis?

(A) Akinesia
(B) Akathisia
(C) Acute dystonia
(D) Parkinsonism
(E) Tardive dyskinesia

47

Which of the following Axis I diagnoses is most common among individuals with bulimia nervosa?

(A) General anxiety disorder
(B) Obsessive compulsive disorder
(C) Alcohol use disorder
(D) Major depressive disorder
(E) Intermittent explosive disorder

48

A 31-year-old man is admitted to an inpatient psychiatric unit after a suicide attempt. Past records show a history of dependence on multiple substances. He sleeps poorly and the next day paces around the unit, restless and grumpy. He is tachycardic at 112 beats per minutes, his palms and forehead are sweaty and his tongue is showing a course tremor. When asked, the patient says he feels anxious. The most likely diagnosis is:

(A) alcohol withdrawal.
(B) nicotine withdrawal.
(C) opioid withdrawal.
(D) cannabis withdrawal.
(E) methamphetamine withdrawal.

49

A 28-year-old woman with an identical twin is diagnosed with major depressive disorder. She asks you to comment on the chance her sister will develop the same illness. Which of the following is the best response regarding the genetic basis of depression?

(A) "Major depression is a genetic illness. Your sister will definitely develop it as well."
(B) "While schizophrenia is quite heritable, there is only a slightly increased risk that your sister will become depressed."
(C) "The likelihood of identical twins sharing an affective illness is high."
(D) "Although there may be some genetic basis for affective illness, it is one's childhood environment that determines whether illness will manifest."
(E) "Your sister's risk of developing depression is the same as any other sibling."

50

For the detection and identification of delirium in medically ill patients, the best strategy to employ is:

(A) enhanced EEG monitoring.
(B) serum and urine lab tests.
(C) revised MMSE.
(D) specific neuroimaging.
(E) observation and rating scales.

51

A 58-year-old man with a history of alcohol dependence and mild dementia presents to the hospital for a liver biopsy due to suspected alcoholic hepatitis. He complains of severe anxiety about having the procedure done and requests "something for my nerves." Which of the following benzodiazepines is safest to administer?

(A) Alprazolam
(B) Chlordiazepoxide
(C) Diazepam
(D) Oxazepam
(E) Clonazepam

52

A 35-year-old patient with schizophrenia has had 4 serious suicide attempts over the past year despite consistent treatment with haloperidol decanoate. Given the patient's recent suicide attempts, what would be the BEST next medication trial?

(A) Olanzapine
(B) Quetiapine
(C) Fluphenazine decanoate
(D) Long-acting risperidone
(E) Clozapine

53

Cognitive behavioral therapy (CBT) is an effective, specific treatment for generalized anxiety disorder (GAD). Emerging evidence suggests that which ONE of the following is similarly effective in treatment for GAD?

(A) Dialectical behavioral therapy (DBT)
(B) Interpersonal psychotherapy (IPT)
(C) Psychoanalysis
(D) Short-term psychodynamic psychotherapy
(E) Supportive psychotherapy

54

A 13-year old boy is seen for outbursts of aggression when he is denied access to food. He is known to be mentally retarded. His mother reports that as an infant he had poor muscle tone and a weak suck reflex. He is morbidly obese, short for his age and has significantly underdeveloped genitalia. His mother reports that he constantly eats to the point they have put locks on the kitchen cabinets and refrigerator. Despite this he will search for food in garbage cans. Lately, when he is denied food, he will have outbursts of anger in which he hits himself or others and throws objects. Which of the following BEST describes the genetic abnormality responsible for this boy's condition?

(A) Williams syndrome
(B) Angelman's syndrome
(C) Prader-Willi syndrome
(D) Klinefelter's syndrome
(E) Down syndrome

55

Which of the following statements represents the most reasonable conclusion that can be drawn from the National Institute of Mental Health's (NIMH) Clinical Antipsychotic Trials of Intervention Effectiveness (CATIE) study?

- (A) Second generation antipsychotics offer no benefit in schizophrenia over first generation antipsychotics.
- (B) Clinicians should consider both first and second generation antipsychotics when treating schizophrenia.
- (C) Antipsychotic medications appear to be less efficacious than previously thought.
- (D) The second generation antipsychotics demonstrate little difference from one another.
- (E) When given in idealized settings, most antipsychotics are roughly equivalent in efficacy.

56

Post-stroke depression is most commonly associated with cerebrovascular disease involving the:

- (A) anterior communicating artery.
- (B) anterior cerebral artery.
- (C) middle cerebral artery.
- (D) posterior communicating artery.
- (E) basilar artery.

57

Which symptom of PTSD has been improved by medications that suppress noradrenergic activity?

- (A) Hypervigilance
- (B) Inability to recall an important aspect of the trauma
- (C) Markedly diminished interest
- (D) Feelings of detachment
- (E) Avoidance of activities related to the trauma

58

A 19-year-old college student comes to the clinic with a complaint of feeling "depressed and worried." He states that he may fail his English class because he is nervous about the public speaking assignment. When he thinks about it, he feels nervous, his heart races, his palms become sweaty, and he becomes short of breath. He endorses a depressed mood because "I feel like I'm wasting my parents' money." He skipped his last three English classes because he knew it would be his turn to give a speech. He attends his other classes with no difficulty. The most likely diagnosis is:

- (A) panic disorder.
- (B) normal shyness.
- (C) social phobia.
- (D) agoraphobia.
- (E) major depressive disorder.

59

A 47-year-old woman is brought for a psychiatric evaluation to assess recent changes in her behavior. Over the past six months, she has become increasingly disinhibited and impulsive in her behavior. Physical examination reveals mild dysarthria, dysphagia, and drooling. Slit lamp examination of the eyes indicates the presence of Kayser-Fleischer rings. Which of the following BEST describes the genetic basis for her illness?

- (A) Autosomal recessive
- (B) Co-dominant
- (C) Mitochondrial
- (D) Polygenetic
- (E) X-linked dominant

60

A patient unconsciously perceives the therapist as having attributes associated with unpleasant interactions in the past. However, the therapist does not respond like the figure from the past, and over time, the old feelings become muted and the patient no longer needs to replay new relationships according to the old emotional script. Which of the following terms define this positive change in psychotherapy?

- (A) Exposure and response prevention
- (B) Corrective emotional experience
- (C) Re-enactment of transference
- (D) Shaping
- (E) Strengthening ego defenses

61

Which of the following is a risk factor for the development of psychosis while using cocaine?

(A) Being female
(B) A greater duration of use during an episode
(C) Non-intravenous use
(D) An elevated body mass index
(E) Being a first time user of cocaine

62

A 38-year-old man presents for treatment of PTSD after surviving a bridge collapse. He was driving on the crowded bridge when it suddenly collapsed, killing over 50 individuals and seriously injuring more. As part of the treatment, the therapist asks the patient to imagine that he is safely driving over a bridge. Which of the following best describes this therapeutic intervention?

(A) Aversion therapy
(B) Dialectical behavioral therapy
(C) Exposure therapy
(D) Insight-oriented psychotherapy
(E) Interpersonal therapy

63

Which of the following characteristics is/are present in patients with locked-in syndrome?

(A) Persistent vegetative state
(B) Ability to experience a range of feelings
(C) Inability to recognize objects and people
(D) Severe depression and desire to die

64

Which of the following interventions has been empirically validated through controlled and randomized trials as effective specifically for adolescents with conduct disorder?

(A) Dialectical behavioral therapy
(B) Cognitive behavioral therapy
(C) Interpersonal therapy
(D) Multisystemic therapy
(E) Psychoeducational therapy

65

Which of the following is the mechanism of action of memantine, a medication used to slow cognitive decline in Alzheimer's dementia?

(A) Cholinesterase inhibitor
(B) Dopamine receptor blocker
(C) Serotonergic reuptake inhibitor
(D) NMDA receptor antagonist
(E) GABA mimetic

66

Which of the following genetic syndromes is caused by a 22q deletion and is clinically manifested by learning disabilities, palatal anomalies, cardiac defects and often schizophrenia?

(A) Fragile X syndrome
(B) Velocardiofacial syndrome
(C) Down syndrome
(D) Cri du chat syndrome
(E) Angelman syndrome

67

Which of the following refers to an ethical decision making approach that involves referring to similar, prior cases including legal precedents and applying reasoning from these cases to the case at hand?

(A) Casuistry
(B) Ethical principles
(C) Expert opinion
(D) General ethical theory
(E) Tradition and current practice standards

68

A 38-year-old woman with treatment resistant schizophrenia is prescribed clozapine. Two weeks after beginning the medication, the woman begins to experience episodes of tachycardia with a heart rate over 120 beats per minute. Electrocardiogram reveals sustained sinus tachycardia with non-specific ST-T wave changes and T-wave flattening while standing and supine. Which of the following medications is most likely to alleviate her tachycardia without increasing chances of a serious adverse effect?

(A) Atenolol
(B) Fludrocortisone
(C) Propranolol
(D) Verapamil

69

The course of dementia in individuals with 16 or more years of education differs from those with lower educational attainment in which way?

(A) Lower cognitive reserve
(B) Ability to maintain higher levels of cognitive functioning in early dementia
(C) Lower levels of cognitive function in early dementia
(D) Less disease burden when dementia is diagnosed
(E) Gentler slope of decline after dementia is diagnosed

70

A 34-year-old woman with bipolar disorder has a body mass index of 31.2. To minimize the risk of aggravating this factor, which of the following medications would be most appropriate?

(A) Lithium
(B) Clozapine
(C) Lamotrigine
(D) Olanzapine
(E) Divalproex

71

According to the ethics primer of the American Psychiatric Association, which one of the following scenarios would most likely be considered a violation of the psychotherapeutic frame?

(A) A patient is late to his psychotherapy session due to an upcoming deadline at work, but the therapist still charges the full amount for the session.
(B) The therapist loses his office keys, but lives across the street. Rather than cancel his patients, he asks his wife and children to stay out for the day and sets up a temporary office in his living room.
(C) A patient does not bring his check book to his final session of the month, when payment is due. The therapist interprets this act as an expression of ambivalence about the treatment, and suggests this to the patient.
(D) The therapist is diagnosed with end-stage cancer, and informs his patient that due to serious illness, he will be terminating his practice over the next month.
(E) A grateful former patient wishes to donate money to the hospital with which his therapist is affiliated. Not wanting to handle the transaction himself, the therapist refers the patient to the hospital's development office.

72

Genetic linkage analysis studies provide information about which one of the following aspects of a gene:

(A) Post-transitional processing
(B) Location
(C) Function
(D) Endophenotype
(E) Population frequency

73

A 17-year-old man is brought to the emergency department after fighting with his girlfriend and ingesting a bottle of alprazolam. En route to the hospital, the girlfriend lost control of the car causing the patient to hit his head against the windshield with loss of consciousness. Examination reveals the patient to be in stupor, with respiratory depression and coma. He has a 4 cm laceration over the right frontal area which is profusely bleeding. Which of the facts of the patient's presentation represents the greatest contraindication to the use of flumazenil?

(A) Age of patient
(B) CNS depression
(C) Benzodiazepine use
(D) Possible traumatic brain injury

74

A 42-year-old man is started on pharmacotherapy for treatment of major depressive disorder. Two weeks later he presents with complaints of dry mouth, impaired ability to focus at close range, constipation, urinary hesitation, tachycardia, and sexual dysfunction. Which of the following medications is most likely to have caused this presentation?

(A) Duloxetine
(B) Fluoxetine
(C) Imipramine
(D) Mirtazapine
(E) Venlafaxine

75

Which of the following medications has been the only one to demonstrate a decrease in suicide risk?

- (A) Valproic acid
- (B) Lithium
- (C) Carbamazepine
- (D) Lamotrigine
- (E) Gabapentin

76

A 34 year-old woman, who has been treated with an antidepressant for the past month, complains that she no longer gets relief from her back pain when she takes codeine which has been prescribed by her orthopedist. Which one of the following antidepressants would be most likely to produce such an effect?

- (A) Escitalopram
- (B) Sertraline
- (C) Paroxetine
- (D) Mirtazapine
- (E) Bupropion

77

Children of European descent with an early history of abuse have been found to be more likely to develop subsequent depression when they have a genetic polymorphism of which of the following neurotransmitter transporters?

- (A) Norepinephrine
- (B) Dopamine
- (C) Serotonin
- (D) Glutamate
- (E) GABA

78

A 45-year-old woman was a witness to a motor vehicle accident that resulted in a number of fatalities. The images and the sounds of the accident greatly distressed her. The day after the accident she was seen by her family physician. The most appropriate next treatment step is:

- (A) education and support about possible reactions that may occur
- (B) immediate referral to a mental health treatment program
- (C) treatment with an antidepressant
- (D) benzodiazepines as needed for sleep
- (E) critical incident debriefing

79

A 48-year-old man with depression has been resistant to treatment with a variety of antidepressants. The decision is made to try him on a monoamine oxidase inhibitor. In order to avoid serotonin syndrome, a washout period of at least five weeks is MOST indicated if he has been taking which antidepressant?

- (A) Bupropion
- (B) Clomipramine
- (C) Fluoxetine
- (D) Paroxetine
- (E) Venlafaxine

80

Which of the following medications used to treat excessive daytime sleepiness associated with narcolepsy has also been abused as a "date-rape" drug?

- (A) Sodium oxybate
- (B) Modafinil
- (C) Methylphenidate
- (D) Selegiline
- (E) Dextroamphetamine

81

A patient recounts a story about getting angry with a store clerk. The therapist asks a factual question about the circumstance, inspiring rage in the patient, who finds him to be uncaring and seeking to blame her. The therapist says, "I wonder if what you're feeling right now is just like the feeling you had in the store, when you attributed the same uncaring attitude toward the clerk. These kinds of misreadings seem to make you very upset in many different settings." Which of the following most accurately describes this type of intervention?

(A) Genetic interpretation
(B) Transference interpretation
(C) Clarification
(D) Observation
(E) Empathic validation

82

Consideration of genotyping for human leukocyte antigen allele HLA-B 1502 has been recommended by the FDA prior to starting carbamazepine on patients with which of the following ancestries?

(A) European
(B) African
(C) Asian
(D) Hispanic
(E) Native American

83

An 84-year-old woman with a history of Alzheimer's disease presents to an emergency department after a fall. She had been experiencing difficulty sleeping at night for several months and was increasingly combative and suspicious of her daughter, with whom she lived. In developing a plan of treatment for this patient, which of the following principles is most appropriate to incorporate?

(A) Adjust doses of medication slowly with long intervals between dose increments
(B) Prescribe small doses of several different medications rather than using one medication
(C) Use a long-acting injectable medication to aid adherence
(D) Use an initial loading dose of medication to speed response

84

A 28-year-old woman with bipolar I disorder is pregnant for the first time. Throughout the pregnancy, she has been maintained on a mood stabilizer. At the time of birth, the baby is noted to have a cardiovascular defect consistent with Ebstein's anomaly. The mood stabilizer the woman was taking was most likely:

(A) Carbamazepine
(B) Haloperidol
(C) Lithium
(D) Lorazepam
(E) Valproate

85

According to simple Mendelian inheritance, if a disease gene is recessive, what is the likelihood of developing the disease if one parent has two dominant genes and the other two recessive genes?

(A) 0%
(B) 25%
(C) 50%
(D) 75%
(E) 100%

86

Which of the following is the medication most often associated with an increased risk of falls in persons age 80 or older?

(A) Antihypertensives
(B) Benzodiazepines
(C) Antidepressants
(D) Histamine H1 receptor antagonists
(E) Atypical antipsychotics

87

Patients who are being treated with exposure therapy for anxiety disorders are:

(A) encouraged to think about non-threatening situations during the treatment.
(B) encouraged to focus on their fears and allow feelings of anxiety to occur.
(C) required to conduct the therapy in real life or fully realistic situations.
(D) required to develop a protocol and start with the most feared stimulus first.
(E) required to be on an appropriate type and dose of anti-anxiety medication.

88

What were the findings of the Treatment for Adolescents with Depression Study (TADS), with regard to efficacy of treatment?

(A) Fluoxetine alone was most effective.
(B) Cognitive behavioral therapy alone was most effective.
(C) Fluoxetine plus cognitive behavioral therapy was most effective.
(D) Interpersonal therapy alone was most effective.
(E) Fluoxetine plus interpersonal therapy was most effective.

89

A 76-year-old woman with a long history of generalized anxiety disorder presents to a psychiatrist. She is interested in the possibility of pharmacotherapy for this disorder. She has a history of hypertension, for which she takes amlodipine, but otherwise is in good health. The most accurate advice regarding the use of pharmacotherapy for this patient is that medications are:

(A) generally not effective in treating anxiety in elderly patients.
(B) contraindicated due to the increased side effects in older adults.
(C) less effective than psychotherapy for anxiety in older adults.
(D) not recommended due to the high potential for drug-drug interactions.
(E) a first line treatment for anxiety in the elderly.

90

You are treating a 16-year-old patient for ADHD who has multiple café au lait spots visible on both arms and legs. A diagnosis of neurofibromatosis is made by a neurology consultant. Which one of the following modes of genetic transmission is seen in this illness?

(A) Autosomal dominant
(B) Autosomal recessive
(C) Non-Mendelian inheritance
(D) X-linked recessive
(E) X-linked dominant

91

Which of the following combination treatments has the best evidence for producing a short term benefit of more rapid stabilization for the acute symptom treatment of panic disorder?

(A) CBT and SSRI
(B) Benzodiazepine and SSRI
(C) CBT and benzodiazepine
(D) SSRI and buspirone

92

A 22-year-old man presents repeatedly over a year with concerns that he is suffering from AIDS. He has never been found to be HIV positive, but is not convinced despite having negative tests. He does not meet the criteria for major depressive disorder, generalized anxiety disorder, or obsessive-compulsive disorder. Which of the following is the most likely diagnosis?

(A) Body dysmorphic disorder
(B) Hypochondriasis
(C) Conversion disorder
(D) Somatization disorder
(E) Undifferentiated somatoform disorder

93

Which of the following neurotransmitters has the largest body of evidence associating it with the reinforcing effects of various types of drugs of abuse?

(A) Acetylcholine
(B) Dopamine
(C) GABA
(D) Glutamate
(E) Serotonin

94

Which of the following is the preferred method to confirm a clinical diagnosis of narcolepsy?

(A) Functional magnetic resonance imaging (fMRI)
(B) Apnea monitoring
(C) Multiple sleep latency test (MSLT)
(D) Human leukocyte antigen (HLA) testing
(E) CSF hypocretin levels

95

Which of the following psychotherapeutic interventions represents the best approach for a patient with germ obsessions who washes his hands every time he touches something he considers dirty?

(A) Having the patient place his hands in a container of mud
(B) Having the patient snap his wrist with a rubber band when he washes his hands
(C) Pointing out to the patient that the germ phobia is an example of distorted thinking
(D) Having the patient touch a dirty object, then not allowing him to wash his hands   *exp resp prevention*
(E) Providing the patient with coping cards to remind him that the hand washing is unnecessary

96

A military veteran is diagnosed with PTSD after his wife encourages him to seek treatment due to problems adjusting to civilian life. It is clear that survivor guilt is a major source of distress. Which of the following is the best intervention for this issue?

(A) Vocational counseling
(B) Couples therapy
(C) Individual psychotherapy
(D) Fluoxetine
(E) Risperidone

97

Which of the following cultural groups is most likely to want to be informed of a terminal prognosis?

(A) Mexican Americans
(B) Korean Americans
(C) African Americans
(D) Japanese Americans
(E) Navajo Americans

98

When diagnosing major depressive disorder in young children, which of the following signs or symptoms is MORE likely to be present than would be expected in an adolescent or adult?

(A) Diurnal variation in mood
(B) Hypersomnia
(C) Melancholia
(D) Poor self-esteem
(E) Somatic complaints

99

A mutation on which of the following chromosomes has been associated with early-onset Alzheimer's dementia?

(A) Chromosome 2
(B) Chromosome 19
(C) Chromosome 21
(D) Y chromosome
(E) X chromosome

100

A 16-year-old girl is brought by her parents for an evaluation as part of the admission process for a weight reduction program. The adolescent agrees that she is overweight and that she would like to lose weight. Which of the following would be MOST indicative that she will be successful in the program?

(A) BMI < 30
(B) No family history of eating disorders
(C) Mother successfully lost weight
(D) She is willing to take medication
(E) She is willing to change her eating habits

101

A 25-year-old woman complains about shortness of breath, chest pain and diaphoresis. She has had multiple attacks in the past 3 weeks. Her medical work-up is negative. Which of the following medications is the best choice considering efficacy and side-effect profile?

(A) Propranolol
(B) Desipramine
(C) Bupropion
(D) Sertraline
(E) Alprazolam

102

The "parent of origin" effect is defined as transmission of a risk for disease based on whether an autosome has been transmitted by the mother or father. As one example of this phenomenon in psychiatric genetics, duplications of chromosome 15q inherited from the mother, but not the father, have been found to account for a small but significant proportion of cases of which of the following disorders?

(A) Schizophrenia
(B) Bipolar disorder
(C) Obsessive-compulsive disorder
(D) Alcohol dependence
(E) Autism

103

A 14-year-old girl presents with significant weight loss. She reports that about one year ago she became concerned that she was overweight and began self-inducing vomiting. Since then, she has continued to use purgatives in addition to misusing laxatives, diuretics and enemas as a means of weight control after binging. She is intensely afraid of becoming fat. She is in the 65th percentile for weight based on height, appears cachetic, but insists she is obese. She has not experienced menses for six months. Which of the following symptoms will MOST likely be elicited from the patient?

(A) A need for orderliness and control
(B) Competitiveness
(C) Obsessional thinking
(D) Perfectionism
(E) Co-morbid impulsivity

104

Cognitive deficits in schizophrenia have been associated with a decrease in $GABA_A$ receptors in which of the following brain areas?

(A) Lateral amygdala
(B) Medial amygdala
(C) Dorsolateral prefrontal cortex
(D) Medial prefrontal cortex
(E) Nucleus accumbens

105

A 19-year-old man presents for an outpatient evaluation of increasing concerns about germs and contamination that are now resulting in several hours per day of hand washing and cleaning rituals to relieve anxiety. He is started on sertraline, the dose of which is increased 50 mg every other day until reaching 200 mg daily. After one week of treatment at this dose, he has not experienced any relief of the symptoms. However, the medication is well-tolerated without significant side effects. In developing further plan of treatment, which of the following is the appropriate total length of time to continue sertraline before changing to another pharmacologic agent?

(A) 2 weeks
(B) 4 weeks
(C) 6 weeks
(D) 8 weeks
(E) 10 weeks

106

A psychiatric consult is requested for a patient who has burns over 60% of his body. The patient has begun refusing dressing changes despite pre-treatment with morphine. Pain control is adequate except during dressing changes. Upon examination, the patient reports that the pain is too severe to tolerate, and he does not feel that the morphine is adequately controlling his pain. The psychiatrist should recommend which of the following agents as an additional medication prior to dressing changes?

(A) Long-acting morphine
(B) Methadone
(C) Meperidine
(D) Fentanyl
(E) Codeine

107

A 36-year-old moderately obese man is seen for evaluation of depressed mood, difficulty falling asleep, poor appetite, and diminished concentration at work, all of which been worsening over the past few weeks. When treatment options are discussed he reports particular concerns about sexual side effects. Considering the patient's concerns, which one of the following medications would be most appropriate to suggest as an initial treatment?

(A) Bupropion
(B) Fluoxetine
(C) Mirtazapine
(D) Nortriptyline
(E) Venlafaxine

108

Which of the following disorders has the most evidence supporting familial aggregation of the disorder?

(A) Posttraumatic stress disorder
(B) Adjustment disorder, mixed features
(C) Panic disorder
(D) Social phobia
(E) Specific phobia

109

Which of the following medical complications is most likely to be seen in a patient with bulimia nervosa?

(A) Decreased serum amylase
(B) Hyperchloremia
(C) Metabolic acidosis
(D) Hypokalemia
(E) Hyperthyroxinemia

110

Evidence to date from OCD genetic studies indicate that its inheritance is best characterized by which pattern?

(A) Automsomal dominant
(B) Autosomal recessive
(C) Sex-linked recessive
(D) Complex
(E) Mendelian

111

A 72-year-old woman is referred to a psychiatrist because the family has noticed increasing apathy. In evaluating the patient, which of the following would be the most useful first step for revealing the likely underlying pathology?

(A) An empirical trial of an antidepressant
(B) An MRI of the brain
(C) History and a full mental status examination
(D) Thyroid function testing
(E) Neuropsychological evaluation

112

Which of the following is believed to be the chief factor in predicting outcome of psychodynamic psychotherapy?

(A) Transference
(B) Countertransference
(C) Therapeutic alliance
(D) Resistance
(E) On time payments

113

An adolescent girl becomes anxious and "panicky" at the thought of spiders. She cannot join her high school classmates for lunch outside due to the fear that she "will run into a spider." The most appropriate diagnosis is:

(A) agoraphobia.
(B) acute stress disorder.
(C) generalized anxiety disorder.
(D) specific phobia.
(E) social phobia.

114

A 31 year old female describes dramatic fluctuations in mood and self-esteem. Which one of the following features would be most helpful in distinguishing bipolar II disorder from borderline personality disorder during a period of elevated mood?

(A) Suicidal ideation with depressed mood
(B) Psychosis while mood is elevated or irritable
(C) Impulsivity while mood is elevated or irritable
(D) A history of continued functioning through mood fluctuations
(E) Mood fluctuations are observed by others

115

Which of the following psychiatric conditions is most commonly associated with self neglect in the geriatric population?

(A) Depression
(B) Generalized anxiety disorder
(C) Panic disorder
(D) Schizophrenia
(E) Personality disorder

116

According to the AMA Code of Medical Ethics, which of the following educationally related gifts from a pharmaceutical company is ethically acceptable?

(A) Money to help defray hotel costs during a CME event
(B) Scholarships awarded to individual residents to attend educational conferences
(C) Reimbursement of travel for a guest faculty speaker
(D) Money to compensate a psychiatrist for time spent at a CME event

117

Which of the following statements best describes the association between PTSD and the subsequent emergence of drug use problems?

(A) Young adults with PTSD due to earlier life-time traumas, with no prior drug use disorders, are about five times more likely to develop drug related problems subsequently compared to traumatized young adults without PTSD.
(B) Experiencing significant trauma without the presence of PTSD is sufficient to subsequently increase the prevalence of drug use disorders substantially.
(C) After controlling for factors such as sex, age and ethnicity, PTSD confers no additional increased risk of subsequent drug use disorders.
(D) After controlling for factors such as childhood conduct problems and risk taking, PTSD confers no additional increased risk of subsequent drug use disorders.
(E) After controlling for factors such as family SES and years of education, PTSD confers no additional increased risk of subsequent drug use disorders.

118

Borderline personality disorder is marked by pervasive instability of self-image, emotions and impulsivity. Which of the following is a DSM diagnostic criteria for this diagnosis?

(A) Consistent irresponsibility
(B) Lack of remorse after injuring others
(C) Requiring excessive admiration
(D) Sense of entitlement
(E) Unstable sense of self

119

Which of the following should be the initial treatment of hypochondriasis?

(A) Cognitive behavioral therapy
(B) Treatment of incidental physical exam findings
(C) Scheduling regular physical examinations
(D) Discussing the false nature of the illness
(E) Pharmacotherapy with SSRIs

120

A 33-year-old man with schizophrenia and alcohol dependence acknowledges that when he drinks beer the police tend to arrest him and bring him to the psychiatric hospital. He agrees to "take medicine to help [him] not drink so much." Due to issues of noncompliance, his current medication is a long-acting injectable antipsychotic. He lives on his own and keeps his clinic appointments, but has had difficulties adhering to oral medication regimens. The best medication to augment the treatment of his alcohol dependence would be:

(A) acamprosate.
(B) clozapine.
(C) disulfiram.
(D) naltrexone.
(E) ondansetron.

121

Avoidant personality disorder is marked by social inhibition, sense of inadequacy and hypersensitivity. Which of the following is a DSM criterion for this disorder?

(A) Requiring excessive admiration
(B) Difficulty making everyday decisions
(C) Excessive devotion to work to the exclusion of friendships
(D) Preoccupation with being socially criticized
(E) Reluctance to delegate tasks or to work with others

122

Which of the following statements gives the most appropriate guidance for patients and their families regarding driving by patients with dementia?

(A) Families have no responsibility for getting involved in driving decisions of patients with mild cognitive impairment.

(B) All patients with mild cognitive impairment should be reported to their State Motor Vehicle Departments for mandatory tracking.

(C) Clinicians should advise all patients with mild cognitive impairment to stop driving and to turn in their driver's licenses.

(D) Mildly impaired patients should be advised to stop driving at night.

(E) Patients and families should be informed that even mild dementia increases the risk of vehicular accidents.

123

An 8-year-old boy presents with a one-month history of stomachaches and headaches every morning just before going to school. When interviewed, he reports having persistent nightmares of being kidnapped and worries about his father having an accident. The most likely diagnosis is:

(A) normal childhood.
(B) agoraphobia.
(C) separation anxiety.
(D) generalized anxiety disorder.
(E) panic disorder.

124

A 65-year-old man has metastatic head-and-neck cancer that leaves him with a ptosis, facial nerve palsy, and an inability to eat solid foods. He complains of feeling hopeless, that life has lost all meaning, and that he wants to die immediately. He does not meet criteria for major depression. The best descriptor for this triad of symptoms is:

(A) anticipatory grief.
(B) demoralization.
(C) mourning.
(D) denial.
(E) bargaining.

125

A 73-year-old woman was prescribed 10 mg of paroxetine for anxiety one week ago. She now presents to the physician's office with confusion. Lab work-up reveals low serum sodium and low plasma osmolarity. Her urine sodium and osmolarity are high. The physician should consider a diagnosis of:

(A) hypothyroidism.
(B) SIADH (Syndrome of Inappropriate Antidiuretic Hormone).
(C) hyperparathyroidism.
(D) renal failure.
(E) dehydration.

126

A 37 year old male software designer is brought to the psychiatrist's office by his brother, who reports that the patient has become increasingly suspicious over the last year. Last week, a shopping mall security guard observed him recording license plate numbers. The guard inquired, the patient explained that he was doing statistical research on license plates, and there was no further incident. He told his brother later that he thought he had noticed these cars parked in front of his home, and might be part of scoping the neighborhood in advance of a crime. The brother is now concerned that it is only a matter of time for the patient to get into his first legal skirmish as a result of this kind of behavior. The patient reports that since his teens, he has needed to be very observant of others to protect himself. He says he has never been a victim of assault or theft only because of his constant vigilance. He experienced several days of auditory hallucinations when he was about 20 years old; "voices" were making deprecatory comments, but he cannot recall further details . These symptoms remitted entirely, and he reports no other psychotic symptoms.

He has worked at the same software company for ten years and while he has been promoted several times, most recently 3 months ago, he thinks he was slighted by his supervisor who gave a better position to a colleague. He is satisfied with his single status. Which ONE of the following disorders is the most likely diagnosis?

(A) Paranoid personality disorder
(B) Delusional disorder
(C) Schizoid personality disorder
(D) Schizophrenia, paranoid type
(E) Schizotypal personality disorder

127

A 6-year-old girl is referred by her teacher because of "acting out" behaviors at school, including inappropriate touching of peers and insistence on sitting on adults' laps. During the session, she tells the psychiatrist that her father touches her "secret place." The father explains that he bathes the girl at night and is simply making sure she is clean everywhere. Which of the following is the most appropriate action for the psychiatrist?

(A) Advise the father not to give baths and see if the behavior resolves.
(B) Tell the teacher to call child protective services.
(C) Relay the findings to the teacher and tell her child protective services will not be necessary.
(D) Try to gather more history to see if this constitutes sexual abuse.
(E) Make a call to child protective services.

128

Patients with acute stress disorder have been shown in controlled trials to be least likely to subsequently develop posttraumatic stress disorder when treated with:

(A) cognitive restructuring therapy.
(B) exposure therapy.
(C) systematic debriefing.
(D) couples therapy.
(E) internet-based CBT.

129

According to the results of the Clinical Antipsychotic Trials of Intervention Effectiveness (CATIE) study, approximately what percentage of patients had continued on their initial antipsychotic medications by 18 months?

(A) 10%
(B) 25%
(C) 50%
(D) 75%
(E) 90%

130

Temperament traits of Harm Avoidance, Novelty Seeking, Reward Dependence, and Persistence are defined as heritable differences underlying automatic responses to danger, novelty, social approval, and intermittent reward, respectively. Which of the following statements about the temperament traits in the general population is MOST accurate?

(A) The phenotypic expression of these traits is primarily due to the experiences of the individual.
(B) They are normally distributed quantitative traits.
(C) They are modifiable based on the goodness of fit with the parent.
(D) They are inconsistently manifested in different cultures.
(E) They are similar to fluid intelligence in that they show demonstrable changes with aging.

131

A 37-year-old single man's sex life centers on donning women's lingerie before engaging in sexual activities with willing female partners. He considers himself heterosexual and has never had any interest in having sex with men. He is distressed about his sexual behavior and is now seeking treatment. Which of the following best describes his behavior?

(A) Transvestic fetishism
(B) Gender identity disorder
(C) Frotteurism
(D) Exhibitionism

132

A 28-year-old woman presents to the clinic concerned about having ADHD. She has noticed that for the last three days she has been "hyper." She stays up until 4 a.m. to rehearse her presentations and awakens easily at 7 a.m. She also now works as late as 9 p.m., whereas she would usually stop at 6 p.m. She finds herself easily distracted and strays from her routine presentation. She experiences these symptoms about three times a year. Talking with her husband reveals that these periods are always followed by a deep depression during which she will rarely get out of bed, does not eat, and will not see clients for about two weeks. Her presentation is most consistent with:

(A) cyclothymia.
(B) bipolar I disorder.
(C) bipolar II disorder.
(D) ADHD – inattentive type.
(E) ADHD – hyperactive/impulsive type.

133

A 19-year-old woman with anorexia presents with shortness of breath and symptoms consistent with heart failure. She admits to using large amounts of ipecac. Which of the following test results would be most consistent with ipecac-induced toxicity?

(A) Decrease in the serum CK value
(B) Decrease in lactate dehydrogenase
(C) Shortening of the QTC interval
(D) Enlarged heart
(E) Bradycardia

134

An assessment of a 25-year old woman as a candidate for psychotherapy reveals that she is able to delay gratification in order to attain personal goals but remains egocentric and defensive. She is noted to have frequent distress when attachments and desires are frustrated. She functions well under good conditions but frequently experiences problems under stress. Based upon the *stages in the development of self-awareness and well being* this woman is MOST likely at what stage?

(A) Stage 0: unaware
(B) Stage 1: average adult cognition
(C) Stage 2: metacognition
(D) Stage 3: contemplation

135

Which of the following techniques or therapies has been shown, in a randomized controlled trial, to be most helpful in the treatment of acute stress disorder?

(A) Cognitive restructuring
(B) Individual psychological debriefing
(C) Exposure-based therapy
(D) EMDR (eye movement desensitization and reprocessing)
(E) Group debriefing

136

Which of the following medications should be the first line treatment for generalized anxiety disorder?

(A) Diazepam
(B) Lorazepam
(C) Buspirone
(D) Paroxetine
(E) Hydroxyzine

137

After performing a thorough history and physical, a psychiatrist suspects that the patient has bipolar I disorder, rapid-cycling. Which of the following tests should be ordered to rule out an underlying medical etiology?

(A) CSF 5-HIAA
(B) 24 hour urine
(C) Thyroid function tests
(D) Liver function tests
(E) Dexamethasone suppression test

138

The symptom domain most strongly correlated with functional impairment in schizophrenia is:

(A) positive symptoms.
(B) negative symptoms.
(C) cognitive impairment.
(D) mood disturbance.

139

A 37-year-old woman, in dynamic psychotherapy for borderline personality disorder, has been expressing an unrealistic overvaluation of the therapist. After many months of this expressed high regard, she suddenly becomes enraged after the therapist fails to return her call, and now declares the therapist to be "the worst ever." Which of the following would be the most appropriate way to handle the patient's new reaction?

(A) Avoid directly responding and instead encourage the patient to further express her emotions.
(B) Apologize for the missed call and then suggest they move on with the current work.
(C) Acknowledge the failing and then question how the patient's opinion could change so dramatically.
(D) Propose that they clarify an appropriate call-back policy to avoid future mishaps.
(E) Suggest to the patient that such inevitable mistakes are an important part of the therapy.

140

Which of the following is the most accurate information to give families regarding the risk of using antipsychotics to treat agitation in elderly patients with moderate dementia of the Alzheimer's type?

(A) There is an increased risk of mortality, but only for the antipsychotics risperidone and olanzapine.
(B) Increased mortality in the elderly has been associated with both atypical and conventional antipsychotics.
(C) Although suggested by earlier studies, subsequent studies have not found a significant risk of mortality with atypical antipsychotics.
(D) The risk is unknown, as inadequate data exists to make any conclusive statements.
(E) Although newer antipsychotics may have a risk, typical antipsychotics appear to be safe.

141

The use of stimulants to treat ADHD is relatively contraindicated if the child has which of the following co-morbid conditions?

(A) Tic disorder
(B) Pre-existing cardiovascular disease
(C) Seizure disorder
(D) Anxiety disorder
(E) Bipolar disorder

142

A patient describes a dinner party at which he felt increasing anxiety and a sense that people were avoiding him. He discussed this with his wife and she became irritated with him, noting that it would help if he could look people in the eye and not wear the same worn-out suit jacket to every party. He tried to explain that this was his lucky jacket and it protected them both from car accidents, but she just shook her head. Based on this, which of the following personality disorders is most likely?

(A) Schizoid
(B) Schizotypal
(C) Antisocial
(D) Borderline
(E) Narcissistic

143

What is the leading cause of disability in the world for persons 15–44 years of age?

(A) Bipolar disorder
(B) Schizophrenia
(C) Self-inflicted injuries
(D) Unipolar major depression
(E) Alcohol use

144

A busy 33-year-old female executive decides that she will end 10 years of smoking. She tried once before, but was unsuccessful. She travels several times a month, and agrees to use a nicotine inhaler, along with brief telephone counseling appointments. When is she most likely to relapse?

(A) On the quit date
(B) During the first few days of the quit date
(C) One week after the quit date
(D) Two weeks after the quit date

145

Clinical efficacy of typical (first generation) antipsychotic medications is highly correlated with binding to which of the following receptors?

(A) Dopamine, D1
(B) Dopamine, D2
(C) Serotonin, 5-HT2a
(D) Muscarinic, M4
(E) Adrenoceptors, α_2

146

Which of the following is a single locus (monogenic) disorder?

(A) Alzheimer's disease
(B) Bipolar disorder
(C) Autism
(D) Huntington's disease
(E) Obsessive-compulsive disorder

147

Which of the following is considered the treatment of choice for the core deficit of children with Asperger's syndrome?

(A) Speech and language therapy
(B) Self-care assistance
(C) Social skills training
(D) Structured educational intervention
(E) Vocational rehabilitation

148

Medications from which one of the following classes have the greatest potential for worsening symptoms of borderline personality disorder?

(A) Selective serotonin reuptake inhibitors
(B) Monoamine oxidase inhibitors
(C) Anticonvulsants
(D) Atypical antipsychotics
(E) Benzodiazepines

149

In order to be given the diagnosis of mild cognitive impairment (MCI), a patient must have:

(A) a memory impairment.
(B) a cognitive complaint in at least one domain.
(C) cognitive complaints in multiple domains.
(D) compromised general cognitive function.
(E) cognitive and memory complaints meeting criteria for mild dementia.

150

A 42-year-old patient requests treatment for anxiety and interpersonal difficulties. The patient reports feelings of social inadequacy and sensitivity to rejection for the past 20 years. The patient does not attend social events or interact with others as a result of this anxiety, worries excessively about being criticized by others, and feels inferior to others. This has caused occupational problems since the patient is only able to function in jobs that have virtually no social interaction. The patient is unhappy that he has no friends and has never been romantically involved. Which of the following is the most likely diagnosis?

(A) Schizoid personality disorder
(B) Generalized anxiety disorder
(C) Avoidant personality disorder
(D) Social anxiety disorder
(E) Obsessive-compulsive disorder

151

The parents of a 10-year-old boy who has had both motor and vocal tics for over a year are wondering whether he will remain symptomatic as an adult. Which of the following statements MOST accurately describes the probable outcome of children with these symptoms?

(A) 50% of children are not symptomatic by age 18.
(B) Symptoms continue to increase in adolescence and adulthood.
(C) The motor tics resolve but the vocal tics persist.
(D) The tics decrease in adolescence but then increase again in adulthood.

152

Increased risk of developing diabetes mellitus and dyslipidemia have most commonly been linked to:

(A) perphenazine.
(B) quetiapine.
(C) risperidone.
(D) ziprasidone.
(E) olanzapine.

153

Patients in a study were asked to exert behavioral inhibition when confronted with negative stimuli. fMRI investigations demonstrated decreased activation of the subgenual anterior cingulate cortex and the posterior medial orbitofrontal cortex, and increased activity in the left and right extended amygdala and ventral striatum relative to controls. These FMRI findings were associated with which of the following diagnoses?

(A) Narcissistic personality disorder
(B) Attention-deficit/hyperactivity disorder (ADHD)
(C) Paranoid personality disorder
(D) Borderline personality disorder
(E) Schizophrenia

154

Binge eating disorder is characterized by:

(A) feelings of being unable to control one's intake of food.
(B) consumption of a large amount of food over a 24-hour period.
(C) purging after eating a large amount of food.
(D) increasing amounts of exercise.
(E) progressive weight loss.

155

A patient who has been diagnosed with PTSD reports nightmares and sleep disruption. Which one of the following medications has been shown to be effective for the treatment of trauma-related nightmares and sleep disruption in patients with PTSD?

(A) Topiramate
(B) Sertraline
(C) Prazosin
(D) Gabapentin
(E) Propranolol

156

A 3-day-postpartum mother with no prior psychiatric diagnosis is concerned about feeling depressed. She endorses a decrease in energy, difficulty sleeping despite being tired, decreased appetite, and frequent mood swings saying, "One minute I'm fine, the next minute I'm crying." Which of the following is the most appropriate treatment?

(A) Psychoeducation
(B) Cognitive behavioral therapy
(C) Pharmacotherapy
(D) Hospitalization
(E) Psychodynamic psychotherapy

157

A 44-year-old woman presents with a general history of alcohol abuse and significant depressive and anxiety symptoms over 20 years. It is unclear whether the substance use was in response to the affective symptoms or if the affective symptoms were substance-induced. Which of the following procedures would help make this determination?

(A) Administer the MacAndrew Alcoholism Scale—Revised (MAC-R).
(B) Conduct a detailed mental status exam, focusing on form of thought.
(C) Draw a timeline of all substances used and all psychiatric symptoms.
(D) Measure the percent carbohydrate-deficient transferrin.
(E) Obtain serial urine toxicology tests.

158

A depressed 62-year-old man being treated with an SSRI is admitted to the hospital with motoric immobility, posturing, grimacing, echolalia and echopraxia. Intravenous administration of lorazepam and amobarbital leads to no relief. Which of the following treatments should be considered?

(A) Add a second antidepressant.
(B) Begin a mood stabilizer.
(C) Initiate electroconvulsive therapy.
(D) Add dantrolene.
(E) Administer intravenous haloperidol.

159

Which of the following antidepressants is the best choice for a patient who wants to avoid orgasm dysfunction as a side effect?

(A) Bupropion
(B) Sertraline
(C) Venlafaxine
(D) Escitalopram
(E) Fluoxetine

160

A 20-year-old female college student presents to the counseling center with concerns about her alcohol use. She describes two occasions in the past year when she attended parties and had "way too much to drink." Following these occasions she feels "lousy," postpones studying, and then must stay up late to study for tests. When she's gone to most other parties she's had four or five drinks with no ill effects. There are no other substance-related symptoms. She expresses some concern about her drinking and asks for recommendations. The best intervention at this point would be to:

(A) provide a brief intervention.
(B) prescribe disulfiram.
(C) recommend attending Alcoholics Anonymous.
(D) prescribe naltrexone.
(E) prescribe acamprosate.

161

Which of the following medications has the greatest body of evidence supporting its use as a monotherapy for acute bipolar depression?

(A) Bupropion
(B) Lamotrigine
(C) Valproate
(D) Olanzapine
(E) Quetiapine

162

A patient reports feeling that he has always had to please others, and that, if he is not liked by everyone, he will never be successful. Which of the following statements would be characteristic of a cognitive behavioral approach to the patient's problem?

(A) "Let's draw out your circle of friends and examine which ones you feel you must please."
(B) "Feeling you must please others is acting more out of an emotional mind than a rational mind."
(C) "Tell me about your experience that you can only be successful by pleasing others."
(D) "Is it possible that feeling you're not being liked by everyone is a way to ease the pressure of having to be successful?"

163

A 32-year-old woman presents with a history of frequent, unanticipated panic attacks. Which of the following medications is most likely to be of benefit for treating her disorder?

(A) Bupropion
(B) Aripiprazole
(C) Gabapentin
(D) Clonazepam
(E) Buspirone

164

Which of the following is the best established psychosocial intervention for the treatment of panic disorder?

(A) Dialectical behavioral therapy
(B) Interpersonal psychotherapy
(C) Psychodynamic psychotherapy
(D) Marital and family therapy
(E) Cognitive-behavioral therapy

165

A patient with a history of substance dependence and depression treated with tranylcypromine presents to the emergency room with hypertension, tachycardia, chest pain and severe occipital headache. The patient says he had a relapse of his drug use. Which of the following substances is the most likely contributor to his clinical presentation at this time?

(A) Vodka
(B) Methamphetamine
(C) PCP
(D) Marijuana
(E) Inhalants

166

Trazodone exerts its hypnotic effects by interaction with which of the following neurotransmitter receptors?

(A) Dopamine
(B) GABA
(C) Histamine
(D) Alpha$_2$
(E) Acetylcholine

167

Based on the results of Phase 1 of the Clinical Antipsychotic Trials of Intervention Effectiveness (CATIE) study, which of the following antipsychotic medications is most likely to be associated with the development of metabolic complications?

(A) Olanzapine
(B) Quetiapine
(C) Risperidone
(D) Ziprasidone
(E) Perphenazine

168

Which of the following SSRIs is designated as FDA pregnancy category D?

(A) Fluoxetine
(B) Paroxetine
(C) Sertraline
(D) Citalopram
(E) Escitalopram

169

According to the National Comorbidity Survey (NCS), which of the following experiences is most frequently associated with PTSD in women in the U.S.?

(A) Being in a life-threatening accident
(B) Combat exposure
(C) Being involved in a natural disaster
(D) Sexual assault
(E) Witnessing someone being badly injured or killed

170

The core techniques of open-ended questions, affirmation, reflective statements, and summary statements (OARS) are central to which one of the following therapies?

(A) Cognitive behavioral
(B) Interpersonal
(C) Motivational interviewing
(D) Twelve-step facilitation
(E) Prolonged exposure

171

Which of the following is the most common sleep problem in persons with major depressive disorder?

(A) Vivid mood congruent dreams
(B) Hypersomnia
(C) Restless leg syndrome
(D) Insomnia
(E) Sleep phase disorder

172

Which of the following psychotherapeutic techniques has the greatest body of evidence supporting it as a first line treatment for PTSD?

(A) Hypnosis
(B) EMDR (Eye Movement Desensitization and Reprocessing)
(C) Prolonged exposure therapy
(D) Stress inoculation training
(E) Systematic desensitization

173

Which of the following is most characteristic of symptoms of PTSD?

(A) Persist long after the precipitating event is over
(B) Exist only while the trauma is present
(C) Directly proportional to the magnitude of the trauma
(D) Occur only in response to certain types of trauma
(E) Develop immediately upon experiencing the trauma

174

A 38-year-old woman with a history of estrogen receptor-positive breast cancer is currently taking tamoxifen to reduce the risk of recurrence. However, she has become increasingly tearful, withdrawn, and anergic over the past month. She also notes difficulty with sleep and concentration as well as distressing hot flashes since initiating tamoxifen. Which one of the following medications is most appropriate to treat her symptoms?

(A) Venlafaxine
(B) Paroxetine
(C) Gabapentin
(D) Fluoxetine
(E) Duloxetine

175

In addition to time course, which of the following symptoms is more prominent in ASD compared to PTSD?

(A) Impairment in functioning
(B) Dissociative symptoms
(C) Fear or helplessness response
(D) Reexperiencing

176

Presence of which of the following symptoms is sufficient to meet DSM-IV-TR criteria for alcohol abuse?

(A) A need to drink increasing amounts to become intoxicated
(B) Continued use despite recurrent liver dysfunction
(C) Repeatedly driving while intoxicated
(D) Unsuccessful attempts to quit drinking
(E) Consuming a greater amount of alcohol than planned

177

A psychiatrist is asked by the local school to consult on a 13-year-old boy who has exhibited problems with compulsive eating and failure to make academic progress. The boy's parents report that he has always eaten "everything in sight" and has been delayed in his development. Medical history is remarkable for poor muscle tone and failure to thrive as an infant. Physical examination reveals hypotonia, obesity, hypogonadism, a narrow-appearing forehead, downslanting palpebral fissures, small-appearing hands and feet and downturning of the corners of the mouth. Intelligence testing is consistent with mental retardation. What is the MOST LIKELY cause of the patient's signs and symptoms?

(A) Childhood degenerative disorder
(B) Congenital rubella infection
(C) Homocystinuria
(D) Prader-Willi syndrome
(E) Tuberous sclerosis

178

Which of the following psychosocial treatments for social phobia has the most evidence supporting effectiveness?

(A) Cognitive-behavioral therapy
(B) Interpersonal psychotherapy
(C) Psychodynamic psychotherapy
(D) Family focused therapy
(E) Group psychoeducation

179

A 62-year-old woman presents for assessment and treatment of a three year history of mild but persistent depressive symptoms. One year ago she was named board chairman of her association and also began a new relationship with a very wealthy individual. The relationship is going well emotionally and sexually, but she sometimes feels inadequate in her new social circles. She misses her former partner particularly when she feels socially awkward. After a discussion of treatment options for improving her overall level of functioning and self satisfaction, she and her psychiatrist decide upon a structured, time-limited course of interpersonal psychotherapy (IPT). Which ONE of the following would be the most appropriate focus of the IPT?

(A) Analysis of transference
(B) Delayed grief
(C) Interpersonal deficits
(D) Role dispute
(E) Role transition

180

Which of the following congenital abnormalities is associated with maternal use of carbamazepine in the first trimester of pregnancy?

(A) An increased risk of Ebstein's anomaly, the downward displacement of the tricuspid valve into the right ventricle and variable levels of right ventricular hyperplasia
(B) Craniofacial defects, fingernail hypoplasia, and developmental delay
(C) Fetal development of skin rash in a neonate who has antigen characteristics different from those of the mother
(D) Impaired temperature regulation and apnea

181

When initiating treatment with long-acting injectable haloperidol every 4 weeks, what period of time is required to reach steady-state?

(A) 4 weeks
(B) 8 weeks
(C) 12 weeks
(D) 16 weeks
(E) 20 weeks

182

In addition to pharmacotherapy, psychotherapy plays an important role in treating bipolar disorder. Which ONE of the following circumstances best describes when cognitive behavioral therapy (CBT) is most effective in the adjunctive treatment of bipolar disorder?

(A) Acutely ill, depressed
(B) Acutely ill, manic
(C) After four or more episodes
(D) Moderately or acutely ill states
(E) Recovered from acute episode

183

Behavioral approaches such as the Semans pause maneuver, the start-stop method of Kaplan, and the pause-squeeze technique of Masters and Johnson have been employed to treat which of the following?

(A) Male erectile disorder
(B) Female sexual arousal disorder
(C) Premature ejaculation
(D) Hypoactive sexual desire disorder
(E) Female orgasmic disorder

184

A 25-year-old man with no past history of abnormal involuntary movements is being treated with haloperidol. He should be evaluated for abnormal involuntary movements every

(A) 1 month
(B) 3 months
(C) 6 months
(D) 12 months
(E) 18 months

185

A 19-year old private in the U.S. Army loses his left leg after his vehicle drives over an improvised explosive device. Two months later he reports ongoing recurrent and intrusive recollections of the event, nightmares and flashbacks to the explosion, avoidance of any activities that remind him of the event, irritability and disturbed sleep. Which of the following psychotherapeutic interventions is MOST likely to be effective in alleviating his symptoms?

(A) Biofeedback
(B) Eye movement desensitization and reprocessing
(C) Exposure-based cognitive-behavior therapy
(D) Guided imagery therapy
(E) Hypnotherapy

186

A 40-year-old patient is taking clozapine for treatment-resistant schizophrenia. Assuming no abnormal laboratory results, after what period of time could complete blood count monitoring be reduced to every four weeks?

(A) 3 months
(B) 6 months
(C) 12 months
(D) 18 months
(E) 24 months

187

For patients with functional gastrointestinal disorders, which of the following medications would be most likely to alleviate the visceral pain associated with irritable bowel syndrome?

(A) Bupropion
(B) Clonazepam
(C) Fluoxetine
(D) Quetiapine
(E) Amitriptyline

188

A 56-year old man with major depression is prescribed paroxetine. One month later, he complains of significant nausea. His dose is lowered from 20 to 10 mg, however he continues to feel nauseated. He is motivated to remain on the medication if possible since he feels it has been enormously helpful for his depression. A genotyping of the cytochrome P450 2D6 gene reveals that he has one inactive copy, and one partially inactive copy. Which of the following would be the most appropriate step to take?

(A) Discontinue paroxetine immediately and wait one month.
(B) Attempt even lower doses of paroxetine.
(C) Discontinue paroxetine and begin fluoxetine.
(D) Discontinue paroxetine and begin citalopram.
(E) Continue paroxetine but add ondansetron.

189

Which symptom is characteristically seen in patients with Münchausen syndrome?

(A) Thoughts of death
(B) Pathological lying
(C) Fear of pain
(D) Perceptual disturbances
(E) Feelings of inadequacy

190

A patient with bipolar disorder is receiving maintenance treatment with extended-release divalproex. How many hours should elapse between his last dose and drawing of the trough level of valproic acid?

(A) 4
(B) 8
(C) 12
(D) 18

191

A woman presents for help in coping with stress. During the assessment, it becomes clear that she is excessively preoccupied with her appearance, particularly her face. She spends hours a day examining and caring for her face. She is convinced that her cheekbones are uneven and make her look like a freak. Her appearance is unremarkable. After the assessment is complete, the psychiatrist's best initial approach is to:

(A) reassure the patient about her appearance.
(B) agree that the situation is quite distressing.
(C) point out that her thinking is quite distorted.
(D) agree that her appearance is a problem.
(E) explain the benefits of medication.

192

Which of the following is a common symptom of seasonal affective disorder?

(A) Light sensitivity
(B) Somatic complaints
(C) Insomnia
(D) Overeating
(E) Impulsiveness

193

Which of the following techniques is commonly used in motivational interviewing?

(A) Confrontation
(B) Interpretation of transference
(C) Identification of cognitive distortions
(D) Decision balance
(E) Relaxation training

194

Which of the following factors best differentiates acute stress disorder from PTSD?

(A) Chronicity
(B) Traumatic event severity
(C) Presence of nightmares
(D) Level of functional impairment
(E) Severity of subjective response to the event

195

Which of the following best describes the mechanism of action of flumazenil in the treatment of benzodiazepine overdose?

(A) Flumazenil blocks benzodiazepines from crossing the blood-brain barrier.
(B) Flumazenil competes with benzodiazepines at central synaptic GABA receptor sites.
(C) Flumazenil decreases the influx of chloride ions into GABAergic neurons preventing hyperpolarization.
(D) Flumazenil increases the influx of sodium ions into GABAergic neurons causing depolarization.
(E) Flumazenil increases the rate of oxidative metabolism of benzodiazepines.

196

A 22-year-old woman was involved in a severe motor vehicle accident in which several people were significantly injured. She had difficulty recalling portions of the accident, nightmares and difficulty falling asleep. She refused to drive her car, had difficulty concentrating and felt emotionally numb. She was unable to attend work. Her symptoms spontaneously resolved after a month and she was able to return to work. The most likely diagnosis is:

(A) acute stress disorder.
(B) adjustment disorder.
(C) posttraumatic stress disorder.
(D) panic disorder.
(E) brief psychotic disorder.

197

Which of the following is the most common form of affective illness in families of patients with bipolar disorder?

(A) Bipolar disorder
(B) Unipolar depression
(C) Dysthymia
(D) Premenstrual dysphoric disorder
(E) Cyclothymia

198

The use of bright light treatment has been shown to be efficacious and safe for the treatment of:

(A) dysthymia.
(B) nonseasonal depression.
(C) bipolar disorder.
(D) PTSD.

199

A 42-year-old woman is referred for a polysomnogram to evaluate her complaint of insomnia. During the polysomnogram, she seems to fall asleep within 15 minutes, and her EEG reflects normal sleep throughout the night. When she wakes in the morning in the sleep lab, she reports that she was awake most of the night. Which type of primary insomnia is this patient most likely to have?

(A) Psychophysiological insomnia
(B) Sleep state misperception
(C) Idiopathic insomnia
(D) Obstructive sleep apnea
(E) Delayed sleep-phase syndrome

200

Which of the following is one of the standards used to determine mental capacity in decision making?

(A) Absence of psychosis
(B) Agreement with the medical recommendations
(C) Severity of psychiatric illness
(D) Rational decision making
(E) Presence of abstract thought

201

Which of the following treatments has the best body of evidence in preventing post-stroke depression in older populations?

(A) Escitalopram
(B) Mianserin
(C) Sertraline
(D) Problem solving therapy
(E) Cognitive behavioral therapy

202

A single mother reports that her 12-year-old child has become increasingly defiant with parental requests, at times becoming physically aggressive by kicking doors and hitting walls. She notes that the child does not exhibit these problems with the father. Which of the following is the most appropriate treatment?

(A) Inoculation techniques, such as boot camp
(B) Contingency management
(C) Medication management
(D) Send the child to live with the father temporarily
(E) Brief hospitalization

203

A 22-year-old man with chronic schizophrenia developed gynecomastia after being treated with risperidone for many months. His prolactin level is markedly elevated and you want to switch him to the antipsychotic drug that is less likely to cause this problem. Which one of the following would be the most appropriate choice?

(A) Aripiprazole
(B) Olanzapine
(C) Perphenazine
(D) Haloperidol
(E) Paliperidone

204

A 70-year-old man presents to a clinic with progressive memory loss. Which of the following findings is most representative of cortical dementia in this patient?

(A) Apathy
(B) Aphasia
(C) Decreased attention
(D) Bradyphrenia
(E) Mood lability

205

A psychiatrist is asked to determine if a very ill, delirious and possibly senile patient has the capacity to make a new will. Which of the following features must be present to determine that the patient has the capacity?

(A) Orientation to time and place
(B) Unimpaired attention span
(C) Awareness that she is making a will
(D) Choice of beneficiary that is not frivolous
(E) Ability to recognize family

206

Which of the following types of therapy used to treat schizophrenia is based on the premise that attempting to suppress or control mental events is NOT helpful?

(A) Traditional cognitive-behavioral therapy (CBT)
(B) Compliance therapy
(C) Acceptance and commitment therapy (ACT)
(D) Supportive psychotherapy
(E) Illness education

207

A 45-year-old patient requests a medication to treat symptoms consistent with generalized anxiety disorder. The patient has a history of heavy drinking. Which of the following medications would be most appropriate to prescribe?

(A) Clonazepam
(B) Bupropion
(C) Quetiapine
(D) Diazepam
(E) Venlafaxine

208

A bus driver calls in sick whenever there is inclement weather such as rain or light snow. He has never had an accident while driving, nor does he know anyone personally who had an accident due to inclement weather. He also avoids driving his own car in poor weather and attempts to convince his family members to do the same. He admits he is very cautious about many things, which interferes with his sleep, causes fatigue, and makes him irritable. Which of the following is the most likely diagnosis?

(A) Panic disorder
(B) Social phobia: situational
(C) Posttraumatic stress disorder
(D) OCD
(E) Generalized anxiety disorder

209

A 20-year-old woman was brought to the emergency department by police after disrupting one of her university classes. She was agitated and demanded that her intellectual abilities be acknowledged. She had pressured speech and her affect alternated between periods of euphoria and irritability. Her roommate told the emergency staff that the patient had been very energetic, unable to sleep for several days and had previously been admitted to hospital for similar behavior. Which of the following diagnoses is most likely?

(A) Delirium
(B) Cyclothymia
(C) Bipolar disorder, manic
(D) Bipolar disorder, mixed state
(E) Schizophrenia

210

Children and adolescents are considered a vulnerable population in the conduct of research because they:

(A) cannot consent.
(B) suffer more adverse effects.
(C) are in riskier studies.
(D) cannot assent.
(E) do not benefit.

211

A 53-year-old man presents asking for help with drinking. He reports frequent swelling of his ankles and says that when he goes to the corner store, he has to walk slowly or he'll get too short of breath. He says he's supposed to be taking "some heart pills," but hasn't had any for a number of months and can't remember their names. He has attempted to quit drinking on two prior occasions and was treated with diazepam for "the shakes." He has been drinking one to two pints of rum daily for the past 10 months. His last drink was several hours ago. What would be the most appropriate initial referral?

(A) Medical hospitalization
(B) Partial hospitalization program
(C) Intensive outpatient program
(D) Office-based program
(E) Therapeutic community

212

A 46-year-old man is begun on citalopram 20 mg daily for a major depressive episode. After four weeks he returns to his psychiatrist citing little if any change in his symptoms. Which of the following would be the most appropriate next step in the patient's treatment?

(A) Increase the patient to 40 mg of citalopram.
(B) Discontinue citalopram and begin venlafaxine.
(C) Continue citalopram but add lithium.
(D) Begin vagal nerve stimulation.
(E) Continue citalopram and begin aripiprazole.

213

Which of the following features would be most predictive of a favorable response to lithium maintenance in bipolar disorder?

(A) Euthymic intervals
(B) Rapid cycling
(C) Mixed episodes
(D) Substance abuse
(E) Psychosis

214

Which of the following medications has shown the most evidence for reducing suicide risk in the long-term treatment of bipolar disorder?

(A) Carbamazepine
(B) Divalproex
(C) Gabapentin
(D) Lithium
(E) Olanzapine

215

A 56-year-old man with a history of cancer presents with confusion, pure amnestic syndrome, and affective symptoms. Diagnostic studies are consistent with paraneoplastic limbic encephalitis. Which of the following cancers is the most common cause of this paraneoplastic syndrome?

(A) Pancreatic cancer
(B) Prostate cancer
(C) Renal cancer
(D) Small cell lung cancer
(E) Testicular cancer

216

A 24-year-old man on lithium maintenance therapy develops severe, persistent polyuria and polydipsia. Which of the following medications is most likely to be effective in treating these side effects without requiring administration of supplemental electrolytes?

(A) Amiloride
(B) Furosemide
(C) Hydrochlorothiazide
(D) Metolazone
(E) Torsemide

217

A 17-year-old patient diagnosed with anorexia nervosa at age 14 is brought to a psychiatrist by her parents. They are concerned because she is 65% of her expected body weight. The most appropriate intervention is to:

(A) suggest a group therapy program.
(B) initiate treatment with an antidepressant.
(C) restore the patient's nutritional state.
(D) refer the patient and family for counseling.
(E) provide cognitive therapy.

218

According to the results of the Clinical Antipsychotic Trials of Intervention Effectiveness (CATIE) study, which antipsychotic medication had the lowest all-cause discontinuation rate?

(A) Olanzapine
(B) Quetiapine
(C) Risperidone
(D) Ziprasidone
(E) Perphanazine

219

Which of the following medication combinations for individuals with OCD comorbid with tic disorder is supported best by evidence?

(A) Fluoxetine plus clonazepam
(B) Sertraline plus buspirone
(C) Nefazodone plus naltrexone
(D) Fluvoxamine plus haloperidol

220

Studies of the neurobiological correlates of borderline personality disorder have revealed hyperactivity in which one of the following?

(A) Amygdala
(B) Prefrontal cortex
(C) Tegmental area
(D) Cingulate
[E] Accumbens

221

A 38-year-old patient with major depressive disorder has had a partial response to 80 mgs of citalopram. He states this is the best drug that he has been on, but continues to experience symptoms despite being on the medication for 7 weeks. He continues to occasionally have suicidal thoughts which frighten him because he made a suicide attempt 4 years ago. The best intervention at this time is to augment with:

(A) fluoxetine.
(B) lamotrigine.
(C) lithium.
(D) thyroid.
(E) buspirone.

222

Which of the following medications for bipolar disorder has been associated with polycystic ovarian syndrome (PCOS)?

(A) Topiramate
(B) Divalproex
(C) Carbamazepine
(D) Lamotrigine
(E) Lithium

223

The parents of a 4-year-old boy report that a few hours after he goes to sleep, their son will suddenly get up in the bed and look extremely frightened. His heart races; he is diaphoretic and cries out. He is difficult to awaken and has no recall for the event the next morning. Which of the following is the most appropriate next step in the management of this patient?

(A) Administer a short-acting hypnotic for two weeks.
(B) Have the child go to bed at a later time.
(C) Obtain an electroencephalogram to rule out temporal lobe epilepsy.
(D) Reassure the parents that their son will outgrow the disorder.
(E) Suggest to the parents that they allow their son to sleep with them for a temporary period.

224

A 68-year-old woman being treated for bipolar disorder became semi-comatose and incontinent of urine. Her serum sodium concentration was 110 mmol/L. Which of the following medications is the most likely cause?

(A) Lithium
(B) Divalproex
(C) Oxcarbazepine
(D) Lamotrigine
(E) Olanzapine

225

In bipolar disorder, which of the following characteristics BEST differentiates adultonset bipolar disorder from childhood-onset?

(A) Presence of psychotic features
(B) Prolonged early course
(C) Mixed episodes
(D) Recurrent depression
(E) Treatment resistance

226

A psychiatrist's neighbor tells her that he is having trouble sleeping due to work related stresses. He asks for recommendations and some medication until he can get an appointment with his internist. What ethical problem results if the psychiatrist gives the neighbor the medication?

(A) Prescribing medication creates a doctor-patient relationship.
(B) The assistance may be ineffective, straining the relationship.
(C) Providing free care can foster resentment.
(D) Assisting this neighbor creates an expectation that the psychiatrist will treat other neighbors.

227

A local radio talk show host comes to see you for psychotherapy because you were described as "the best doctor at the clinic" by one of his friends. He spends most of the hour talking about problems he is having with a workmate who he feels is treating him rudely. At the end of the session he asks to be seen at a special time to accommodate his work schedule. When you tell him you will be unavailable at that time, he becomes dismissive and angry. These traits are suggestive of which ONE of the following:

(A) Schizoid
(B) Antisocial
(C) Obsessive-compulsive
(D) Narcissistic
(E) Borderline

228

A 14-year-old patient with anorexia nervosa has achieved a stable weight and nutritional status. Which of the following interventions has the MOST evidence demonstrating effectiveness in the treatment of this disorder?

(A) Family based therapies
(B) Fluoxetine
(C) Individual cognitive behavioral therapy
(D) Individual interpersonal psychotherapy
(E) Olanzapine

229

Which of the following traumatic events is MOST likely to induce PTSD in exposed individuals?

(A) Unexpected death
(B) Natural disasters
(C) Motor vehicle accidents
(D) Witness to violence
(E) Sexual assault

230

A 9-year-old boy is brought by his mother at the insistence of the school for the assessment of behavior problems. The diagnosis of attention-deficit/hyperactivity disorder is made, along with the recommendation to start stimulant medication. The mother is concerned that stimulant medication might put her son at risk for developing substance use problems. Regarding the risk of developing substance use problems, what is known about stimulant treatment for ADHD?

(A) Increased risk of drug dependence only
(B) Increased risk of both alcohol and drug dependence
(C) Decreased risk of drug dependence only
(D) Decreased risk of both alcohol and drug dependence
(E) Unchanged risk for both alcohol and drug dependence

231

Which of the following disorders must be considered in the differential diagnosis of individuals with late onset obsessive-compulsive disorder (after the age of 45 years)?

(A) Huntington's disease
(B) Asperger's syndrome
(C) Delusional disorder
(D) Body dysmorphic disorder
(E) Schizophrenia

232

A psychiatrist has been seeing a terminally ill woman in psychotherapy. The patient has become too ill to come to the office so the psychiatrist elects to make a house call. In committing this boundary crossing, he should:

(A) act in a more social manner.
(B) discuss this variation from usual practice with a lawyer before going.
(C) discuss the implications of this change of venue with the patient.
(D) never go to the patient's home.

233

Which of the following is the most common psychiatric symptom found in patients with fibromyalgia?

(A) Anorexia
(B) Psychosis
(C) Hypersomnia
(D) Mania
(E) Depression

234

Which type of treatment program has the best short-term outcomes for cocaine dependence?

(A) Voucher-based contingency management
(B) Psychodynamic group psychotherapy
(C) Interpersonal psychotherapy
(D) Twelve-step groups (without other counseling)
(E) Cue exposure therapy

235

A patient in therapy has recently been told that his psychiatrist may change jobs and will be transferring his care to another psychiatrist. He has always needed a great deal of reassurance but now calls almost daily asking for opinions on decisions he is trying to make in his life. He often worries his ill wife will die before he does. Each time he is advised to attend day treatment to get further support, he often agrees to do so but does not follow through. Based on this vignette, which of the following personality disorders is most likely?

(A) Dependent
(B) Antisocial
(C) Paranoid
(D) Borderline
(E) Narcissistic

236

During an initial evaluation, a patient complains of multiple episodes of having palpitations, sweating and intense anxiety. Information that would be most supportive of panic disorder is that the episodes occur when the patient:

(A) is reminded of a past assault.
(B) must use a public bathroom.
(C) attends a large party.
(D) is in essentially any setting.
(E) must use an elevator.

237

Which of the following statements most accurately describes the benefits of SSRIs in the treatment of PTSD? SSRIs have been shown to:

(A) ameliorate core PTSD and other associated symptoms.
(B) treat primarily the comorbid psychiatric disorders.
(C) improve primarily hyperarousal symptoms.
(D) improve the effectiveness of alpha 2 adrenergic agonists.
(E) act only to augment psychotherapy in PTSD.

238

Which of the following factors will increase the potential for toxicity with lithium?

(A) Cigarette smoking
(B) Concomitant administration of mirtazapine (Remeron)
(C) Drinking a lot of water
(D) Exercising outdoors on a hot day

239

An individual with a history of opiate dependence admits to daily use of opiates, but a confirmatory urine toxicology screen is negative. Which of the following opiates is the patient most likely using?

(A) Hydrocodone
(B) Morphine
(C) Codeine
(D) Heroin
(E) Opium

240

A 72-year-old man with severe chronic obstructive airway disease complains of anxiety, muscle tension and a general feeling of uneasiness. The most appropriate psychotropic medication for this patient's condition would be:

(A) clonazepam.
(B) diazepam.
(C) alprazolam.
(D) sorazepam.
(E) buspirone.

241

Which of the following statements best describes the mechanism of action of acamprosate, thought to occur in the treatment of alcohol dependence?

(A) Acamprosate blocks the reuptake of chloride ions in central GABAergic neurons.
(B) Acamprosate competes with alcohol for central GABAergic neurons in a dose-dependent fashion.
(C) Acamprosate affects mu opiate receptors blocking the centrally mediated reinforcing effects of alcohol.
(D) Acamprosate inhibits aldehyde dehydrogenase, resulting in the accumulation of toxic levels of acetaldehyde.
(E) Acamposate reduces neuronal hyperactivity during early alcohol recovery.

242

In a recent study, which of the following substances was associated with an increase in the long term risk of developing psychotic disorder?

(A) Alcohol
(B) Cannabis
(C) Nicotine
(D) Opiates
(E) Inhalants

243

A psychiatrist may terminate care of a patient in which of the following circumstances?

(A) Patient has not paid a bill
(B) Patient has failed to be cooperative in treatment
(C) Patient has consultation with another psychiatrist
(D) Patient misses two appointments and does not return the psychiatrist's calls
(E) Patient is hospitalized on an inpatient unit and care is permanently transferred

244

Which of the following medications, commonly used in alcohol treatment to decrease craving, has been shown to be more effective if given after a period of sobriety?

(A) Acamprosate
(B) Disulfiram
(C) Gabapentin
(D) Naltrexone
(E) Topiramate

245

Which of the following is characteristic of social phobia?

(A) Spontaneous uncued panic attacks
(B) Avoiding public speaking because of trembling
(C) Fear of humiliation when speaking in a group setting
(D) Fainting while having blood drawn
(E) Avoiding parties because of fear of contamination

246

A patient with OCD and fears of contamination insists that his family remove their shoes when they enter his living space. Which of the following concepts best describes this behavior?

(A) Repetition compulsion
(B) Displacement
(C) Ritual by proxy
(D) Projection
(E) Reaction formation

247

A 48-year-old woman is brought to the emergency department after being found unconscious. Examination reveals respiratory depression, extreme miosis, stupor, coma and pulmonary edema. The patient's presentation is MOST consistent with an overdose of:

(A) alcohol.
(B) cannabis.
(C) inhalants.
(D) opioids.
(E) sedative-hypnotics.

248

Patients with obsessive-compulsive disorder are most likely to respond to which of the following therapy modalities?

(A) Psychoanalysis
(B) Dynamic psychotherapy
(C) Dialectical behavior therapy
(D) Motivational enhancement therapy
(E) Exposure and response prevention

249

Which of following is the most common fear during the dying process?

(A) Loneliness
(B) Abandonment
(C) Pain
(D) Uncertainty

250

A 38-year-old woman is admitted to the hospital with a severe manic episode. On examination, she is noted to have motor excitement, mutism and stereotypic movements. Which of the following medications would be the most appropriate in treating this patient?

(A) Carbamazepine
(B) Haloperidol
(C) Lamotrigine
(D) Lorazepam
(E) Olanzapine

251

A 35-year-old man with a history of opiate dependence is brought to the emergency department after being found unconscious. Examination reveals respiratory depression, extreme miosis, stupor, coma and pulmonary edema. The emergency department physician administers naloxone 1.0 mg intravenously every three minutes until a maximum dosage of 10 mg has been given. However, the patient remains unresponsive. What would be the most appropriate next step?

(A) Double the next intravenous dose of naloxone.
(B) Increase the frequency with which the naloxone is administered.
(C) Reconsider the diagnosis of an opioid overdose.
(D) Start a continuous infusion of naloxone.
(E) Switch from intravenous naloxone to nasogastric administration of naltrexone.

252

The concept that directs child psychiatrists and health care providers to involve children in decisions about their care commensurate with their developmental capacity is referred to as:

(A) cognitive incapacity.
(B) pediatric assent.
(C) pediatric consent.
(D) remaining autonomy.

253

Which of the following syndromes is the most common form of inherited mental retardation?

(A) Fragile X syndrome
(B) Williams syndrome
(C) Rett syndrome
(D) Prader-Willi syndrome
(E) Angelman syndrome

254

Hypertensive paroxysms associated with diaphoresis, tachycardia, flushing, nausea and significant apprehension suggests the presence of which of the following general medical conditions that mimics anxiety?

(A) Mitral valve problem
(B) Cocaine withdrawal
(C) Coronary insufficiency
(D) Hyperthyroidism
(E) Pheochromocytoma

255

Behavioral therapy for a patient with OCD is most difficult when which of the following symptoms are present?

(A) Observable rituals
(B) Delusions
(C) Contamination fears
(D) Checking behaviors

256

A psychiatrist is seeing a 35-year-old patient with schizophrenia who is accompanied by his mother. During a discussion about possible medication options, the psychiatrist turns to the patient and asks "What would you prefer to do?" This question is an example of which ethical principle?

(A) Altruism
(B) Respect for autonomy
(C) Beneficence
(D) Nonmaleficence

257

Which of the following defines the virtue "veracity"?

(A) Saying only what is true, never misleading the patient, and pacing disclosure to the patient effectively.
(B) Practicing medicine consistent with the highest intellectual and moral standards, both professional and individual.
(C) Recognizing, preventing, and relieving pain, suffering, and distress and acting to prevent and relieve pain, suffering and distress.
(D) Not being excessively swayed by potential feared consequence.
(E) Taking reasonable risks to one's self-interest (in time, convenience, health and even life), to protect the interests of patients.

258

A 25-year-old man has a history of facial and truncal tics since childhood. He presents to an outpatient clinic for evaluation of anxiety and is diagnosed as having OCD. Which of the following patterns of OCD symptoms is he most likely to exhibit?

(A) Obsessions and checking
(B) Cleanliness and washing
(C) Symmetry and ordering
(D) Hoarding

259

The starting dose of lamotrigine should be reduced by half if a patient is taking which of the following medications?

(A) Carbamazepine
(B) Oral contraceptive
(C) Phenobarbital
(D) Divalproex
(E) Phenytoin

260

A 75-year-old man with a history of mild Alzheimer's disease becomes increasingly aggressive at home. In addition, he is noted to have worsening memory and word-finding difficulty, inadequate self-care, and less interest in activities. Which of the patient's symptoms is most likely to be helped by risperidone?

(A) Memory
(B) Word finding
(C) Independent functioning
(D) Aggression
(E) Interest in activities

261

Two teenagers randomly fire their guns at a 54-year-old man in their neighborhood. A week later the patient complains that he can't "get it out of my mind" and is having frequent nightmares about this incident. He is always "on the watch" when he drives down the road and avoids going out alone. The most likely diagnosis for this patient is:

(A) generalized anxiety disorder.
(B) obsessive-compulsive disorder.
(C) acute stress disorder.
(D) social phobia.
(E) posttraumatic stress disorder.

262

A 42-year-old patient complains of a fear of crowded places. This fear is present in any situation in which the patient perceives that escape may be difficult, including riding alone in elevators and cars. As a result of this fear, the patient rarely leaves home. Which of the following is the most likely diagnosis?

(A) Social phobia
(B) Agoraphobia
(C) Specific phobia
(D) Avoidant personality disorder
(E) Panic disorder

263

Which of the following is an objective sleep disturbance that occurs in depression?

(A) Shortened sleep latency
(B) Decreased nighttime arousal
(C) Increased total sleep time
(D) Shortened REM latency
(E) Increased slow wave sleep

264

The main factor of somatization disorder which differentiates it from factitious disorder or malingering is that in somatization disorder:

(A) patients seek to play the sick role.
(B) there are external incentives for the behavior.
(C) complaint of symptoms is exaggerated.
(D) patients often have had multiple hospitalizations.
(E) symptoms are not under voluntary control.

265

A 38-year-old married woman presents to a psychiatrist complaining of difficulty in her sex life. She reports that, for much of her married life, she has had little interest in sexual intercourse with her husband. She has not had any affairs, and she denies any discord in her relationship with her husband aside from the lack of a satisfactory sex life. She does not masturbate and rarely has any sexual fantasies. On the few occasions that she does have intercourse with her husband, she is able to enjoy sex and achieve an orgasm. Which of the following diagnoses is most appropriate?

(A) Dyspareunia
(B) Sexual aversion disorder
(C) Hypoactive sexual desire disorder
(D) Female sexual arousal disorder
(E) Female orgasmic disorder

266

The age at which a clinician should consider the possibility of the early onset subtype of dementia of the Alzheimer's type is:

(A) 35 years.
(B) 45 years or below.
(C) 55 years or below.
(D) 65 years or below.
(E) 75 years or below.

267

A 22-year-old woman is driving her boyfriend home. The car hits a tree and he is killed. Six months after the accident she is still unable to drive, avoids going out, jumps when she hears loud noises and cannot feel any sadness or happiness. What is the most likely diagnosis for this patient?

(A) Adjustment disorder
(B) Agoraphobia
(C) Major depressive disorder
(D) Posttraumatic stress disorder
(E) Acute stress disorder

268

Which of the following actions is most likely to ease the fears of a dying patient and his family?

(A) Postponing the discussion of pain and pain management
(B) Giving the family and patient information on a need to know basis
(C) Telling the patient that only the family's input regarding care will be sought
(D) Educating the patient that he may have discomfort that cannot be alleviated
(E) Obtaining the patient's wishes regarding treatment decisions

269

A 26-year-old bystander of a horrific motor vehicle accident is taken to the ED after reporting that suddenly she had gone blind. She does not appear to focus on anyone who is talking. However, her eyes are noted to track her reflection when a mirror is waved in front of her. After hospital admission, a complete medical and neurological workup is found to be normal. What should be the first intervention for her condition?

(A) Pointing out that she can see as a result of the mirror test
(B) Instituting a reward system for sight improvement
(C) Discussing the stress of the event under amobarbital
(D) Suggesting symptom improvement through hypnosis
(E) Reassuring her that her sight will soon return

270

A 48-year-old obese man presents for an evaluation, at the prompting of his wife. The wife, who has accompanied the patient to the appointment, complains that the patient snores loudly and keeps her awake at night. She states he sometimes seems to be gasping for air. On questioning, the patient admits to falling asleep easily during the day, and even falling asleep while driving on occasion. He also complains of morning headaches and was recently diagnosed with hypertension. Which of the following is the best initial treatment for this patient's condition?

(A) Uvulopalatopharyngoplasty
(B) Temazepam
(C) Biofeedback
(D) Modafinil
(E) Nasal continuous positive airway pressure (CPAP)

271

A 55-year-old patient with alcohol dependence treated with naltrexone 50mg daily has been abstinent from alcohol for the past 2 months. The patient has been advised to undergo surgical knee replacement. What is the minimum duration of time prior to the surgery for which naltrexone must be discontinued in order for opiate analgesia to be effective?

(A) 24 hours
(B) 72 hours
(C) 5 days
(D) 1 week
(E) 2 weeks

272

A 35-year-old patient worries obsessively that he will kill his mother. To alleviate the anxiety, he calls her repeatedly throughout the day to hear her voice and reassure himself that he has not harmed her. He has tried adequate trials of high doses of fluoxetine, paroxetine, lorazepam, and clonazepam, without improvement. Which of the following medications would be most appropriate to prescribe next?

(A) Citalopram
(B) Alprazolam
(C) Bupropion
(D) Lithium
(E) Clomipramine

273

A 60-year-old man with early Parkinson's disease presents to your office at the urging of his wife. She reports that the patient has begun "acting out" his dreams while asleep, and on at least one occasion this "acting out" led to his assaulting her. Polysomnogram is likely to demonstrate motor artifact and/or lack of complete hypotonia during which phase of sleep?

(A) Stage I
(B) Stage II
(C) Stage III
(D) Stage IV
(E) REM sleep

274

Adding which one of the following medicines can increase the risk of toxicity in a patient stabilized on lamotrigine for bipolar maintenance therapy?

(A) Lithium
(B) Valproate
(C) Quetiapine
(D) Topiramate
(E) Olanzapine

275

A 52-year-old man presents with a rapidly progressive dementia, visual symptoms and cerebellar signs. Within a few weeks he is mute and has myoclonus. He dies four months later. Light microscopy of the brain reveals spongiform changes. This presentation is most consistent with which of the following diagnoses?

(A) Creutzfeldt-Jakob disease
(B) HIV infection
(C) Huntington's disease
(D) Progressive supranuclear palsy
(E) Wilson's disease

276

A family is seen in family therapy. During the process, the therapist attempts to increase differentiation, decrease triangulations, resolve cutoffs and improve the ability of the family to manage anxiety. This process is MOST consistent with which family therapeutic approach?

(A) Behavioral/cognitive-behavioral therapy
(B) Systemic family therapy
(C) Psychodynamic-psychoanalytic psychotherapy
(D) Strategic family therapy
(E) Transgenerational family therapy

277

Which of the following is the most common male sexual disorder?

(A) Fetishism
(B) Male orgasmic disorder
(C) Male erectile disorder
(D) Premature ejaculation
(E) Sexual masochism

278

A 72 year old patient is admitted to the hospital with a fever of 101.8° F and a urinary tract infection. The patient believes that it is 1974 and that the hospital room is a kitchen. The nursing staff is concerned because the patient is agitated, trying to get out of bed, and trying to pull out the IV. Which of the following medications is the best choice for the patient's agitation?

(A) Lorazepam
(B) Haloperidol
(C) Diazepam
(D) Thioridazine
(E) Valproate

279

Which of the following stages has been identified by Kübler-Ross as a part of the process for dying patients?

(A) Anger
(B) Suicidal ideation
(C) Intellectualization
(D) Visual hallucinations
(E) Disorientation

280

In partial responders, which of the following classes of medications are effective adjuncts to SSRIs for the core symptoms of PTSD?

(A) Tricyclic antidepressants
(B) Lithium
(C) Anticonvulsants
(D) Benzodiazepines
(E) Atypical antipsychotics

281

The treatment for body dysmorphic disorder that has been shown to be most effective includes which of the following psychotherapeutic techniques?

(A) Mindfulness training
(B) Exposure and response prevention
(C) Group psychotherapy
(D) Social skills training
(E) Biofeedback

282

A 69-year-old woman is hospitalized for pyelonephritis, which is successfully treated with antibiotics. Discharge to her home, where she lives alone, is planned. However, her daughter calls and informs the treatment team that she found several bottles of unused medications in the patient's home. The team wonders whether the patient can safely manage her medications at home, and asks psychiatry to evaluate her capacity. Which of the following potential reasons for medication noncompliance implies that the patient lacks capacity?

(A) The patient was too delirious from her infection to remember to take her medications.
(B) The patient's eyesight is too impaired to read the instructions on her pill bottles.
(C) The patient is unable to understand the reasons the medications were prescribed.
(D) The patient has a long history of noncompliance owing to a general mistrust of doctors.
(E) The patient felt too hopeless and depressed to comply with her medication regimen.

283

A 35-year-old man presents with memory deficits and emotional lability. Head CT reveals atrophy of the caudate. His father died from the same disorder when he was 38 years old. This presentation is most consistent with which of the following disorders?

(A) Alzheimer's disease
(B) Huntington's disease
(C) Progressive multifocal leukodystrophy
(D) Subacute sclerosing panencephalitis
(E) Whipple's disease

284

A 21-year-old patient has been diagnosed as having panic disorder. She reports that she frequently had difficulties with side effects in starting medications in the past. For this patient, which of the following would be the best beginning dose of sertraline?

(A) 25 mg
(B) 50 mg
(C) 75 mg
(D) 100 mg

285

Paranoid personality disorder is marked by pervasive distrust and suspiciousness of others. For this diagnosis, distrust and suspiciousness can be manifested by which ONE of the following?

(A) Choosing solitary activities most of the time
(B) Experiencing social anxiety that persists even with familiarity
(C) Experiencing unusual perceptions such as bodily illusions
(D) Reading hidden, threatening meaning into benign events
(E) Showing emotional detachment

286

A 50-year-old man with a 20-year history of smoking 1–2 packs per day attempts to quit by using the nicotine patch. He relapses to smoking after four days of cessation. He comes for an appointment, saying he knew it was going to be harder than he thought and he's not sure he can go through the process again. The best response would be:

(A) "Most people need more than two tries before they successfully quit."
(B) "You will need to try harder next time."
(C) "With persistence about 75% of smokers successfully quit."
(D) "Let's try the same thing again."
(E) "Most smokers require more intensive treatment to quit."

287

In elderly patients, which of the following conditions is most important to address to prevent depressive symptoms after hip fracture surgery?

(A) Postoperative pain
(B) Requiring assistance with mobility
(C) Using benzodiazepines daily
(D) Using >4 medications

288

A 36-year-old woman with breast cancer completed radiotherapy. However, three months later she continues to complain of disabling fatigue. In evaluating this patient, which of the following symptoms would suggest that the fatigue was directly due to her medical condition rather than depression?

(A) Late insomnia
(B) Impaired concentration
(C) Feelings of limb heaviness
(D) Decreased interest in activities
(E) Weight loss

289

A 24-year-old woman is comatose with generalized myoclonic twitching and is found to have a serum lithium concentration of 4.2 mEq/L. The treatment of choice is:

(A) saline diuresis.
(B) hemodialysis.
(C) exchange transfusion.
(D) plasmapheresis.

290

A 72-year-old man is referred by his primary care doctor to a geriatric psychiatrist for treatment of depression. Two weeks earlier the man had seen his primary care doctor who started citalopram 20 mg daily. The patient continues to report severe depressive symptoms. On interview, it becomes apparent that this is the man's first episode of depression, and he has no history of any prior psychiatric disorder. The psychiatrist should advise that the patient:

(A) discontinue citalopram and begin nortriptyline.
(B) discontinue citalopram and begin venlafaxine.
(C) continue citalopram, but add lithium.
(D) continue the current treatment as prescribed.
(E) increase the citalopram to 40 mg daily.

291

In addition to being effective in treating major depression, interpersonal psychotherapy has been shown to be highly effective in the treatment of which of the following disorders?

(A) Substance abuse
(B) Bulimia nervosa
(C) Obsessive-compulsive disorder
(D) Schizophrenia
(E) Dysthymia

292

A decrease of which neuropeptide has been linked most closely to narcolepsy?

(A) Neurotensin
(B) Oxytocin
(C) Somatostatin
(D) Hypocretin
(E) Melanocyte-stimulating hormone

293

Which of the following antidepressants could be prescribed for a depressed patient who has major concerns about the possible effects of medication on sexual functioning?

(A) Sertraline
(B) Venlafaxine
(C) Paroxetine
(D) Bupropion
(E) Trazodone

294

Which of the diagnostic criteria for PTSD is rarely fully-endorsed in preschool children?

(A) Disturbance of over one month
(B) Re-experiencing
(C) Avoidance/numbing
(D) Increased arousal
(E) Clinically significant impairment

295

When compared to individuals with Parkinson's disease dementia (PD-D), individuals with Alzheimer's disease dementia (AD-D) typically show more severe impairment in:

(A) apraxia.
(B) visual hallucinosis.
(C) depressive symptoms.
(D) visuospatial dysfunction.

296

Generally, restraint and seclusion are considered appropriate treatment interventions when the patient is at imminent risk to harm himself or others AND:

(A) the patient is refusing medication.
(B) no less restrictive alternative is available.
(C) the hospital prefers physical to chemical restraint.
(D) the time period is expected to be brief.
(E) a physician is present to write the order.

297

A bus carrying students from a local high school is swept down the side of the mountain following a mudslide. Despite rescue attempts, all the youth on the bus either die or are seriously wounded. Based on prevalence data, which of the following groups of individuals is most likely to develop PTSD symptoms after the disaster?

(A) Family members
(B) First responders
(C) Guidance counselors
(D) Classmates
(E) Teachers

298

In association with research leading up to DSM-5, the core features of personality disorders are being re-examined. Investigators are assessing which characteristics are stable, trait-like and "attitudinal", and which tend to vary with life-stresses over time. For which one of the following personality disorder diagnoses were rigidity and problems delegating found to be the least changeable criteria?

(A) Schizotypal personality disorder
(B) Narcissistic personality disorder
(C) Borderline personality disorder
(D) Avoidant personality disorder
(E) Obsessive-compulsive personality disorder

299

Which of the following antiepileptic drugs has been shown to be effective in treating binge eating disorder associated with obesity in short-term, placebo-controlled studies?

(A) Topiramate
(B) Lamotrigine
(C) Oxcarbazepine
(D) Valproate
(E) Tiagabine

300

A 32-year-old man is admitted to the hospital with a severe episode of bipolar disorder, mixed. Which of the following would be the best first-line pharmacologic treatment for him?

(A) Lithium alone
(B) Lithium plus a benzodiazepine
(C) Lithium plus an antidepressant
(D) Lithium plus an antipsychotic
(E) Lithium plus valproate

301

Which of the following medications has the strongest body of evidence for the treatment of bulimia nervosa?

(A) Bupropion
(B) Fluoxetine
(C) Duloxetine
(D) Paroxetine
(E) Venlafaxine

302

Which of the following patterns is most likely to be seen on an EEG of a delirious patient?

(A) Generalized slowing
(B) Increased alpha
(C) Decreased theta
(D) Triphasic sharp waves
(E) Focal high frequency spikes

303

Which of the following types of psychotherapy focuses on a patient's current social functioning within one of four problem areas (reaction, interpersonal disputes, role transition, or interpersonal deficits)?

(A) Supportive psychotherapy
(B) Interpersonal psychotherapy
(C) Cognitive therapy
(D) Psychodynamic psychotherapy
(E) Psychoanalytic psychotherapy

304

A patient with a long history of successful treatment with 20 mg of fluoxetine has been found to be HIV+ and has initiated antiretroviral therapy. The patient sees you because of a return of symptoms of depression. Which of the following is the most likely pharmacologic cause?

(A) As the patient gained weight from an increased appetite, more of the imipramine became bound to fat cells.
(B) The protease inhibitor caused lipodystrophy which decreased fluoxetine levels.
(C) The protease inhibitor began to compete with fluoxetine for protein-binding sites.
(D) The protease inhibitor induced the activity of an enzyme that enhanced the metabolism of fluoxetine and norfluoxetine.
(E) The protease inhibitor has a direct interaction on the fluoxetine, causing it to lose efficacy.

305

A 24-year-old man is arrested after repeated episodes of rubbing his genitals against women's buttocks while riding on the subway. The most likely paraphilic diagnosis is which of the following?

(A) Fetishism
(B) Frotteurism
(C) Exhibitionism
(D) Voyeurism
(E) Sexual masochism

306

Which ONE of the following is the most consistently agreed upon characteristic of supportive psychotherapy?

(A) It is a form of psychodynamic psychotherapy.
(B) It is based on the use of transference or other interpretation.
(C) It is best for patients with Axis II disorders.
(D) Its practice requires only common sense, interpersonal skills, and a capacity for empathy.
(E) It serves primarily to strengthen patient's self-esteem.

307

Which of the following treatments has the greatest body of evidence demonstrating efficacy for treatment of specific phobia?

(A) Eye movement desensitization and reprocessing (EMDR)
(B) In vivo exposure therapy
(C) Hypnotherapy
(D) Pharmacotherapy
(E) Imaginal exposure therapy

308

A 23-year-old man is the sole survivor of a fire aboard a crowded plane. In the immediate aftermath of exposure to the trauma, which of the following interventions is most likely to be successful in preventing psychological sequelae?

(A) Encourage him to imagine positive emotions.
(B) Have the man ventilate about how he is feeling.
(C) Normalize the stress reaction.
(D) Prescribe a short-acting benzodiazepine.
(E) Use critical incident debriefing.

309

Following survival from a tornado that killed 38 people in a local community, a woman is provided with education and training of coping skills that includes deep muscle relaxation, breathing control, assertiveness, role playing, covert modeling, thought stopping, positive thinking, and self-talks. The intervention described is:

(A) aversion therapy.
(B) insight-oriented psychotherapy.
(C) interpersonal therapy.
(D) stress inoculation training.

310

Which of the following symptoms is most consistent with a medication side effect rather than progression of Huntington's disease?

(A) Flowing movements
(B) Postural instability
(C) Effects on swallowing
(D) Akathisia
(E) Facial apraxia

311

The hormone that masculinizes the human brain during uterine life is:

(A) testosterone.
(B) dihydrotestosterone.
(C) estrone.
(D) estradiol.
(E) progesterone.

312

Which of the following cognitive abilities is preserved in normal aging?

(A) Working memory
(B) Perceptual-motor skills
(C) Vocabulary
(D) Fluency
(E) Logical problem solving

313

Explicit feelings of shame, shame proneness, and self-stigma associated with higher ratings of anger and hostility have been empirically demonstrated to be increased in patients with which of the following disorders?

(A) Social phobia
(B) Borderline personality disorder
(C) Histrionic personality disorder
(D) Dysthymia
(E) Paranoid personality disorder

314

Following a massive hurricane, the occupants of a city are placed in a temporary refugee camp until other housing can be obtained. Which of the following ways of organizing the refugee camp is likely to be most successful in preventing PTSD?

(A) Bring in citizen leaders from nearby cities to run the camp.
(B) Develop the camp into a village with a village council.
(C) Have the military oversee operation of the camp.
(D) Organize the camp along racial, religious, and ethnic divisions.
(E) Provide individuals with their own tents.

315

Which of the following signs and symptoms is most reliable in distinguishing between delirium and dementia?

(A) Orientation
(B) Short-term memory
(C) Long-term memory
(D) Sleep pattern
(E) Level of consciousness

316

A 64-year-old patient is hospitalized for an injury that occurred while he was inebriated. Three days after admission the patient is disoriented, hallucinating, and has a grand mal seizure. His blood pressure is 160/100, with a pulse of 105. Which of the following medications is most appropriate for managing this patient's condition?

(A) Haloperidol
(B) Sertraline
(C) Quetiapine
(D) Lorazepam
(E) Propranolol

317

Which of the following chromosomal abnormalities is associated with an increased risk of early onset Alzheimer's dementia?

(A) Angelman syndrome (Deletion of the 15q11-q13 region of chromosome 15)
(B) Down syndrome (trisomy 21)
(C) Turner syndrome (monosomy X)
(D) Klinefelter syndrome (46, xy/47, xxy mosaicism)

318

Which of the following is the most common psychiatric diagnosis among patients with cancer who have no prior psychiatric history?

(A) Posttraumatic stress disorder
(B) Major depressive disorder
(C) Acute stress disorder
(D) Adjustment disorder
(E) Generalized anxiety disorder

319

A 40-year-old woman with bipolar I disorder complains of a lengthy, paralyzing period of depression following an episode of mania that led to hospitalization. Her symptoms have not responded to treatment with lamotrigine alone. Which of the following medications has the best evidence for efficacy as monotherapy to treat this patient's depression?

(A) Aripiprazole
(B) Haloperidol
(C) Quetiapine
(D) Valproic acid

320

A 28-year-old man presents with the chief complaint of excessive daytime sleepiness. He reports the sudden onset of brief periods of daytime sleep that are very restful. On a few occasions, he has experienced brief muscle paralysis after laughter. Recently, he has had two episodes of temporary paralysis when he awakens during the morning accompanied by vivid visual hallucinations. A polysomnogram is most likely to show which of the following?

(A) Episodes of decreased blood oxygen saturation in spite of ventilatory effort
(B) Sleep-onset REM periods within 15 minutes of falling asleep
(C) Increased sleep spindles and K-complexes in stage 2 non-REM sleep
(D) Multiple awakenings during stage 3 and 4 of non-REM sleep
(E) Prolonged episodes of REM sleep in the first half of the night

321

Which of the following is most likely to be predictive of a good prognosis in schizophrenia?

(A) Early age at onset of symptoms
(B) Presence of predominantly negative symptoms
(C) Acute onset with underlying precipitating factors
(D) Presence of neurological signs and symptoms
(E) Low IQ

322

Which of the following medications is considered to be a first-line pharmacological treatment for delirium?

(A) Lorazepam
(B) Haloperidol
(C) Quetiapine
(D) Trazodone
(E) Hydroxyzine

323

A 67-year-old woman presents with visual hallucinations, memory loss, apathy and extrapyramidal symptoms. The patient's extrapyramidal symptoms increase markedly when given olanzapine 2.5 mg. This presentation is most consistent with:

(A) vascular dementia.
(B) dementia of the Alzheimer's type.
(C) Lewy body dementia.
(D) dementia due to HIV.
(E) dementia due to Huntington's disease.

324

A 70-year-old woman presents with a history of a fixed belief that her arms and legs are infested with bugs that are crawling and biting her. She has no known associated medical condition and is physically healthy. Which of the following is best supported as a treatment of her condition?

(A) Methylphenidate
(B) Imipramine
(C) Pimozide
(D) Selegiline
(E) Fluoxetine

325

For the treatment of vaginismus, which of the following interventions in combination with education and counseling would be most effective?

(A) A short-acting benzodiazepine prior to intercourse
(B) Guided imagery during intercourse
(C) Limiting intercourse to the female superior position
(D) Use of a vibrator applied to the clitoris to induce orgasm
(E) Vaginal dilation exercises using plastic dilators

326

Which antidepressant group is most likely to induce significant anticholinergic side effects that should be considered when treating late-life depression?

(A) Serotonin norepinephrine reuptake inhibitors
(B) Monoamine oxidase inhibitors
(C) Selective serotonin reuptake inhibitors
(D) Reversible monoamine oxidase inhibitors
(E) Tricyclic antidepressants

327

A 69-year old man with chronic obstructive pulmonary disease, cirrhosis of the liver, benign prostatic hypertrophy and alcohol dependence is prescribed acamprosate as part of his comprehensive treatment plan for his alcoholism. Which of the following laboratory tests would be most appropriate to obtain in order to determine the best starting dose of acamprosate?

(A) Alanine aminotransferase
(B) Electrolytes
(C) Creatinine clearance
(D) Serum Osmolality
(E) Serum Total Protein

328

Social rhythm therapy for bipolar disorder is based on which of the following types of psychotherapy?

(A) Cognitive-behavioral therapy
(B) Family therapy
(C) Group therapy
(D) Interpersonal therapy
(E) Psychodynamic psychotherapy

329

A 15-year-old girl is diagnosed with anorexia nervosa. She has had symptoms for 18 months. Her medical status is stable and she maintains an acceptable weight. The treatment that would be most beneficial for ongoing care is:

(A) behavioral management.
(B) psychodynamic psychotherapy.
(C) cognitive-behavioral therapy.
(D) family therapy.
(E) dialectical behavior therapy.

330

Which one of the following medications is associated with causing Ebstein's anomaly in the newborn if taken regularly by pregnant women?

(A) Lithium
(B) Valproic acid
(C) Carbamazepine
(D) Lamotrigine
(E) Aripiprazole

331

A 42-year-old woman receiving chemotherapy for non-Hodgkin's lymphoma develops anorexia-cachexia syndrome. She is started on a medication to address her symptoms. A few weeks later she returns with reports of an increase in her sense of well-being, and decreased pain and nausea. However, she has gained no weight and has new onset muscle weakness. Which of the following agents is most likely responsible?

(A) Corticosteroids
(B) Cyproheptadine
(C) Medroxyprogesterone acetate
(D) Metoclopramide
(E) Ondansetron

332

A 42-year man is being treated with cognitive-behavior therapy (CBT) for depression. He describes several mistakes he made at work, and voices the belief that "no matter what I try, I always fail." This is an example of:

(A) automatic thought.
(B) maladaptive schema.
(C) full consciousness.
(D) modified cognition.
(E) unconscious conflict.

333

Which of the following mood stabilizers is FDA-approved for acute mania in children older than 12 years?

(A) Lithium
(B) Sodium valproate
(C) Carbamazepine
(D) Lamotrigine
(E) Topiramate

334

A 66-year-old man being treated for bipolar disorder is noted to have asymptomatic hypercalcemia and elevated levels of parathyroid hormone. Which of the following medications is the most likely cause?

(A) Divalproex
(B) Lamotrigine
(C) Lithium
(D) Topiramate
(E) Olanzapine

335

A 28-year-old hospitalized patient is started on an antipsychotic medication for schizophrenia. Within 3 weeks, the patient complains of chest pain, shortness of breath, and swelling of the lower extremities. Which medication is the patient most likely taking?

(A) Fluphenazine
(B) Quetiapine
(C) Risperidone
(D) Aripiprazole
(E) Clozapine

336

A requirement for initiating hospice care is that the patient must have:

(A) a cognitive-impairing terminal illness.
(B) a health care power-of-attorney.
(C) a prognosis of ≤ 6 months to live.
(D) no family members able to provide care.
(E) Medicare and/or Medicaid benefits.

337

A 38-year-old patient with schizophrenia is observed holding her arms in bizarre positions for hours at a time. On interview, the patient does not answer any questions, but rather repeats everything the psychiatrist says. Which of the following is the most appropriate initial treatment?

(A) Lorazepam
(B) Propranolol
(C) Diphenhydramine
(D) Phenobarbital
(E) Botulinum toxin

338

Procedural justice in the process of civil commitment refers to:

(A) physician decision-making that supports a beneficial outcome for patients.
(B) a style of communication that alleviates patients' experience of coercion.
(C) the inclusion of a patient's family in commitment decisions.
(D) judicial decision-making that takes into account patients' therapeutic options.
(E) choosing the least restrictive alternative for patients.

339

A review of the current evidence suggests that the BEST explanation for an increase in the rate of autism spectrum disorders is:

(A) exposure to childhood vaccines.
(B) rates of genetic mutations.
(C) exposure to environmental toxins.
(D) screening and diagnosis.
(E) survival of premature infants.

340

A 22-year-old male college student has a positive HIV test. History reveals he had unprotected sex with multiple partners. His CBC is consistent with anemia. Which of the following factors places him at highest risk for eventually developing an HIV dementia?

(A) Age
(B) Anemia
(C) Educational level
(D) Gender
(E) Multiple sexual partners

341

The symptom that is most suggestive that an individual has generalized anxiety disorder is worrying about:

(A) specific behaviors.
(B) physical symptoms.
(C) embarrassment.
(D) all experiences.
(E) past events.

342

A 7-year-old boy with an anxiety disorder is in cognitive behavior therapy. The parents ask how they should approach getting the child to do activities that he is fearful about, such as socializing with peers and participating in competitive situations. Which of the following is the MOST appropriate response?

(A) Wait until the anxiety and fearfulness have been resolved.
(B) Start when the child understands his anxieties.
(C) Gradually approach with reinforcement for trying.
(D) Find appropriate non-anxiety-producing substitutes.
(E) Make fun activities contingent on doing anxiety-provoking things.

343

A patient presents with a well-defined history of recurrent hypomanic episodes but denies ever having had depressive symptoms or full manic episodes. According to DSM-IV-TR criteria, the most appropriate diagnosis would be:

(A) cyclothymic disorder.
(B) schizoaffective disorder.
(C) bipolar I disorder.
(D) bipolar II disorder.
(E) bipolar disorder, not otherwise specified.

344

Which of the following is a required criterion for the diagnosis of depression with melancholic features?

(A) Mood worse in the late afternoon
(B) Middle or late insomnia
(C) Significant hyperphagia or weight gain
(D) Mood changes similar to those found in bereavement
(E) Loss of pleasure in all, or almost all, activities

345

A 10-year-old boy is referred for psychiatric assessment after setting his family's home on fire. His mother smoked cigarettes during the pregnancy. The patient grew up in an extremely impoverished neighborhood with his mother as his sole caregiver. His mother describes the boy as being extremely oppositional and defiant as a preschooler. She has primarily used corporal punishment including beating him with a belt and electric cords. Since starting school he has had multiple suspensions for fighting with peers and teachers. Intelligence testing is consistent with borderline intellectual functioning. Which of these factors from the patient's history is MOST predictive of a poor outcome in this patient's conduct disorder?

(A) Early age at onset of symptoms.
(B) Exposure to toxins in utero.
(C) Lack of a father figure in his life.
(D) Impaired intellectual functioning.

346

During the assessment of a $3\frac{1}{2}$ -year-old boy who has been referred for biting other children at preschool, the mother discloses that the boy's stepfather has been physically abusive towards her. The child may have witnessed some of the abusive episodes. Which of the following MUST be done prior to the end of the session?

(A) Explain that the child is at risk for PTSD.
(B) Refer the mother for her own treatment.
(C) Find contact information for shelters.
(D) Explore whether the child has been abused.
(E) Explore mother's reasons for staying with the stepfather.

347

Which of the following signs differentiate patients with pseudodementia from patients who are severely demented?

(A) Less attention to self care
(B) Cognitive impairment
(C) Complaints of memory loss
(D) Less attention to environment
(E) Memory storage and retrieval

348

A 32-year-old woman who does not want to take medication complains about shortness of breath, chest pain and diaphoresis. She has had multiple attacks in the past 3 weeks. Her medical work-up is negative. Which of the following treatments has the strongest evidence supporting it as first choice for this patient?

(A) Dialectical behavioral therapy
(B) Family therapy
(C) Group therapy
(D) Patient support groups
(E) Cognitive-behavioral therapy

349

A 74-year-old man with known dementia is admitted to the hospital for workup and treatment of a presumed delirium. He scores a 21 on the Mini Mental State Exam (MMSE) on admission, and a 15 two days later. Nursing notes from his hospitalization indicate that there are times when he is completely alert and other times when he is nearly stuporous. Without appearing bothered, he has occasionally described seeing brightly colored birds perching on the windowsill of his room. A thorough delirium workup reveals no cause for his waxing and waning mental status findings. This description is most consistent with which dementing process?

(A) Vascular dementia
(B) Alzheimer dementia
(C) Frontotemporal dementia
(D) Lewy body dementia
(E) Korsakoff dementia

350

Which of the following features differentiates autism from Asperger's syndrome?

(A) Obsessive and compulsive behaviors
(B) Failure to develop peer relationships appropriate to the developmental level
(C) Inflexible adherence to specific non functional routines
(D) Single words used by age 2, phrases by age 3
(E) Stereotyped and repetitive motor mannerisms

351

Which of the following psychosocial treatments for depression has the most robust data supporting its use?

(A) Cognitive-behavioral therapy
(B) Dialectical behavioral therapy
(C) Group therapy
(D) Psychodynamic psychotherapy
(E) Supportive therapy

352

A 25-year-old patient with schizophrenia is admitted to the hospital with auditory hallucinations and persecutory delusions. The psychiatrist initiates haloperidol 5mg orally twice per day. After 48 hours of receiving medication, the patient becomes increasingly irritable, agitated, and is noted to be restless and pacing. The patient's blood pressure is 130/85 with a pulse of 88. The next step in management of this patient's symptoms should be to:

(A) increase the haloperidol to 10mg orally twice per day.
(B) administer benztropine 1mg orally twice per day.
(C) administer a one-time dose of haloperidol 5mg intramuscularly.
(D) administer a one-time dose of diphenhydramine 25mg intramuscularly.
(E) initiate propranolol 20mg orally three times per day.

353

Which of the following doses of haloperidol decanoate has been shown to have the lowest rate of symptomatic exacerbation, yet minimal increased risk of adverse effect or subjective discomfort?

(A) 25 mg/month
(B) 50 mg/month
(C) 100 mg/month
(D) 200 mg/month

354

Which of the following medications has the potential for a significantly increased risk of hemorrhagic pancreatitis?

(A) Clozapine
(B) Divalproex
(C) Nefazodone
(D) Pemoline
(E) Thioridazine

355

Which of the following situations is the individual with social phobia likely to avoid?

(A) Crossing bridges
(B) Eating in public
(C) Being in closed spaces
(D) Proximity to spiders
(E) Sitting in movie theatres

356

A 32-year-old woman with a history of early childhood abuse and abandonment begins dynamic psychotherapy. Although the initial stages of treatment proceed well, after three months her psychiatrist notices that she is becoming more critical of the therapy and frequently questions the value of it. In addition, she is dismissive of the psychiatrist and begins to question whether the psychiatrist is adequately trained. As a result, the psychiatrist begins to dread the sessions, and occasionally begins the sessions late. This mode of interaction is best described as a type of:

(A) Projective identification
(B) Displacement
(C) Sublimation
(D) Paranoid-schizoid position
(E) Ambivalent/resistant pattern

357

The parents of a 16-year-old year old boy ask if he can be treated to prevent the development of schizophrenia. For the last year, the boy has been more irritable, staying in his room most of the time playing music. His grades have declined. His uncle was diagnosed with schizophrenia at the age of 17. Which of the following statements BEST describes the current knowledge about the early identification and treatment of individuals who will become schizophrenic?

(A) Many adolescents with these symptoms will not become schizophrenic.
(B) Treatment with low dose atypical antipsychotics will prevent schizophrenia.
(C) Long term use of atypical antipsychotics does not have major adverse effects.
(D) Psychosocial interventions are more effective than medication treatment.

358

Which of the following is a common adverse effect of monoamine oxidase inhibitors therapy?

(A) Serotonin syndrome
(B) Hypertensive crisis
(C) Priapism
(D) Orthostatic hypotension
(E) Weight loss

359

A patient who was recently diagnosed with panic disorder complains 2 days after starting citalopram that she continues to be very anxious about having another panic attack. Even her sleep has been disrupted. Which of the following would treat her anxiety best?

(A) Increase the citalopram.
(B) Add lithium.
(C) Lower citalopram.
(D) Add clonazepam.
(E) Add trazodone.

360

A 32-year-old woman presents to the emergency department after being raped. She appears confused and extremely frightened. She mentions a history of prior rapes. Which of the following psychotherapies, if administered soon after the event, has the best body of evidence in preventing the patient from progressing to a posttraumatic stress disorder?

(A) Supportive psychotherapy
(B) Psychological debriefing
(C) Hypnosis
(D) Cognitive-behavioral therapy
(E) Single session exposure therapy

361

A 28-year-old patient with schizophrenia is prescribed an atypical antipsychotic medication. A baseline fasting plasma glucose level is obtained and is within normal limits. After what period of time should this test be repeated?

(A) 2 weeks, and then quarterly
(B) 3 months, and then annually
(C) 6 months, and then annually
(D) Every 6 months
(E) Annually

362

Which of the following reflects the APA's position on psychiatrists' participation in legally authorized executions?

(A) Sanctioning of participation is determined by state associations.
(B) Psychiatrists should not participate in executions.
(C) Participation is left up to the discretion of the psychiatrist.
(D) Psychiatrists may only perform a mental status exam prior to execution.
(E) Psychiatrists may participate if they are only in a supervisory role.

363

A 20-year-old college student presents to the mental health clinic because he is worried about an exam that he must take in two days. He has chronic problems with concentration and sleep, and complains that he is easily fatigued. He states that he is tired of the pressure he always feels. He adds that he has been to the medical clinic as well because he feared that his frequent muscle tension and headaches meant he had a neurological disease. Which of the following is the most likely diagnosis?

(A) Major depression
(B) Hypochondriasis
(C) Generalized anxiety disorder
(D) Adjustment disorder
(E) Somatization disorder

364

Which medication has the most evidence supporting its use as an augmenting agent for treatment of a major depression?

(A) Divalproex sodium
(B) Lamotrigine
(C) Lithium
(D) Lorazepam
(E) Phenelzine

365

EMDR (eye movement desensitization and reprocessing) has several features that distinguish it from the other cognitive behavioral treatments for PTSD. In addition to the directed eye movements, which of the following also distinguishes EMDR?

(A) Having patients think about the trauma rather than verbalize it
(B) Encouraging patients to learn to identify cognitive distortions
(C) Utilizing and emphasizing exposures to the traumatic material
(D) Teaching relaxation and imaging techniques to manage anxiety
(E) Employing homework assignments to reinforce session work

366

A 28-year-old woman with bipolar II disorder has been using an oral contraceptive for birth control. She currently presents with a hypomanic episode. Which of the following medications would be best to treat her hypomania without impairing the efficacy of the oral contraceptive?

(A) Carbamazepine
(B) Lithium
(C) Oxcarbamazepine
(D) Topirimate

367

Which psychotherapeutic modality involves teaching patients to tolerate distress, regulate their emotions, reduce vulnerability to cues, and avoid or distract without problem behavior, while concomitantly reducing reinforcement of maladaptive behavior?

(A) Psychoanalytic psychotherapy
(B) Cognitive behavioral therapy
(C) Interpersonal psychotherapy
(D) Dialectical behavior therapy
(E) Supportive therapy

368

Which of the following drug classes is the preferred initial pharmacotherapy for social anxiety disorder (generalized)?

(A) Tricyclic antidepressant (TCA)
(B) Monoamine oxidase inhibitor (MAOI)
(C) Benzodiazepine (BDZ)
(D) Selective serotonin reuptake inhibitor (SSRI)
(E) Beta-blockers

369

Which of the following factors is most likely to be associated with bacterial soft tissue infections in drug users?

(A) Cleaning the skin before injection
(B) Being HIV negative
(C) Being an experienced injector
(D) Intravenous injection
(E) Subcutaneous injection

370

A 40-year-old patient complains of episodes of intense fear with associated somatic symptoms that have a sudden onset and peak within minutes. Which of the following is the essential feature required for a diagnosis of panic *disorder*?

(A) Anticipatory anxiety and avoidance of public speaking
(B) Unexpected, "out-of-the-blue" nature of the episodes
(C) Presence of 4 or more characteristic symptoms during episodes
(D) Episodes precipitated by memories of a past trauma
(E) Episodes triggered by contact with "contaminated" objects

371

A 53-year-old man with a history of alcohol dependence has been abstinent from alcohol for three months. Although he continues to attend peer support groups, he reports that he has recently begun drinking one to two drinks approximately every other day, and is fearful that his relapse will worsen. Which of the following medications would be the most appropriate first-line pharmacological intervention for this patient?

(A) Naltrexone
(B) Acamprosate
(C) Bupropion
(D) Fluoxetine
(E) Disulfiram

372

A 20-year-old patient with schizophrenia receiving antipsychotic treatment complains of breast tenderness, galactorrhea, and amenorrhea. Which of the following medications is the patient most likely taking?

(A) Aripiprazole
(B) Risperidone
(C) Quetiapine
(D) Clozapine
(E) Ziprasidone

373

Which of the following statements most accurately reflects the position of the *APA's Principles of Medical Ethics* on faculty psychiatrists having sex with trainees?

(A) There is no established APA position on sexual relationships with trainees.
(B) Sexual relationships with trainees are absolutely unethical.
(C) Sexual relationships are permissible when both parties are consenting adults.
(D) Sexual behavior in faculty/trainee relationships may negatively impact patient care.

374

In which of the following situations would a high potency benzodiazepine be the preferred initial pharmacotherapy for panic disorder?

(A) Co-morbid major depression
(B) Need for rapid onset of action
(C) Anticipation of long-term treatment
(D) Associated agoraphobia
(E) Co-morbid cardiovascular disease

375

Which of the following substance abuse therapist attributes has the greatest and most consistent impact on patient retention and reduced substance use?

(A) Therapists skilled at limit setting
(B) Therapists who were successfully treated for substance dependence
(C) Therapists who have a first degree relative who was substance dependent
(D) Therapists with strong interpersonal skills
(E) Therapists who are knowledgeable about both biological and psychosocial interventions

376

The daughter of an 89-year-old man with severe dementia requests that her father be deemed incompetent. The ultimate decision to determine competence is made by the:

(A) daughter.
(B) court.
(C) psychiatrist.
(D) treating physician.
(E) health care power-of-attorney.

377

Anger is most closely associated with which of the following temperament traits?

(A) Harm Avoidance
(B) Novelty Seeking
(C) Reward Dependence
(D) Persistence

378

An 80-year-old man is brought to the emergency room after suffering a grand mal seizure. His serum sodium concentration is 107mmol/L. Which of the following medications is most likely to have caused the hyponatremia?

(A) Topiramate
(B) Lamotrigine
(C) Gabapentin
(D) Oxcarbazepine
(E) Valproate

379

In children with major depressive disorder, which of the following is MORE likely to occur in boys than girls?

(A) Feelings of anxiety
(B) Acting-out behaviors
(C) Poorer self-esteem
(D) Severe symptoms of depression
(E) Shorter period of recovery

380

A 21-year-old patient dropped out of college and has been unable to attend social gatherings as a result of extreme fear of embarrassing herself. She has failed to respond to therapeutic trials of paroxetine, fluvoxamine, sertraline, clonazepam, and buspirone. Which of the following medications would be most appropriate to prescribe next?

(A) Fluoxetine
(B) Propranolol
(C) Phenelzine
(D) Lithium
(E) Risperidone

381

Which of the following psychotropic medications has been associated with polycystic ovarian syndrome?

(A) Lithium
(B) Divalproex
(C) Methylphenidate
(D) Citalopram
(E) Aripiprazole

382

A 58-year-old patient with diabetic peripheral neuropathic pain presents with major depressive disorder. Which of the following antidepressants is most likely to have beneficial effects on both conditions?

(A) Bupropion
(B) Duloxetine
(C) Escitalopram
(D) Nefazodone
(E) Mirtazapine

383

When initiating treatment with risperidone long-acting injection, oral risperidone should be concomitantly prescribed for what length of time?

(A) 1 week
(B) 3 weeks
(C) 6 weeks
(D) 8 weeks
(E) 12 weeks

384

Which of the following personality disorders most closely resembles social phobia?

(A) Schizoid
(B) Borderline
(C) Avoidant
(D) Dependent
(E) Histrionic

385

Which antidepressant has been shown to be most efficacious in the treatment of depression in patients with HIV/AIDS with chronic diarrhea?

(A) Fluoxetine
(B) Mirtazapine
(C) Paroxetine
(D) Sertraline
(E) Venlafaxine

386

Which of the following is the best predictor of a recurrence of depression in someone with major depressive disorder?

(A) Family history of depression
(B) Prior episodes of depression
(C) Prior suicidal attempt
(D) Co-morbid Axis I disorder
(E) Co-morbid medical condition

387

A patient has been successfully treated with an SSRI for acute panic episodes. What is the minimum length of time recommended for maintenance pharmacotherapy for this patient?

(A) 2–4 months
(B) 6–12 months
(C) 18 months
(D) Over 24 months

388

Which of the following is a required gateway symptom for a major depressive disorder?

(A) Insomnia or hypersomnia
(B) Recurrent thoughts of death
(C) Feelings of worthlessness
(D) Psychomotor agitation or retardation
(E) Loss of interest or pleasure

389

In contrast to delusional disorders, schizophrenia is characterized by:

(A) disorganized speech.
(B) grandiosity.
(C) mood episodes.
(D) paranoid beliefs.
(E) physiological effects of a general medical condition.

390

Which of the following symptoms of PTSD is classified as an avoidance symptom?

(A) Difficulty falling asleep
(B) Recurrent nightmares
(C) Exaggerated startle response
(D) Sense of foreshortened future
(E) Difficulty concentrating

391

The personality disorder most closely associated with social anxiety disorder is which of the following?

(A) Schizoid
(B) Obsessive-compulsive
(C) Histrionic
(D) Avoidant
(E) Borderline

392

In order to make a diagnosis of bulimia nervosa, the symptoms must have duration of at least:

(A) 1 month.
(B) 3 months.
(C) 6 months.
(D) 9 months.
(E) 12 months.

393

A 65-year-old man whose wife died 3 months ago presents to the clinic, accompanied by his daughter. The daughter states that the couple had been married for 40 years, and that he now feels utterly worthless without his wife. Since her death, he has stayed in the house, letting the newspapers pile up, and he doesn't answer the phone. He stopped his weekly fishing trips with his neighbor, a pastime of his for 20 years. He denies suicidal ideation, but states that he wishes to join his wife. He has had a weight loss of 30 pounds over the past 3 months and has stopped taking his hypertension medications. What is the most likely diagnosis?

(A) Bereavement
(B) Adjustment disorder with depressed mood
(C) Major depressive disorder
(D) Depressive disorder, NOS
(E) Dysthymic disorder

394

In dialectical behavior therapy (DBT), the term "dialectical" refers to which of the following therapeutic principles?

(A) Psychic integration of good and bad objects
(B) A simultaneous emphasis on validation and change
(C) Efforts to treat both the manic and depressed phases of bipolar disorder
(D) A simultaneous focus on both thoughts and behaviors
(E) A dual focus on one's feelings and their impact on others

395

Which of the following approaches to neurotransmitter modulation would be most appropriate in treating a patient with Tourette's disorder?

(A) Dopaminergic modulation at the striatum and serotonergic modulation at the orbitofrontal cortex
(B) Dopaminergic modulation at the striatum
(C) Serotonergic modulation at the orbitofrontal cortex
(D) Noradrenergic modulation

396

Features that support the diagnosis of somatization disorder include involvement of multiple organ systems, early onset, absence of expected lab abnormalities, and:

(A) chronic course without development of physical signs.
(B) distinct, clearly delineated symptoms of limited duration.
(C) symptoms that are different from those of organic disorders.
(D) symptoms that do not cause functional impairment.
(E) signs not acknowledged or recognized by the patient.

397

Demographic and clinical factors associated with suicide in patients with schizophrenia include:

(A) older age.
(B) female gender.
(C) higher cognitive function.
(D) lower socioeconomic status.
(E) good social support.

398

Which of the following therapeutic strategies for OCD maintains treatment success for the longest period of time after active therapy is discontinued?

(A) Psychoeducation
(B) Record keeping
(C) A selective serotonin reuptake inhibitor
(D) Exposure and response prevention
(E) Supportive psychotherapy

399

The highest level of decision making capacity is required for which of the following actions?

(A) Making a will
(B) Appointing a substitute decision maker
(C) Agreeing to participate in a research study
(D) Making a decision about treatment
(E) Consenting to phlebotomy

400

Which of the following agents has been shown to be effective in the treatment of trauma-related nightmares and sleep disruption?

(A) Phenelzine
(B) Prazosin
(C) Bupropion
(D) Cyproheptadine
(E) Diphenhydramine

Section 2: Answers and Explanations

1

An 18-year-old woman is brought to the emergency department after collapsing at a party. She appears delirious and confused, with a temperature of 104°F. The friends who brought her to the emergency room say that she might have taken some pills. She was talking about feeling blissful and dancing a lot until she collapsed. Which of the following is the most likely drug ingested?

(A) Methylenedioxymethamphetamine (MDMA)
(B) Ketamine
(C) Flunitrazepam
(D) Gamma-hydroxybutyrate (GHB)

The correct answer is option **A**: Methylenedioxymethamphetamine

(MDMA) Methylenedioxymethamphetamine (MDMA), ketamine and gamma-hydroxybutyrate (GHB), commonly known as "club drugs," are frequently used at rave parties. They are also known as Ecstasy, Special K and liquid Ecstasy, respectively. MDMA intoxication can produce severe adverse effects including altered mental status, convulsions, hypo- or hyperthermia, cardiovascular instability, hepatotoxicity and even death. This severity of intoxication is uncommon, however, in community settings.

Ketamine has a high therapeutic index, and typically produces distorted perceptions of time, surroundings and one's body. GHB can produce a sense of disinhibition, somewhat like alcohol. While overdose can produce an altered mental status, hyperthermia is rare. Flunitrazepam, a short-acting benzodiazepine, can induce amnesia and has been called a "date rape drug."

McDowell DM: MDMA, Ketamine, GHB and the "Club Drug" Scene, in The American Psychiatric Publishing Textbook of Substance Abuse Treatment. Edited by Galanter M, Kleber HD. Washington, DC, American Psychiatric Press, Inc. 2004, pp 321–333.

Weaver MF, Schnoll SH: Hallucinogens and Club Drugs, in The American Psychiatric Publishing Textbook of Substance Abuse Treatment. Edited by Galanter M, Kleber HD. Arlington, VA, American Psychiatric Publishing, 2008, pp 191–200.

2

Which one of these terms defines the most common form of genetic variation observed in the genome?

(A) Short tandem repeat
(B) Single nucleotide polymorphism
(C) Haplotype
(D) Allele
(E) Variable number of tandem repeat

The correct response is option **B**: Single nucleotide polymorphism

Single nucleotide polymorphisms (SNPs) are DNA sequence variations occurring when a single nucleotide (A, T, C, or G) in the genome (or other shared sequence) differs between members of a species or between paired chromosomes in an individual. A SNP, therefore, involves a single base difference at a particular site in the genome. In two-thirds of the cases, a cytosine (C)–to–thymidine (T) exchange occurs. Although many SNPs do not produce physical changes in people, scientists believe that other SNPs may predispose people to disease and even influence their response to drug regimens. A haplotype is the sequence of alleles along an adjacent series of polymorphic sites on a single chromosome. An allele is one member of a pair of genes located at a specific position on a specific chromosome.

SNPs: Variations on a theme. http://www.ncbi.nlm.nih.gov/About/primer/snps.html.

Burmeister M: Genetics of Psychiatric Disorders: A Primer. Focus 2006 4:324–325

3

In adults, which of the following anxiety disorders is diagnosed in equal numbers in men and women?

    (A) Generalized anxiety disorder
    (B) Panic disorder
    (C) Specific phobia
    (D) Obsessive-compulsive disorder (OCD)
    (E) Obsessive-compulsive personality disorder

The correct response is option **D**: Obsessive-compulsive disorder (OCD)

OCD is equally common in adult men and women. However in children, boys are more often diagnosed with OCD than girls. GAD is diagnosed more frequently in women. Panic disorder without agoraphobia has a 2:1 female: male ratio and panic disorder with agoraphobia has a 3:1 female: male ratio. Twice as many women are diagnosed with specific phobia as men. Obsessive-compulsive personality disorder is diagnosed in men twice as often as in women.

Diagnostic and Statistical Manual of Mental Disorders, Fourth Edition, Text Revision (DSM-IV-TR). Washington, DC, American Psychiatric Association, 2000, pp 436, 446, 459, 474, 728.

4

Which of the following SSRIs is most likely to be "self-tapering," thereby decreasing the chances of withdrawal effects?

    (A) Citalopram
    (B) Escitalopram
    (C) Fluoxetine
    (D) Paroxetine
    (E) Sertraline

The correct response is option **C**: Fluoxetine

Fluoxetine has a half-life of 4–6 days, citalopram 35 hours, escitalopram 27–32 hours, and sertraline 26 hours. Paroxetine has the shortest half-life of 21 hours, and is most the common SSRI associated with a discontinuation syndrome. The withdrawal symptoms resemble "flu" like syndrome. Fluoxetine, on the other hand, has a half-life of 4 to 6 days. The elimination half-life of norfluoxetine, its main metabolite, is even longer (4–16 days).

Sadock BJ, Sadock VA, Ruiz P (eds): Kaplan & Sadock's Comprehensive Textbook of Psychiatry, 9th ed. Philadelphia, Lippincott Williams & Wilkins, 2009, p 3199

Sadock BJ and Sadock VA (eds): Kaplan & Sadock's Synopsis of Psychiatry, 10th ed. Philadelphia, Lippincott Williams & Wilkins, 2007, 1090–1091.

Rosenbaum JF & Tollefson GD. In Schatzberg AF Nemeroff CB (eds). Essentials of Clinical Psychopharmacology. 2nd ed. Washington, DC: American Psychiatric Publishing, Inc., 2006. p. 33

5

Dialectical behavior therapy (DBT) was developed specifically for the treatment symptoms associated with which one of the following personality disorders?

    (A) Antisocial
    (B) Borderline
    (C) Avoidant
    (D) Obsessive-compulsive
    (E) Histrionic

The correct response is option **B**: Borderline

Dialectical behavior therapy was developed initially by Marsha M. Linehan, Ph.D. as a treatment for parasuicidal behaviors associated with borderline personality disorder. Subsequently, it has been used to treat a variety of conditions including emotional disregulation associated with eating disorders, adult ADHD, and major depressive disorder. DBT involves skills training, individual therapy, telephone consultation, and use of a consultation team.

Sadock BJ, Sadock VA (eds): Kaplan & Sadock's Comprehensive Textbook of Psychiatry, 9th ed. Philadelphia, Lippincott Williams & Wilkins, 2009, pp 2884–2893

Robins CJ, Chapman AL: Dialectical behavior therapy: current status, recent developments, and future directions. J Pers Disord. 2004; 18:73–89

Linehan MM: Dialectical behavior therapy for borderline personality disorder. Theory and method. Bull Menninger Clin. 1987; 51: 261–76

6

The most common cause of treatment failure in HIV/ AIDS patients on antiretroviral medications is that most patients:

(A) have infections that are resistant to most available medications.
(B) fail to maintain the required adherence to the medication regime.
(C) do not start treatment until the infection is in the terminal stages.
(D) refuse to participate in medical treatment and take medications.
(E) have such severe side effects that medications cannot be used.

The correct response is option **B**: fail to maintain the required adherence to the medication regime.

A major approach to the prevention of HIV disease progression is the optimization of adherence to antiretroviral regimens. Despite the considerable advances in the treatment of HIV/AIDS, treatment regimes remain complicated and difficult to maintain with many patients having inadequate responses due to a lack of adherence to the medications.

Forstein M, Cournos F, Douaihy A, Goodkin K, Wainberg ML, Wapenyi KH. Guideline Watch: Practice Guideline for the Treatment of Patients with HIV/AIDS. American Psychiatric Association; 2006. p. 3 http://www.psychiatryonline.com/content.aspx?aid=147976

Goodkin K. Psychiatric aspects of HIV spectrum disease. FOCUS. 2009; 3:303–310

7

Advanced paternal age is a well established risk factor for which of the following psychiatric illnesses?

(A) Schizophrenia
(B) Substance dependence
(C) Major depressive disorder
(D) Generalized anxiety disorder

The correct response is option **A**: Schizophrenia

Studies have linked schizophrenia, as well as autism and bipolar disorder, to advanced paternal age, defined differently in different studies, but generally between ages 40 and 50.

Brown AS et al: Paternal age and risk of schizophrenia in adult offspring, Am J Psychiatry 2002; 159:1528–1533

Dalman C: Advanced paternal age increases risk of bipolar disorder in offspring, Evid. Based Ment. Health 2009;12;59 doi:10.1136/ebmh.12.2.59

Reichenberg A et al: Advancing paternal age and autism, Arch Gen Psychiatry. 2006;63:1026–1032.

Sipos A et al: Paternal age and schizophrenia: a population based cohort study, BMJ, doi:10.1136/bmj.38243.672396.55 (published 22 October 2004)

8

A 21-year-old woman presents with questions about her risk of developing schizophrenia. She is worried because her 18-year-old brother has recently been diagnosed with schizophrenia and required hospitalization for psychosis. There are no other family members who have a history of schizophrenia. Having a sibling with schizophrenia increases a person's risk of developing schizophrenia by approximately what amount?

(A) the sibling is no more likely to develop schizophrenia
(B) the risk of developing schizophrenia for a sibling is 50%
(C) the risk of developing schizophrenia for a sibling is 10 fold
(D) the risk of developing schizophrenia is 30 fold
(E) it is almost certain the sibling will develop schizophrenia

The correct response is option **C**: the risk of developing schizophrenia is 10 fold.

The risk of developing schizophrenia for a sibling of a patient with schizophrenia is estimated at 10%. More than 25 studies have consistently reported elevated risk for schizophrenia in first degree relatives of individuals with schizophrenia (parents, mean = 5.6%; sibs, 10.1%; children, 12.8%) This is a 10-fold increase above the general population lifetime risk of 1%.

Hales RE, Yudofsky SC (eds): The American Psychiatric Publishing Textbook of Psychiatry, 5th ed. Washington, DC, American Psychiatric Publishing, 2008. p 208.

Shih RA, Belmonte PL, Zandi PP. A review of the evidence from family, twin and adoption studies for a genetic contribution to adult psychiatric disorders. International Review of Psychiatry 2004.16:4,260–283 open access http://dx.doi.org/10.1080/09540260400014401

NIMH Genetics Workgroup. Report of the NIMH Genetic's Workgroup: Summary of Research. Biological Psychiatry. 1999; 45: 573–602.

An 18-year-old female has high scores on scales of the personality traits of Harm Avoidance and Reward Dependence. Based on these personality traits, she is at HIGHEST risk for developing which one of the following disorders?

(A) Anorexia nervosa
(B) Major depressive disorder
(C) Obsessive-compulsive disorder
(D) Schizophrenia
(E) Social anxiety disorder

The correct response is option **E**: Social Anxiety Disorder

Personality traits are consistently associated with different clinical disorders that a clinician may use the information in the differential diagnostic process. Anorexia nervosa is associated with high Harm Avoidance and Persistence; major depressive disorder with high Harm Avoidance and low Self-Directedness; obsessive-compulsive disorder with high Harm Avoidance and low Novelty Seeking; and social anxiety disorder with high Harm Avoidance and Reward Dependence.

Sadock BJ, Sadock VA (eds): Kaplan and Sadock's Comprehensive Textbook of Psychiatry, 9th ed. Philadelphia, Lippinicott Williams & Wilkins, 2009, pp. 2211–2212.

Faytout M, Tignol J, Swendsen J, Grabot D, Aouizerate B, Lépine JP. Social phobia, fear of negative evaluation and harm avoidance. Eur Psychiatry. 2007 Mar;22(2):75–9. Epub 2006 Nov 13.

Mörtberg E, Bejerot S, Aberg Wistedt A. Temperament and character dimensions in patients with social phobia: patterns of change following treatments? Psychiatry Res. 2007 Jul 30;152(1):81–90. Epub 2007 Feb 27.

A 40-year-old man with a 20-year history of heroin dependence and high tolerance is admitted to the hospital for IV antibiotic treatment of bacterial endocarditis. To prevent opioid withdrawal, considering his opioid tolerance, he is prescribed a moderately high dose of buprenorphine. He is just beginning to experience withdrawal symptoms before the first buprenorphine dose, but shortly thereafter, his anxiety, muscle aches and rhinorrhea worsen. At this point the best option would be to:

(A) increase the dose of buprenorphine.
(B) decrease the dose of buprenorphine.
(C) change to methadone.
(D) add a benzodiazepine.
(E) add naltrexone.

The correct response is option **C**: change to methadone.

Because buprenorphine is only a partial agonist at the mu opioid receptor, when given in high doses to someone with high tolerance in early withdrawal, it can induce withdrawal. Increasing the dose may worsen withdrawal, while decreasing the dose may not provide adequate mu coverage. The best option is to change to the full agonist methadone, which has a linear dose-response curve, allowing for easier dose titration and alleviation of withdrawal symptoms. Naltrexone, a full mu antagonist, will worsen the withdrawal symptoms. The benzodiazepine is likely to have minimal effect, having no activity at the mu receptor.

Center for Substance Abuse Treatment: Clinical Guidelines for the Use of Buprenorphine in the Treatment of Opioid Addiction. Treatment Improvement Protocol (TIP) Series 40. DHHS Publication No. (SMA) 04-3939. Rockville, MD: Substance Abuse and Mental Health Services Administration, 2004. http://www.buprenorphine.samhsa.gov/publications.html.

Pechnick RN, Glasner-Edwards S, Hrymoc M, Wilkins, JN. Preclinical development and clinical implementation of treatments for substance abuse disorders. FOCUS: Substance Abuse: Spring 2007; 2:151–162.

A 35-year-old man with obsessive-compulsive disorder presents for treatment. He would prefer not using medication due to possible side effects. Which of the following psychotherapies would be the treatment of choice for his disorder?

- (A) Supportive psychotherapy
- (B) Exposure with response prevention
- (C) Hypnotherapy
- (D) Interpersonal therapy
- (E) Psychodynamic psychotherapy

The correct response is option **B**: Exposure with response prevention

Exposure with response prevention (ERP) is the psychotherapeutic treatment of choice for obsessive-compulsive disorder. In ERP, patients are exposed to the feared stimuli and obsessions while rituals that typically serve to reduce anxiety are prevented.

Sadock BJ, Sadock VA, Ruiz P (eds): Kaplan and Sadock's Comprehensive Textbook of Psychiatry, 9th ed. Philadelphia, Lippinicott Williams & Wilkins, 2009, p 2790

Koran LM: Obsessive-compulsive disorder: An update for the clinician. Focus 2007; 5(3):299–313

American Psychiatric Association Practice Guideline for the Treatment of Patients with Obsessive-Compulsive Disorder. 2007. http://psychiatryonline.com/pracGuide/pracGuideHome.aspx

12

An adolescent with mild mental retardation continues to be significantly depressed despite actively participating in psychotherapy for several months. Which of the following is the best clinical option?

- (A) Start treatment with an atypical antipsychotic
- (B) Start treatment with an SSRI
- (C) Change psychotherapeutic approaches
- (D) Implement intense behavioral management

The correct response is option **B**: Start treatment with an SSRI.

Generally, symptoms in mentally retarded individuals are treated with the same medications that are used in non-mentally retarded individuals. Mentally retarded children and adolescents may have less of a response or have more side effects. For depression, an SSRI would be the first choice with ongoing monitoring for adverse effects. Starting an antidepressant as an adjunct to psychotherapy after the adolescent has failed to respond to psychotherapy alone is a standard approach to the treatment of adolescent depression.

AACAP practice parameter for the assessment and treatment of children and adolescents with depressive disorders. J Am Acad Child Adolesc Psychiatry. 2007. Reprinted in FOCUS: Child and Adolescent Psychiatry. Summer 2008; 6(3):387

AACAP practice parameter for the assessment and treatment of children, adolescents, and adults with mental retardation and comorbid mental disorders. J Am Acad Child Adolesc Psychiatry. 1999; 38:1609

Handen B, Gilchrist R. Practitioner review: psychopharmacology in children and adolescents with mental retardation. Journal of Child Psychology & Psychiatry and Allied Disciplines. 2006; 47: 871–82

13

Personalities characterized by the traits of persistence, perfectionism, and decreased flexibility in "set shifting," i.e. the ability to move back and forth between tasks, operations or mental sets, are associated with which of the following disorders?

- (A) Alcohol dependence in full-sustained remission
- (B) Delusional disorder
- (C) Anorexia nervosa
- (D) Early Alzheimer's disease
- (E) Traumatic brain injury

The correct response is option **C**: Anorexia nervosa

Persistence and perfectionism are associated with obsessive-compulsive personality traits and disorders, occurring in many patients with anorexia nervosa. When patients with anorexia nervosa were compared to normal controls on neuropsychological tests of "set shifting," functions primarily linked to the prefrontal cortex, patients with anorexia nervosa and their healthy sisters both took significantly longer on set-shifting tasks than the normal controls and did not differ from each other. Recovered women did not differ from unrecovered women on these tasks. Specifically in reaction to tasks requiring behavioral response shifts, these patients showed brain patterns that differed significantly from the comparison. These findings are consistent with other features of obsessive-compulsive personalities found in these populations. Such features have been linked to abnormalities in the serotonergic system, implicated in the regulation of impulsivity and cognitive inflexibility, reported in anorexia nervosa.

Zastrow A, Kaiser S, Stippich C, Walther S, Herzog W, Tchanturia K, Belger A, Weisbrod M, Treasure J, Friederich HC. Neural correlates of impaired cognitive-behavioral flexibility in anorexia nervosa. Am J Psychiatry. 2009 May; 166(5):608–16.

Holliday J, Tchanturia K, Landau S, Collier D, Treasure J. Is impaired set-shifting an endophenotype of anorexia nervosa? Am J Psychiatry, December 2005; 162:2269–2275

14

Which of the following treatments is considered the best approach to managing a patient with panic disorder, unresponsive to initial treatments with an SSRI and a benzodiazepine?

- (A) SNRI
- (B) Buspirone
- (C) Atypical antipsychotic
- (D) Another SSRI
- (E) CBT

The correct response is option **E**: CBT

Based on current evidence, CBT is the psychosocial treatment that would be indicated most often. According to The American Psychiatric Association Practice Guideline for the Treatment of Patients with Panic Disorder the effects of cognitive behavioral therapy (CBT) have been shown to be at least as efficacious as those of first-line pharmacotherapies. CBT for panic disorder has continued to demonstrate short and long term efficacy in clinical trials and may present less risk or relapse than pharmacological treatment.

Bystritsky A. Diagnosis and treatment of anxiety. FOCUS Summer 2004; 3:333–342

American Psychiatric Association Practice Guideline for the Treatment of Patients with Panic Disorder (2009). http://psychiatryonline.com/pracGuide/pracGuideHome.aspx

15

A 27-year-old man has borderline personality disorder, primarily manifested by an inability to control his urges to hurt himself. As a result, when frustrated, he will frequently superficially cut his wrists. Which of the following medications has been found to be most helpful in curbing this behavior?

(A) Olanzapine
(B) Fluoxetine
(C) Clonazepam
(D) Divalproex
(E) Naloxone

The correct response is option **B**: Fluoxetine

Although psychotherapy remains the primary treatment for borderline personality disorder, an increasing body of literature suggests that pharmacotherapy may have a role. Pharmacotherary should be symptom-focused; the symptomatic targets of therapy are grouped into three clusters: cognitive-perceptual symptoms, affective dysregulation, and impulsive behavioral dyscontrol. For impulsive behavioral dyscontrol such as that exhibited by the patient in this question, SSRI's have the strongest data for efficacy among the SSRI's, fluoxetine has been most often studied. Low dose neuroleptics have some efficacy as well and are considered second line treatment, often in conjunction with an SSRI. Although atypical neuroleptics are becoming more commonly used in clinical practice, they have rarely been studied and the bulk of data is for typical neuroleptics. Among the anticonvulsants, divalproex has been most often studied—it has shown some efficacy for affective instability, but the results for impulsivity have been equivocal. Benzodiazepines, although widely employed, have little evidence to support their use, and although some preliminary case studies have reported good results with opiate antagonists, the only controlled trial so far showed no difference from placebo.

Oldham JM, Bender DS, Skodol AE, Dyck IR, Sanislow CA, Yen S, Grilo CM, Shea MT, Zanarini MC, Gunderson JG, McGlashan TH. Testing an APA practice guideline: Symptom-targeted medication utilization for patients with borderline personality disorder. J Psychiatr Pract 2004 May;10(3):156–61. Reprinted in FOCUS 2005;3:484–488

American Psychiatric Association. Practice guideline for the treatment of patients with borderline personality disorder. Am J Psychiatry 2001;158(Suppl):1–52

16

A visibly pregnant 29-year-old woman presents seeking treatment for oxycodone dependence. Because of her pregnancy, she wants to stop using all drugs and does not want to take any medications. She went through untreated opiate withdrawal in the past when she couldn't get any pills, and while it was very uncomfortable, she thinks she could do it again with intensive social support and counseling. At this point the best treatment recommendation would be to initiate:

(A) methadone maintenance.
(B) methadone-assisted withdrawal.
(C) clonidine-naltrexone assisted withdrawal.
(D) buprenorphine maintenance.
(E) daily clinic visits to provide support.

The correct response is option **A**: Methadone maintenance

Notwithstanding the patient's initial thoughts of avoiding medications, opioid withdrawal should be avoided in pregnancy due to the greater risk of adverse fetal outcomes compared to methadone maintenance. Withdrawing the mother completely from opioids raises the risk of relapse and that the fetus will be harmed. Non-pharmacological treatment alone will likely expose the fetus to continued illicit drug use and multiple withdrawals. Naltrexone should never be given to a pregnant woman because of the risk of spontaneous abortion, stillbirth and other adverse events. There is a long history of the safety of methadone maintenance for both mother and fetus/neonate. Early clinical experience suggests that buprenorphine may have similar safety, but there is insufficient evidence to recommend its initiation in known pregnancy.

American Psychiatric Association Practice Guideline for the Treatment of Patients with Substance Use Disorders, 2nd Edition (2006), http://psychiatryonline.com/pracGuide/pracGuideHome.aspx.

Galanter M, Kleber HD (eds): Textbook of Substance Abuse Treatment, 4th ed. Arlington, VA, American Psychiatric Publishing, 2008, pp 281–82.

17

A 38-year-old female patient with schizophrenia has been treated with haloperidol and risperidone at different times in the past. Currently, she exhibits a non-rhythmical hyperkinetic movement disorder of the lips and jaw. The movement disorder most likely consistent with this finding is:

(A) akathisia (motor restlessness).
(B) Parkinsonian's tremor.
(C) tardive dyskinesia.
(D) tardive dystonia.

The correct response is option **C**: Tardive dyskinesia

Tardive dyskinesia is a non-rhythmical movement disorder first presenting in the mouth area. Parkinson's tremor is a perioral tremor (and therefore is rhythmical). Akathisia usually manifests in the lower limbs, leg shifting from one foot to the other, or pacing. Tardive dystonia usually presents in the head and neck (e.g. sideways movement of the head associated with hypertonicity of muscles).

Kay J, Tasman A. Essentials of Psychiatry. John Wiley and Sons, Hoboken, NJ. 2006, pp 952–954.

18

Which one of the following dimensions assessed on the Temperament and Character Inventory (TCI) is MOST likely to increase with age?

(A) Cooperativeness
(B) Harm avoidance
(C) Persistence
(D) Reward dependence
(E) Self-transcendence

The correct response is option **A**: Cooperativeness

Personality disorder is associated with younger age. This indicates maturation with increasing age. In general, three dimensions of personality change substantially with age. Novelty Seeking decreases; Cooperativeness increases; and Self-Directedness increases.

Sadock BJ, Sadock VA (eds): Kaplan and Sadock's Comprehensive Textbook of Psychiatry, 9th ed. Philadelphia, Lippincott Williams & Wilkins, 2009, p. 2233.

19

A 74-year-old man presents with a history of rapidly progressive cognitive decline with ataxia, multifocal myoclonic jerks and visual field cut. MRI reveals increased T2 and FLAIR signal intensity in the basal ganglia. Which of the following is the most likely diagnosis?

(A) Alzheimer's dementia
(B) Huntington's chorea
(C) Creutzfeldt-Jakob disease
(D) Vascular dementia
(E) Lewy body disease

The correct response is option **C**: Creutzfeldt-Jakob disease

Creutzfeldt-Jakob disease is the most common among the prion-related neurodegenerative disorders, and is characterized by rapid cognitive decline with ataxia; multifocal myoclonic jerks, and startle myoclonus. Other clinical features include weakness, neuropathy, chorea, hallucinations, visual field cuts, language disturbances and seizures. MRI of the head can show very specific abnormalities and can aid in the diagnosis. Increased T2 and FLAIR signal intensity in the basal ganglia is reported. Alzheimer's disease is characterized by a gradual onset of cognitive decline along with impairment of executive function or ataxia, apraxia or agnosia. Vascular Dementia is often associated with a stepwise deterioration and presence of strokes. Lewy body dementia is often characterized by progressive cognitive decline, extrapyramidal symptoms and visual hallucinations. Huntington's chorea is characterized by choreifrom, dyskinetic movements and may be associated with cognitive decline.

Yudofsky SC, Hales RE (eds): The American Psychiatric Publishing Textbook of Neuropsychiatry and Behavioral Sciences, 5th ed. Washington DC: American Psychiatric Publishing Inc; 2008. pp. 955–957

20

Recent genome-wide association studies (GWAS) have implicated regions of which chromosome in autism spectrum disorders (ASD)?

(A) Chromosome 1
(B) Chromosome 5
(C) Chromosome 8
(D) Chromosome 22

The correct response is option **B**: Chromosome 5

The first published GWAS of ASD found evidence of a genome-wide significant association signal on chromosome 5p14. This original genome-wide association signal was replicated in a large case–control sample. The second association data identified genome wide significant association on chromosome 5p15.

Collectively, the two reported ASD GWAS studies point to regions of chromosome 5p that may include common genetic variants that contribute to ASD risk. Additional studies will be required.

Campbell DB: Advances and challenges in the genetics of autism. FOCUS Summer 2010 8(3):339–349

21

A 16-year-old woman presents with fatigue and dehydration. On physical examination she is noted to have swollen salivary glands and calluses on her knuckles. She is also hypokalemic. These findings are most consistent with which of the following diagnoses?

(A) Chronic fatigue syndrome
(B) Bulimia nervosa
(C) Obsessive-compulsive disorder
(D) Anorexia nervosa
(E) Rumination disorder

The correct response is option **B**: Bulimia nervosa

Bulimia nervosa, purging type, is characterized by frequent episodes of binge eating and "self-induced vomiting or the misuse of laxatives, diuretics or enemas." Swollen salivary glands, calluses on knuckles, and hypokalemia are complications of excessive self-induced vomiting.

American Psychiatric Association: Diagnostic and Statistical Manual of Mental Disorders, 4th Edition, Text Revision (DSM-IV-TR). Washington DC, American Psychiatric Association. 2000; pp 589–594

Mehler PS. Bulimia nervosa. N Engl J Med. 2003; 349:875–881

Hales RE, Yudofsky SC, Gabbard GO (eds): The American Psychiatric Publishing Textbook of Psychiatry, 5th ed. Washington, DC, American Psychiatric Publishing, Inc., 2008. pp 983–984

22

A 21-year old college student is seen in the University counseling center because of relationship problems. He has had one serious relationship with a woman that lasted about six months. He terminated the relationship because he discovered that the woman was seeing someone else. Although he wants to engage in a new relationship, he is extremely reluctant stating: "Women just can't be trusted." Which of the following BEST describes this thinking error?

(A) Arbitrary inference
(B) Dichotomous thinking
(C) Magnification
(D) Overgeneralization
(E) Selective abstraction

The correct response is option **D**: Overgeneralization

Overgeneralization is the process that occurs when someone believes in and follows a general rule on the basis of limited examples. Arbitrary inference is reaching a conclusion in the absence of any evidence that would support the idea (e.g., assuming you will lose your job because your boss sends you an email asking to meet). Dichotomous thinking is "all or nothing" thinking in which a person reduces situations to "black versus white." Magnification is when an individual assigns subjective "weights" to their interpretation of situations, resulting, for example, in giving negative events greater weight than positive occurrences. Lastly, selective abstraction is focusing on a detail taken out of context.

Sadock BJ, Sadock VA, Ruiz P (eds): Kaplan and Sadock's Comprehensive Textbook of Psychiatry, 9th ed. Philadelphia, Lippincott Williams & Wilkins, 2009, pp 2858–2859

Textbook of Psychotherapeutic Treatments.Gabbard GO (ed). Arlington, VA, American Psychiatric Publishing Inc, 2009, p 173

23

A 40 year old patient is diagnosed with Alzheimer's disease. Which of the following genes is associated with this very early form of Alzheimer's disease?

(A) Presenilin 1
(B) Presenilin 2
(C) Apo E2
(D) Apo E3
(E) Apo E4

The correct response is option **A**: Presenilin 1

Only 10 percent of Alzheimer's cases are considered to be hereditary. Of these, 70 to 80 percent are attributable to mutations in the presenilin 1 gene, found on chromosome 14, which causes onset of symptoms at 40–50 years of age. Mutations in presenilin 2 are rare causes of early onset familial Alzheimer's disease. A mutation in presenilin 2 is associated with onset at approximately age 50. Apolipoprotein E2 (Apo E2) protects Tau protein from phosphorylation and thus from the neurofibrillary tangles associated with the disease, whereas Apo E3 and Apo E4 are not associated as strongly with this protection. The E3 and E4 alleles account for 10–50% of the risk of sporadic AD with onset of symptoms at 60 years of age.

Sadock BJ, Sadock VA (eds): Kaplan & Sadock's Synopsis of Psychiatry: Behavioral Sciences/Clinical Psychiatry, 10th ed. Philadelphia, Lippincott Williams & Wilkins, 2007, p 129

Alzheimer's Disease Genetics Fact Sheet, NIH Publication No. 08-6424, November 2008, http://www.nia.nih.gov/alzheimers/publications/geneticsfs.htm

Bettens K, Sleegers K, Van Broeckhoven C: Current status on Alzheimer disease molecular genetics: from past, to present, to future. Hum Mol Genet. 2010 Apr 15;19(R1):R4–R11. Epub 2010 Apr 13.

Jayadev S, Leverenz JB, Steinbart E, Stahl J, Klunk W, Yu CE, Bird TD. Alzheimer's disease phenotypes and genotypes associated with mutations in presenilin 2. Brain. 2010 Apr;133(Pt 4):1143–54.

24

During an interview of a patient with a substance abuse disorder, the therapist asks the patient about the pros and cons of specific behaviors, explores the patient's goals and associated ambivalence about reaching those goals, and listens reflectively to the patient's response. This treatment approach is most consistent with:

(A) cognitive-behavioral therapy.
(B) contingency management.
(C) interpersonal therapy.
(D) motivational enhancement therapy.
(E) psychodynamic psychotherapy.

The correct response is option **D**: Motivational enhancement therapy

Motivational enhancement therapy (MET) combines techniques from cognitive, client-centered, systems, and social-psychological persuasion approaches. MET is characterized by an empathic approach in which the therapist helps to motivate the patient by exploring readiness for change. This treatment modality is effective even for patients who are not highly motivated to change.

American Psychiatric Association Practice Guideline for the Treatment of Patients with Substance Use Disorders, 2nd Edition (2006), http://psychiatryonline.com/pracGuide/pracGuideHome.aspx

25

Which of the following antidepressants has the greatest body of evidence for efficacy in treating major depressive disorder in children and adolescents?

    (A) Citalopram
    (B) Fluoxetine
    (C) Fluvoxamine
    (D) Sertraline
    (E) Paroxetine

The correct response is option **B**: Fluoxetine

Fluoxetine has the greatest body of evidence for treating child and adolescent depression (ages 8 to ≤18). Studies have shown mixed results for other SSRIs. Studies have also shown some evidence of efficacy in other SSRIs, but the strongest evidence of efficacy in RTC exists for fluoxetine.

Cheung AH, Emslie GJ, Mayes TL. The use of antidepressants to treat depression in children and adolescents. Can Med Assoc J 2006; 174:193–200. http://www.pubmedcentral.nih.gov/articlerender.fcgi?tool_pubmed&pubmedid_16415467

Boylan K, Romero S, Birmaher B. Psychopharmacologic treatment of pediatric major depressive disorder. Psychopharmacol 2007; 191:27–38

Vasa RA, Carlino AR, Pine DS. Pharmacotherapy of depressed children and adolescents: current issues and potential directions. Biol Psychiatry 2006; 59:1021–1028

AACAP practice parameter for the assessment and treatment of children and adolescents with depressive disorders. J Am Acad Child Adolesc Psychiatry. 2007. FOCUS. American Psychiatric Publishing, Inc., Arlington (VA). Reprinted in 2008; 6(3):389

26

A city is attacked by terrorists intermittently over a three-week period. There is no indication that the attacks will stop. Which of the following interventions is most likely to be effective in lowering the risk of developing PTSD in the months following exposure?

    (A) Educating the public about symptoms of PTSD
    (B) Evacuating the most vulnerable population
    (C) Limiting exposure to media coverage of the attacks
    (D) Providing psychological debriefing to survivors
    (E) Reestablishing a relative sense of safety

The correct response is option **E**: Reestablishing a relative sense of safety

Negative post-trauma reactions tend to persist under conditions of ongoing threat or danger, as studies in a variety of cultures have shown. To the extent that safety is introduced, these reactions show a gradual reduction over time. Moreover, even where threat continues, those who can maintain or re-establish a relative sense of safety have considerably lower risk of developing PTSD in the months following exposure than those who do not.

Hobfoll SE, Watson P, Bell CC, Bryant RA, Brymer MJ, Friedman MJ, Friedman M, Gersons BP, de Jong JT, Layne CM, Maguen S, Neria Y, Norwood AE, Pynoos RS, Reissman D, Ruzek JI, Shalev AY, Solomon Z, Steinberg AM, Ursano RJ. Five essential elements of immediate and mid-term mass trauma intervention: empirical evidence. Psychiatry. 2007; 70(4):283–315. Reprinted in FOCUS. 2009; 2:221–242

27

Defining high-risk situations, covert antecedents, and stimulus control techniques are a focus of which of the following therapeutic modalities?

(A) Brief psychodynamic psychotherapy
(B) Cognitive behavioral therapy
(C) Supportive therapy
(D) Interpersonal therapy
(E) Relapse prevention therapy

The correct response is option **E**: Relapse prevention therapy

Relapse prevention therapy focuses on factors or situations that can precipitate or contribute to relapse to substance use. These factors include immediate determinants, such as high-risk situations, and covert antecedents, such as seemingly irrelevant decisions. Stimulus control techniques are employed to help with management of cravings and/or urges. Brief psychodynamic psychotherapy focuses on the role unconscious processes play in the patient's present behavior. Cognitive behavioral therapy focuses on patterns of thinking and underlying beliefs that are maladaptive. Supportive therapy encompasses a variety of techniques but tends to focus on maximizing a patient's adaptive coping mechanisms. Interpersonal psychotherapy focuses on the connections between a person's symptoms and their interactions with others.

Larimer ME, Palmer RS, Marlatt GA: Relapse prevention: an overview of Marlatt's cognitive-behavioral model. Alcohol Research and Health 1999; 23:151–60

28

A 42-year-old patient with schizophrenia presents to the emergency department with confusion and agitation following an overdose of antipsychotic medication. The patient has a temperature of 101.7 degrees Fahrenheit, blood pressure of 140/80 mm Hg, and pulse of 112. Physical examination reveals hot, dry skin, dilated pupils, and decreased bowel sounds. This patient's symptoms are most likely caused by medication effects at which of the following receptors?

(A) Muscarinic cholinergic
(B) Nicotinic cholinergic
(C) α1-adrenergic
(D) Histaminergic
(E) Dopaminergic

The correct response is option **A**: Muscarinic cholinergic

Antipsychotic medications have effects at muscarinic cholinergic, α1-adrenergic, histaminergic, and dopaminergic receptors. This patient's symptoms are most consistent with anticholinergic toxicity, and therefore are most likely to be caused by blockade at the muscarinic cholinergic receptors.

Schatzberg AF, Nemeroff CB (eds): Essentials of Clinical Psychopharmacology, 2nd ed. Arlington, VA, American Psychiatric Publishing, Inc., 2006. p 218

29

Which of the following therapies for borderline personality disorder incorporates psychoeducation about the illness, emotional management skills training, and behavior skills training?

(A) Mentalization based therapy
(B) Schema-focused therapy
(C) Trauma-focused cognitive-behavior therapy
(D) Eye movement desensitization and reprocessing
(E) Systems Training for Emotional Predictability and Problem Solving

The correct response is option **E**: Systems Training for Emotional Predictability and Problem Solving

The STEPPS program combines cognitive behavioral elements with skills training. It is done only in groups and is meant to complement ongoing therapy. Mentalization based therapy, though useful in borderline personality disorder, is a psychoanalytic treatment. Schema-focused therapy is a cognitive therapy for borderline personality disorder. Trauma-focused CBT and EMDR are treatments for PTSD.

Blum N et al: Systems Training for Emotional Predictability and Problem Solving (STEPPS) for outpatients with borderline personality disorder: A randomized controlled trial and 1-year follow-up. Am J Psychiatry 2008; 165:469

Hales RE, Yudofsky SC, Gabbard GO: The American Psychiatric Publishing Textbook of Psychiatry, 5th ed, Arlington, VA: American Psychiatric Publishing, Inc., 2008, pp 580, 842

When managing a chronically suicidal patient, respecting the patient's preference to remain at home and not be admitted to the psychiatric unit for additional care reflects which of the following ethical principles?

(A) Autonomy
(B) Beneficence
(C) Non-Maleficence
(D) Egalitarianism

The correct response is option **A**: Autonomy

A decision to respect a patient's preference reflects a decision to respect a patient's decision-making or *autonomous* judgment of the possible benefits and adverse consequences for the decisions made. Beneficence-based obligations seek to provide beneficial outcomes to patients and to avoid possible adverse consequences of patients' decision-making. Physicians have obligations of beneficence and obligations to respect patients' autonomy or preferences. Many chronically suicidal patients are safely managed at home. Non-maleficence refers to not causing harm by a decision made. Justice-based considerations are less relevant here. Egalitarian justice is an obligation to provide benefits in equal proportion to individual's needs.

Roberts LW. Ethical principles and skills in the care of mental illness. FOCUS: Forensic and Ethical Issues Fall 2003; 4:340.

Sadock BJ, Sadock VA, Ruiz P (eds): Kaplan & Sadock's Comprehensive Textbook of Psychiatry, 9th ed. Philadelphia, Lippincott Williams & Wilkins, 2009, p 4441.

A 12-year-old boy is hospitalized after a serious suicide attempt. His parents report that they noticed a difference in his behavior about a year ago. He became increasingly withdrawn; was preoccupied with mythical creatures; his academic performance declined significantly, he had difficulty sleeping and a decreased appetite. Over the past two months, he has seemed progressively worse. He has demonstrated both persecutory and somatic delusions; has reported he hears voices telling him to "beware–they are watching you–you're a naughty little boy." Today he heard a voice telling him that he was "rotting inside" and in response, he attempted to hang himself. On examination he denies a mood disturbance. His thinking is illogical and non-linear. What is the most likely diagnosis?

(A) Bipolar disorder
(B) Attention-deficit/hyperactivity disorder
(C) Schizophrenia
(D) Major depressive disorder
(E) Asperger's syndrome

The correct response is option **C**: Schizophrenia

Auditory hallucinations are the most frequently reported positive symptom of childhood-onset schizophrenia. It is estimated that 80–100% of children with schizophrenia age 13 years or younger report hallucinations. The other symptoms in the vignette occur less frequently. The lack of mood disturbance eliminates the possibility of bipolar disorder or major depressive disorder. This patient's symptoms (e.g., delusions, auditory hallucinations) and presentation (onset of symptoms at 11 years old) are inconsistent with ADHD and Asperger's syndrome.

Dulcan MK, Weiner JM. Essentials of Child and Adolescent Psychiatry. Arlington (VA): American Psychiatric Publishing, Inc., 2006. pp. 238–240 238–240.

Hales RE, Yudofsky SC, and Gabbard GO (eds). The American Psychiatric Publishing Textbook of Psychiatry. 5th ed. Arlington (VA), American Psychiatric Publishing, Inc., 2008. pp. 836, 882–892

Individuals with two copies of which one of the following genes develop Alzheimer's disease eight times more frequently than those without it?

(A) APOE E1
(B) APOE E2
(C) APOE E3
(D) APOE E4
(E) APOE E5

The correct response is option **D**: APOE E4

Of the three allelic varieties of the APOE gene, APOE E2 may provide some protection against developing Alzheimer's disease (AD). The most common allele, APOE E3, may be risk neutral, while APOE E4 is associated with increased susceptibility to the disease. Individuals with a single copy of the E4 gene may have Alzheimer's disease three times more frequently as compared to individuals with no E4 gene. Furthermore, individuals with two E4 genes have the disease eight times more frequently than do those with no E4 gene. According to NIH, "APOE ε4 occurs in about 40 percent of all people who develop late-onset AD and is present in about 25 to 30 percent of the population. People with AD are more likely to have an APOE ε4 allele than people who do not develop AD. However, many people with AD do not have an APOE ε4 allele." Diagnostic testing for this gene is not currently recommended since it is found in persons without dementia.

Alzheimer's Disease Genetics Fact Sheet, NIH Publication No. 08-6424, November 2008, http://www.nia.nih.gov/alzheimers/publications/geneticsfs.htm

Sadock BJ, Sadock VA (eds): Kaplan & Sadock's Comprehensive Textbook of Psychiatry, 9th ed. Philadelphia, Lippincott Williams & Wilkins, 2009, pp 4059–4060

In addition to the neuroticism, extraversion, openness, and conscientious facets of personality, the fifth facet of personality being considered as an alternative or complement to the classification for personality disorders in the revision of the Diagnostic and Statistical Manual of Mental Disorders (DSM) is which ONE of the following?

(A) Agreeableness
(B) Brightness
(C) Happiness
(D) Humor
(E) Optimism

The correct response is option **A**: Agreeableness

One proposal for the revision of DSM is to reconceptualize personality disorders via dimensions. The Five-Factor Model (FFM) has received much attention, either as a supplement or replacement for the diagnosis of personality disorders. The FFM describes personality in a continuous manner along 30 traits or facets, grouped into five general categories, rather than the current DSM method of defining unique personality disorders by specific criteria.

Rottman BM, Ahn W, Sanislow CA, Kim NS: Can clinicians recognize DSM-IV personality disorders from five-factor model descriptions of patient cases? Am J Psychiatry 2009; 166:427–433

Clark LA: Assessment and diagnosis of personality disorder: perennial issues and emerging reconceptualization. Annu Rev Psychol 2007; 58:227–257

Diagnostic and Statistical Manual of Mental Disorders, Fourth Edition, Text Revision (DSM-IV-TR). Washington, DC, American Psychiatric Association, 2000.

34

A 32-year-old man with a history of bipolar I disorder has been off all medication for over six months. He currently presents with symptoms consistent with a moderately severe major depressive episode. Which of the following has the best evidence as a pharmacologic treatment for him?

(A) Clonazepam and lithium
(B) Olanzapine and fluoxetine
(C) Lithium and paroxetine
(D) Valproate and fluoxetine
(E) Bupropion alone

The correct response is option **B**: Olanzapine and fluoxetine

Of the pharmacological options given, only the olanzapine and fluoxetine combination has substantial evidence for efficacy in randomized placebo-controlled, double-blind trials. In general, antidepressant monotherapy is not recommended because of a potential increase in the likelihood of hypomanic, manic, or mixed episodes occurring. However, some studies have supported the use of paroxetine, venlafaxine or quetiapine alone. Although some clinicians will initiate simultaneous treatment with lithium and an antidepressant, this is generally reserved for more severely ill patients or when other approaches, such as initiation and optimization of lithium, have not produced a clinical response.

American Psychiatric Association Practice Guideline for the Treatment of Patients with Bipolar Disorder, 2nd ed (2002). Reprinted in FOCUS: Bipolar Disorder, Winter 2003; 1:64–110.

Hirschfeld RMA: "Guideline Watch: Practice Guideline for the Treatment of Patients with Bipolar Disorder, 2nd Edition" APA Practice Guidelines November 2005. Reprinted in FOCUS: Bipolar Disorder, Winter 2007;5;1:34–39.

35

Which of the following psychiatric disorders confers the highest genetic relative risk for first degree relatives?

(A) Panic disorder
(B) Alcoholism
(C) Major depression
(D) Bipolar disorder
(E) Schizophrenia

The correct response is option **D**: Bipolar disorder

All of the above disorders have a significant relative risk (the risk to a relative of an affected individual compared to the overall incidence of the disorder). However, bipolar disorder has the highest at 24.5, followed by schizophrenia at 18.5, panic at 9.6, alcoholism at 7.4 and major depression at 3.0.

Hales RE, Yudofsky SC, Gabbard GO (eds): The American Psychiatric Publishing Textbook of Psychiatry, 5th ed, 2008 pp 196–197

36

A 35-year-old woman began taking citalopram, 20 mg, daily about three months ago when she presented with symptoms consistent with panic disorder. On the current regimen, her symptoms are under control. Until her recent episode of illness she has had no other history of psychiatric symptoms and there is no family history of psychiatric illness. How long should she continue this medication?

(A) Four weeks
(B) Three months
(C) One year
(D) Three years
(E) Indefinitely

The correct response is option **C**: One year

Pharmacotherapy should generally be continued for 1 year or more after acute response to promote further symptom reduction and decrease risk of recurrence. Incorporating maintenance treatment (e.g., monthly "booster" sessions focused on relapse prevention) into psychosocial treatments for panic disorder also may help maintain positive response, although more systematic investigation of this issue is needed.

American Psychiatric Association Practice Guideline for the treatment of Patients with Panic Disorder (2009). http://psychiatryonline.com/pracGuide/pracGuideHome.aspx

37

Based upon the results of the National Institute of Mental Health funded multi-site Multimodal Treatment Study of Children with Attention Deficit-Hyperactivity Disorder (MTA), which of the following interventions was proven to be the MOST effective in treating the majority of children with ADHD?

(A) Medication alone
(B) Medication with an intensive summer treatment program
(C) Medication with community referral
(D) Medication with parent training
(E) Medication with school consultation

The correct response is option **A**: Medication alone

Although it would seem logical that combined treatments would improve outcomes for the child with ADHD, this was not supported by the MTA study. The MTA study randomly assigned children ages 7–9 years with ADHD (combined type) to either 1) medication treatment (primarily psychostimulants) 2) a comprehensive psychosocial treatment package including parent training, intensive summer treatment program, and school consultation 3) the combined psychosocial package and medication, or 4) community referral as a control group. Children randomly assigned to the medication treatment arm overall had significantly improved outcomes compared with children receiving psychosocial treatment alone or those referred out for community care. Subjects receiving the combined medication and psychosocial treatment fared little better in general than subjects receiving medication treatment alone. The advantage of combination therapy over medication treatment alone was small.

AACAP practice parameter for the assessment and treatment of children and adolescents with attention-deficit/hyperactivity disorder. J Am Child Adolesc Psychiatry. 2007. Reprinted in FOCUS. 2008; 6(3):409.

Dulcan MK, Weiner JM. Essentials of Child and Adolescent Psychiatry. Arlington, VA, American Psychiatric Publishing, Inc., 2006. pp 341–342.

The MTA Cooperative Goup. A 14-month randomized clinical trial of treatment strategies for attention-deficit/hyperactivity disorder. Arch Gen Psychiatry 1999; 56(12):1073–86

38

Which of the following personality disorders is most common in the biological relatives of patients with schizophrenia?

(A) Schizoid
(B) Paranoid
(C) Schizotypal
(D) Histrionic
(E) Antisocial

The correct response is option **C**: Schizotypal

There is a greater presence of schizotypal patients in families with a history of schizophrenia than in control groups. There is less correlation between paranoid or schizoid PD in families with schizophrenia. Cluster B disorders, including histrionic and antisocial PD, have different genetic associations. Specifically, antisocial PD is associated with alcohol use disorders, and histrionic with somatization disorder (Briquet's syndrome).

Sadock BJ, Sadock VA (eds): Kaplan & Sadock's Synopsis of Psychiatry: Behavioral Sciences/Clinical Psychiatry, 10th ed. Philadelphia, Lippincott Williams & Wilkins, 2007, p 791.

39

Which of the following symptoms is a diagnostic feature of atypical depression?

(A) Insomnia
(B) Weight loss
(C) Suicidal ideation
(D) Mood reactivity
(E) Inappropriate guilt

The correct response is option **D**: Mood reactivity

The Atypical Features specifier in DSM-IV-TR can be applied to major depressive episodes in depression or bipolar disorder, or to dysthymic disorder. But the criteria that differentiate atypical depression from those disorders require mood reactivity as well as two or more of the following: weight gain or appetite increase; hypersomnia; leaden paralysis; rejection sensitivity (a long-standing pattern).

Diagnostic and Statistical Manual of Mental Disorders, 4th ed. Text Revision (DSM-IV-TR). Washington, DC, American Psychiatric Association, 2000, pp 420–422

40

A 33-year-old man whose bipolar I disorder has been well controlled on medication, presents to the emergency department with severe left upper quadrant pain radiating to his back, nausea and vomiting. Which medication is most likely contributing to these symptoms?

(A) Lamotrigine
(B) Lithium
(C) Olanzapine
(D) Valproate
(E) Ziprasidone

The correct response is option **D**: Valproate

Rare, idiosyncratic, but potentially fatal adverse events with valproate include irreversible hepatic failure, hemorrhagic pancreatitis, and agranulocytosis. Thus, patients taking valproate should be instructed to contact their psychiatrist or primary care physician immediately if they develop symptoms of these conditions. The symptoms and laboratory findings are consistent with a diagnosis of acute pancreatitis. Based on reports of pancreatitis associated with valproate use, a black box warning was added to its package insert in 2000. While routine monitoring of pancreatic function is not necessary, clinical manifestations suggestive of acute pancreatitis should be evaluated promptly and fully.

American Psychiatric Association Practice Guideline for the Treatment of Patients with Bipolar Disorder, 2nd Edition (2002). Reprinted in FOCUS: Bipolar Disorder, 2003; 1:84–85.

Pellock JM, Wilder BJ, Deaton R, Sommerville KW: Acute pancreatitis coincident with valproate use: a critical review. Epilepsia 2002; 43:1421–1424.

Yazdani K, Lippmann M, Gala I: Fatal pancreatitis associated with valproic acid. Medicine 2002; 81:305–310.

41

A sniper attacks a city hall building, killing 13 individuals and significantly injuring another 12 before he takes his own life. Therapists from the local mental health clinic are dispatched to the scene to provide psychological debriefing to prevent PTSD symptoms. Using an evidence-based framework, what is the most likely impact of this intervention on direct survivors?

    (A) It will be ineffective or harmful to the direct survivors.
    (B) It will decrease the probability of developing PTSD symptoms.
    (C) It will decrease the severity of PTSD symptoms.
    (D) It will decrease the time period for recovery from PTSD symptoms.
    (E) It will delay the onset of PTSD symptoms.

The correct response is option **A**: It will be ineffective or harmful to the direct survivors.

Restoring social and behavioral functioning after disasters and situations of mass casualty has been extensively explored over the last few decades. No evidence-based consensus has been reached to date with regard to effective interventions. Recent findings indicate that commonly utilized interventions, such as psychological debriefing, do not prevent PTSD, may not be effective in preventing long-term distress and dysfunction, and may even be harmful to direct survivors of disasters.

Hobfoll SE, Watson P, Bell CC, Bryant RA, Brymer MJ, Friedman MJ, Gersons BP, de Jong JT, Layne CM, Maguen S, Neria Y, Norwood AE, Pynoos RS, Reissman D, Ruzek JI, Shalev AY, Solomon Z, Steinberg AM, Ursano RJ. Five essential elements of immediate and mid-term mass trauma intervention: empirical evidence. Psychiatry. 2007; 70(4):284. Reprinted in FOCUS. 2009; 2:221–242

42

You are asked to write 22 questions for a board-type examination in less than four weeks. Your first thought is, "I will never be able to get all those questions written in such a short time!" You ignore the fact that you seem to have been able to be successful at this several times before. From a cognitive therapy perspective, what is the best description of this type of thinking?

    (A) Magnification
    (B) Minimization
    (C) Personalization
    (D) Selective abstraction
    (E) Catastrophic thinking

The correct response is option **E**: Catastrophic thinking

Catastrophic thinking involves predicting the worst possible outcome while ignoring more likely eventualities. Magnification is over-valuing, and minimization is under-valuing the significance of a personal attribute, a life event, or a future possibility. Personalization is linking external occurrences to oneself when there is little reason to do so. Selective abstraction is drawing a conclusion based only on a small portion of available data.

Hales RE, Yudofsky SC, Gabbard GO (eds): The American Psychiatric Publishing Textbook of Psychiatry, 5th ed. Arlington VA, American Psychiatric Publishing Inc, 2008, p 1214

43

A patient with four or more mood disturbances within a single year that meet both the duration and symptom criteria for major depressive, mixed, manic and/or hypomanic episodes demarcated by remission or switch to opposite polarity, meets the DSM IV criteria for which of the following disorders?

(A) Bipolar disorder with rapid cycling specifier
(B) Bipolar disorder, Not Otherwise Specified
(C) Cyclothymic disorder
(D) Schizoaffective disorder (bipolar type)

The correct response is option **A**: Bipolar disorder with rapid cycling specifier

The rapid cycling specifier, the presence of four or more distinct mood episodes per year, can be applied to both bipolar I and bipolar II disorder. Cyclothymic disorder is characterized by numerous periods of hypomanic symptoms that do not meet criteria for manic episode and numerous periods of depressive symptoms that do not meet criteria for major depressive episode. NOS refers to patients that do not meet criteria for any specific mood disorder. Schizoaffective disorder (bipolar type) meets the criteria for schizoaffective disorder, and a manic episode or mixed episode is part of the presentation.

American Psychiatric Association: Diagnostic and Statistical Manual of mental Disorder 4th edition text revision. Washington DC, American Psychiatric Association, 2000 pp 320–321, 398–399, 427–428.
Schneck CD, Miklowitz DJ, Calabrese JR, Allen MH, Thomas MR, Wisniewski SR, Miyahara S, Shelton MD, Ketter, TA, Goldberg, JF, Bowden CL, Sachs GS. Phenomenology of rapid-cycling bipolar disorder: data from the first 500 participants in the Systematic Treatment Enhancement Program Am J Psychiatry 2004; 161:1902–1908.

44

Which of the following disorders has been shown to have the greatest degree of heritability?

(A) Schizophrenia
(B) Autism
(C) Bipolar disorder
(D) Alcoholism
(E) Attention-deficit/hyperactivity disorder (ADHD)

The correct response is option **B**: Autism

Heritability is the proportion of variance in familial risk attributed to genes. It is 90% for autism compared to at least 75% for bipolar disorder and schizophrenia, 60% for ADHD, and 40% for alcoholism.

Sadock BJ, Sadock VA (eds): Kaplan & Sadock's Comprehensive Textbook of Psychiatry, 9th ed. Philadelphia, Lippincott Williams & Wilkins, 2009, pp 304

45

A 42-year-old man presents to a psychiatrist 6 months after a motor vehicle accident. He has difficulty sleeping because he has frequent nightmares about the accident. He has not been able to drive since the accident, and his wife usually drives for him. Even then, he finds it very difficult to be in a car, often panicking if another car is near them on the road. Which of the following medications would be the most appropriate for this man?

(A) Propranolol
(B) Nortriptyline
(C) Clonazepam
(D) Olanzapine
(E) Sertraline

The correct response is option **E**: Sertraline

Although a number of medications have shown some efficacy for posttraumatic stress disorder, the American Psychiatric Association's Practice Guideline for the Treatment of Patients with Acute Stress Disorder and Posttraumatic Stress Disorder and the 2009 Guideline Watch recommend selective serotonin reuptake inhibitors as the first-line medication treatment for patients with PTSD. The other medications listed are generally not considered first-line medications as they have less data to support their use.

American Psychiatric Association Practice Guideline for the Treatment of Patients with Acute Stress Disorder and Posttraumatic Stress Disorder. Am J Psychiatry. 2004; 161(11 Suppl):3–31 http://www.psychiatryonline.com/pracGuide/pracGuideTopic_11.aspx
Benedek DM, Friedman MJ, Zatzick D, Ursano RJ. Guideline Watch (March 2009): Practice Guideline for the Treatment of Patients with Acute Stress Disorder and Posttraumatic Stress Disorder. FOCUS. 2009; 2:204–213 http://www.psychiatryonline.com/content.aspx?aid=156498.

46

A patient presents with involuntary frowning, blinking, grimacing, and choreoathetoid movements of the upper extremities after several years of antipsychotic medication treatment. Which one of the following is the most likely diagnosis?

(A) Akinesia
(B) Akathisia
(C) Acute dystonia
(D) Parkinsonism
(E) Tardive dyskinesia

The correct response is option **E**: Tardive dyskinesia

Tardive dyskinesia is characterized by involuntary movements of the face, trunk, or extremities and usually occurs after prolonged exposure to dopamine blocking agents. Symptoms include facial and oral movements, extremity movements, and trunk movements. The Abnormal Involuntary Movement Scale is used to examine for these side effects.

Hales RE, Yudofsky SC, Gabbard GO (eds.): The American Psychiatric Publishing Textbook of Psychiatry, 5th ed. Arlington VA, American Psychiatric Publishing Inc, 2008, pp 1090–91

47

Which of the following Axis I diagnoses is most common among individuals with bulimia nervosa?

(A) General anxiety disorder
(B) Obsessive compulsive disorder
(C) Alcohol use disorder
(D) Major depressive disorder
(E) Intermittent explosive disorder

The correct response is option **D**: Major depressive disorder

High rates of co-occurring psychiatric illness are found in patients seeking treatment for anorexia and bulimia. Lifetime co-occurring major depression or dysthymia has been reported in 50%–75% of patients with anorexia and bulimia. While the other disorders may co-occur with bulimia nervosa, the prevalence rates are much lower.

Sadock BJ, Sadock VA, Ruiz P (eds): Kaplan & Sadock's Comprehensive Textbook of Psychiatry, 9th ed. Philadelphia, Lippincott Williams & Wilkins, 2009, pp 2140–41
American Psychiatric Association Practice Guideline for the Treatment of Patients with Eating Disorders, 3rd ed. (2005), http://www.psychiatryonline.com/pracGuide/pracGuideTopic_12.aspx

A 31-year-old man is admitted to an inpatient psychiatric unit after a suicide attempt. Past records show a history of dependence on multiple substances. He sleeps poorly and the next day paces around the unit, restless and grumpy. He is tachycardic at 112 beats per minutes, his palms and forehead are sweaty and his tongue is showing a course tremor. When asked, the patient says he feels anxious. The most likely diagnosis is:

(A) alcohol withdrawal.
(B) nicotine withdrawal.
(C) opioid withdrawal.
(D) cannabis withdrawal.
(E) methamphetamine withdrawal.

The correct response is option **A**: Alcohol withdrawal.

The symptoms described are characteristic of alcohol withdrawal. While anxiety, insomnia, and diaphoresis are nonspecific symptoms common with several withdrawal syndromes, a coarse tremor observable in the tongue is particular to alcohol withdrawal. Tachycardia can be a symptom of opioid withdrawal, while mild bradycardia would be more characteristic of nicotine withdrawal. Methamphetamine withdrawal more typically presents with hypersomnia, while the symptoms of cannabis withdrawal are somewhat nonspecific.

Diagnostic and Statistical Manual of Mental Disorders, Fourth Edition, Text Revision (DSM-IV-TR). Washington, DC, American Psychiatric Association, 2000, pp 215–73.

49

A 28-year-old woman with an identical twin is diagnosed with major depressive disorder. She asks you to comment on the chance her sister will develop the same illness. Which of the following is the best response regarding the genetic basis of depression?

(A) "Major depression is a genetic illness. Your sister will definitely develop it as well."
(B) "While schizophrenia is quite heritable, there is only a slightly increased risk that your sister will become depressed."
(C) "The likelihood of identical twins sharing an affective illness is high."
(D) "Although there may be some genetic basis for affective illness, it is one's childhood environment that determines whether illness will manifest."
(E) "Your sister's risk of developing depression is the same as any other sibling."

The correct response is option **C**: "The likelihood of identical twins sharing an affective illness is high."

Both genetic and environmental factors likely contribute to the emergence of affective illness. Twin studies compare resemblance for a condition within types of twin pairs: monozygotic twins (MZ) and dizygotic twins (DZ) who share on average 100% of their DNA like other sibling pairs. Metaanalysis of data reports a summary heritability of 37%. For published studies since 1985, MZ concordance ranged from 30% to 50% and DZ concordance, from 12% to 40%.

Hehema JM: Genetics of depression, FOCUS Summer 2010; 8:316–322.
Smoller JW, Sheidley BR, Tsuang MT. Psychiatric Genetics: Applications in Clinical Practice. American Psychiatric Publishing, Inc.; 1st edition, 2008, p 145

50

For the detection and identification of delirium in medically ill patients, the best strategy to employ is:

(A) enhanced EEG monitoring.
(B) serum and urine lab tests.
(C) revised MMSE.
(D) specific neuroimaging.
(E) observation and rating scales.

The correct response is option **E**: Observation and rating scales

Delirium remains a condition that is often not detected or diagnosed. There have been improvements in screening due to the development of sensitive observation and rating scales such as Delirium Rating Scale—Revised–98, including a version for use with children; the Delirium Observation Screening Scale; and the Confusion Assessment Method for the Intensive Care Unit.

Cook IA. Guideline Watch: Practice Guideline for the Treatment of Patients with Delirium. Washington, DC: American Psychiatric Association; 2004 http://www.psychiatryonline.com/pracGuide/pracGuideTopic_2.aspx

51

A 58-year-old man with a history of alcohol dependence and mild dementia presents to the hospital for a liver biopsy due to suspected alcoholic hepatitis. He complains of severe anxiety about having the procedure done and requests "something for my nerves." Which of the following benzodiazepines is safest to administer?

(A) Alprazolam
(B) Chlordiazepoxide
(C) Diazepam
(D) Oxazepam
(E) Clonazepam

The correct response is option **D**: Oxazepam

For patients who have severe hepatic disease, who are elderly, or have delirium, dementia, or another cognitive disorder, short-acting benzodiazepines such as oxazepam or lorazepam are preferred. Oxazepam, temazepam and lorazepam do not require multi-step biotransformation; they are metabolized by phase II enzymes (glucuronidation) that are not affected by alcohol-related hepatitis.

American Psychiatric Association Practice Guideline for the Treatment of Patients with Substance Use Disorders, 2nd Edition, (2006). p 380–381, http://psychiatryonline.com/pracGuide/pracGuideHome.aspx

52

A 35-year-old patient with schizophrenia has had 4 serious suicide attempts over the past year despite consistent treatment with haloperidol decanoate. Given the patient's recent suicide attempts, what would be the BEST next medication trial?

(A) Olanzapine
(B) Quetiapine
(C) Fluphenazine decanoate
(D) Long-acting risperidone
(E) Clozapine

The correct response is option **E**: Clozapine

Clozapine has been shown to have the greatest therapeutic effect on suicidal behavior associated with schizophrenia, possibly reducing the suicide rate by as much as 75%–85%. For these reasons, clozapine should be preferentially considered for patients with schizophrenia who have a history of chronic and persistent suicidal ideation or behaviors.

Clozaril® package insert, Novartis Pharmaceuticals Corporation, East Hanover, NJ, 2005. http://www.pharma.us.novartis.com/product/pi/pdf/Clozaril.pdf.

American Psychiatric Association Practice Guideline for the Treatment of Patients with Schizophrenia, 2nd ed (2004). pp 576 http://www.psychiatryonline.com/pracGuide/pracGuideHome.aspx.

53

Cognitive behavioral therapy (CBT) is an effective, specific treatment for generalized anxiety disorder (GAD). Emerging evidence suggests that which ONE of the following is similarly effective in treatment for GAD?

(A) Dialectical behavioral therapy (DBT)
(B) Interpersonal psychotherapy (IPT)
(C) Psychoanalysis
(D) Short-term psychodynamic psychotherapy
(E) Supportive psychotherapy

The correct response is option **D**: Short-term psychodynamic psychotherapy

As Leichsenring et al. (2009) reports in their prospective, randomized study of 57 patients with generalized anxiety disorder (GAD), subjects were treated with cognitive behavioral therapy (CBT) or short-term psychodynamic psychotherapy (SPP). Both groups improved significantly in measures of anxiety and depression. However, CBT was more effective in reducing the level of worrying. CBT often targets worrying as a symptom.

Leichsenring F, Salzer S, Jaeger U, Kächele H, Kreische R, Leweke F, et al: Short-term psychodynamic psychotherapy and cognitive-behavioral therapy in generalized anxiety disorder: a randomized, controlled trial. Am J Psychiatry 2009; 166:875–881.

54

A 13-year old boy is seen for outbursts of aggression when he is denied access to food. He is known to be mentally retarded. His mother reports that as an infant he had poor muscle tone and a weak suck reflex. He is morbidly obese, short for his age and has significantly underdeveloped genitalia. His mother reports that he constantly eats to the point they have put locks on the kitchen cabinets and refrigerator. Despite this he will search for food in garbage cans. Lately, when he is denied food, he will have outbursts of anger in which he hits himself or others and throws objects. Which of the following BEST describes the genetic abnormality responsible for this boy's condition?

(A) Williams syndrome
(B) Angelman's syndrome
(C) Prader-Willi syndrome
(D) Klinefelter's syndrome
(E) Down syndrome

The correct response is option **C**: Prader-Willi

The patient's presentation is consistent with Prader–Willi syndrome. Prader–Willi syndrome represents an important genetic principle known as genomic imprinting. The majority of individuals have deletions of a segment of chromosome15. Prader–Willi syndrome emerges most frequently from deletions or absence of 15q12 from paternal origin.

Sadock BJ, Sadock VA (eds): Kaplan and Sadock's Comprehensive Textbook of Psychiatry, 9th ed. Philadelphia, Lippinicott Williams & Wilkins, 2009, p. 583.

55

Which of the following statements represents the most reasonable conclusion that can be drawn from the National Institute of Mental Health's (NIMH) Clinical Antipsychotic Trials of Intervention Effectiveness (CATIE) study?

(A) Second generation antipsychotics offer no benefit in schizophrenia over first generation antipsychotics.
(B) Clinicians should consider both first and second generation antipsychotics when treating schizophrenia.
(C) Antipsychotic medications appear to be less efficacious than previously thought.
(D) The second generation antipsychotics demonstrate little difference from one another.
(E) When given in idealized settings, most antipsychotics are roughly equivalent in efficacy.

The correct response is option **B**: Clinicians should consider both first and second generation antipsychotics when treating schizophrenia.

The CATIE study was designed to compare various antipsychotic medications in real-world treatment settings. The primary outcome concerned time until a switch in medication, thus it is not a study of efficacy. The finding that outcomes were similar for the first generation antipsychotic perphenazine and the second generation antipsychotics was unexpected; however, this does not imply that second generation antipsychotic medication may not have unique benefits. In some patients, individual differences were found in outcome and side effects between the different medications. The best conclusion that can be drawn from these data is that there are significant differences between the medications, and that patients may benefit from either first or second generation medications.

Lieberman JA, Hsiao JK: Interpreting the results of the CATIE study. Psychiatr Serv 2006 Jan;57(1):139

Ragins M: Should the CATIE study be a wake-up call? Psychiatric Services 56: 1489, 2005

Lieberman JA, Stroup TS, McEvoy JP, et al: Effectiveness of antipsychotic drugs in patients with chronic schizophrenia. New England Journal of Medicine 353:1209–1223, 2005

56

Post-stroke depression is most commonly associated with cerebrovascular disease involving the:

(A) anterior communicating artery.
(B) anterior cerebral artery.
(C) middle cerebral artery.
(D) posterior communicating artery.
(E) basilar artery.

The correct response is option **C**: Middle cerebral artery

Post-stroke depression is highly prevalent among elderly patients with hypertension and coronary artery disease. It often involves the vascular territory of the middle cerebral artery and is seen most commonly after left hemispheric stroke. The larger the size of the ischemic area, the more depression is refractory to standard treatment approaches.

Yudofsky SC, Hales RE (eds): The American Psychiatric Publishing Textbook of Neuropsychiatry and Behavioral Sciences, 5th ed. Washington DC: American Psychiatric Publishing Inc; 2008, pp 708–722

57

Which symptom of PTSD has been improved by medications that suppress noradrenergic activity?

(A) Hypervigilance
(B) Inability to recall an important aspect of the trauma
(C) Markedly diminished interest
(D) Feelings of detachment
(E) Avoidance of activities related to the trauma

The correct response is option **A**: Hypervigilance

Treatment with adrenergic-blocking agents, such as clonidine or propranolol, has been shown to decrease symptoms of hyperarousal and intrusive recollections.

Hales RE, Yudofsky SC, Gabbard GO (eds). The American Psychiatric Publishing Textbook of Psychiatry, 5th ed. Arlington, VA, American Psychiatric Publishing, Inc., 2008, p 577

Stein DJ, Hollander E. Textbook of Anxiety Disorders. Washington, DC. American Psychiatric Publishing, Inc., 2002. p 396–397.

Raskind MA, Peskind ER, Kanter ED, Petrie EC, Radant A, Thompson CE, Dobie DJ, Hoff D, Rein RJ, Straits-Tröster K, Thomas RG, McFall MM. Reduction of nightmares and other PTSD symptoms in combat veterans by prazosin: a placebo-controlled study. Am J Psychiatry. 2003 Feb;160(2):371–3.

A 19-year-old college student comes to the clinic with a complaint of feeling "depressed and worried." He states that he may fail his English class because he is nervous about the public speaking assignment. When he thinks about it, he feels nervous, his heart races, his palms become sweaty, and he becomes short of breath. He endorses a depressed mood because "I feel like I'm wasting my parents' money." He skipped his last three English classes because he knew it would be his turn to give a speech. He attends his other classes with no difficulty. The most likely diagnosis is:

(A) panic disorder.
(B) normal shyness.
(C) social phobia.
(D) agoraphobia.
(E) major depressive disorder.

The correct response is option **C**: Social phobia

Panic disorder is unlikely, as the symptoms are limited to the specific situation of the speech. This is more than normal shyness as it is significantly interfering with occupational functioning. It is not agoraphobia because he has no difficulty going to his other classes. His depressive mood is limited to thinking about the current situation, and he shows no other symptoms of depression.

Sadock BJ, Sadock VA, eds: Kaplan & Sadock's Synopsis of Psychiatry, 9th ed. Philadelphia, Lippincott Williams & Wilkins, 2003, p 614.

Diagnostic and Statistical Manual of Mental Disorders, Fourth Edition, Text Revision (DSM-IV-TR). Washington, DC, American Psychiatric Association, 2000, pp 454.

A 47-year-old woman is brought for a psychiatric evaluation to assess recent changes in her behavior. Over the past six months, she has become increasingly disinhibited and impulsive in her behavior. Physical examination reveals mild dysarthria, dysphagia, and drooling. Slit lamp examination of the eyes indicates the presence of Kayser-Fleischer rings. Which of the following BEST describes the genetic basis for her illness?

(A) Autosomal recessive
(B) Co-dominant
(C) Mitochondrial
(D) Polygenetic
(E) X-linked dominant

The correct response is option **A**: Autosomal recessive

The patient's presentation is consistent with Wilson's disease. Wilson's disease is an autosomal recessive disorder caused by mutations in a copper transporting ATPase encoded by the *ATP7B* gene on chromosome 13. A characteristic feature is Kayser-Fleischer rings due to copper deposition in the outer ring of the cornea. The most common reasons for psychiatric referral are behavioral and personality changes, with disinhibition, bizarre or impulsive behavior being present in about a quarter of patients.

Sadock BJ, Sadock VA (eds): Kaplan and Sadock's Comprehensive Textbook of Psychiatry, 9th ed. Philadelphia, Lippincott Williams & Wilkins, 2009, p. 605.

Smoller JW, Sheidley BR, Tsuang MT. Psychiatric Genetics: Applications in Clinical Practice. American Psychiatric Publishing, Inc.; 1st edition, 2008, p. 212.

60

A patient unconsciously perceives the therapist as having attributes associated with unpleasant interactions in the past. However, the therapist does not respond like the figure from the past, and over time, the old feelings become muted and the patient no longer needs to replay new relationships according to the old emotional script. Which of the following terms define this positive change in psychotherapy?

(A) Exposure and response prevention
(B) Corrective emotional experience
(C) Re-enactment of transference
(D) Shaping
(E) Strengthening ego defenses

The correct response is option **B**: Corrective emotional experience

The term *corrective emotional experience* was introduced by Alexander and French as the fundamental therapeutic principle of all psychotherapy. In their definition, the term implies "to re-expose the patient, under more favorable circumstances, to emotional situations which he could not handle in the past. The patient, in order to be helped, must undergo a corrective emotional experience suitable to repair the traumatic influence of previous experiences." Such experiences may occur at any point of the continuum of psychotherapy.

Winston A, Rosenthal RN, Pinsker H: Introduction to Supportive Psychotherapy (Core Competencies in Psychotherapy), 1st ed.. Washington DC, American Psychiatric Publishing Inc, 2004, p 19
Textbook of Psychotherapeutic Treatments. Gabbard GO (ed). Arlington VA, American Psychiatric Publishing Inc, 2009, p 401

61

Which of the following is a risk factor for the development of psychosis while using cocaine?

(A) Being female
(B) A greater duration of use during an episode
(C) Non-intravenous use
(D) An elevated body mass index
(E) Being a first time user of cocaine

The correct response is option **B**: A greater duration of use during an episode

Those who develop psychosis with cocaine are likely to be men, have a greater duration and amount of use, and have a lower body mass index. Intravenous abusers have more paranoia and hallucinations than non-intravenous abusers, and users are sensitized so that psychosis becomes more severe and occurs more rapidly with repeated cocaine use.

Thirthalli J, Benegal V. Psychosis among substance users. Curr Opin Psychiatry. 2006 May;19(3):239–45.

62

A 38-year-old man presents for treatment of PTSD after surviving a bridge collapse. He was driving on the crowded bridge when it suddenly collapsed, killing over 50 individuals and seriously injuring more. As part of the treatment, the therapist asks the patient to imagine that he is safely driving over a bridge. Which of the following best describes this therapeutic intervention?

(A) Aversion therapy
(B) Dialectical behavioral therapy
(C) Exposure therapy
(D) Insight-oriented psychotherapy
(E) Interpersonal therapy

The correct response is option **C**: Exposure therapy

Studies of exposure therapy have found that a key to therapeutic success is to interrupt the posttraumatic stimulus generalization that links harmless images, people, and things to dangerous stimuli associated with the original traumatic threat. This is done through both imagined exposure and real-world, in-vivo exposures in ways that re-link those images, people, and events with safety. Dialectical behavior therapy is used to treat borderline personality disorder, and has not been studied in the area of traumatic stress.

Hobfoll SE, Watson P, Bell CC, Bryant RA, Brymer MJ, Friedman MJ, Friedman M, Gersons BP, de Jong JT, Layne CM, Maguen S, Neria Y, Norwood AE, Pynoos RS, Reissman D, Ruzek JI, Shalev AY, Solomon Z, Steinberg AM, Ursano RJ: Five essential elements of immediate and mid-term mass trauma intervention: empirical evidence. Psychiatry. 2007; 70(4):283–315. Reprinted in FOCUS. 2009; 2:221–242

63

Which of the following characteristics is/are present in patients with locked-in syndrome?

(A) Persistent vegetative state
(B) Ability to experience a range of feelings
(C) Inability to recognize objects and people
(D) Severe depression and desire to die

The correct response is option **B**: Ability to experience a range of feelings

It is important to appreciate that locked-in syndrome has very different clinical and ethical implications than a persistent vegetative state. Locked-in syndrome is typically caused by an injury to the brain stem (e.g. infarct, trauma, hemorrhage). Patients retain full consciousness and can recognize objects and people. The fact that the patient is conscious, however, is unrecognizable to everybody except the person concerned, and except perhaps to those particularly attuned to the patient. A patient in locked-in syndrome cannot interact with others because he or she has lost control of the body except, perhaps, the ability to move the eyes up or down. Patients experience a range of feelings, especially tremendous frustration at being unable to convey feelings, and loneliness. In a persistent vegetative state, however, patients do not retain consciousness. It is important to realize that despite profound disabilities, a patient in a locked-in state does not necessarily want to die. Early goals of management include establishing effective lines of communications.

Smith E, Delargy M. Locked-in syndrome. BMJ 2005; 331:406–409.

Chisholm N, Gillett G. The patient's journey: living with locked-in syndrome. BMJ 2005; 331:94–97.

64

Which of the following interventions has been empirically validated through controlled and randomized trials as effective specifically for adolescents with conduct disorder?

(A) Dialectical behavioral therapy
(B) Cognitive behavioral therapy
(C) Interpersonal therapy
(D) Multisystemic therapy
(E) Psychoeducational therapy

The correct response is option **D**: Multisystemic therapy

The goal of multisystemic therapy is to empower parents with skills and resources and to empower their teenage children with conduct disorder to cope with a variety of problems. Dialectical behavioral therapy is useful for borderline personality disorder. Interpersonal therapy is often used for depression. Cognitive behavioral and psychoeducational therapy are used for a wide range of diagnoses.

Martin A, Volkmar FR (eds): Lewis's Child and Adolescent Psychiatry, 4th ed. Philadelphia, Lippincott Williams & Wilkins, pp 859–860, 2007

65

Which of the following is the mechanism of action of memantine, a medication used to slow cognitive decline in Alzheimer's dementia?

(A) Cholinesterase inhibitor
(B) Dopamine receptor blocker
(C) Serotonergic reuptake inhibitor
(D) NMDA receptor antagonist
(E) GABA mimetic

The correct response is option **D**: NMDA receptor antagonist

Memantine is an NMDA antagonist that blocks glutamate-medicated excitotoxicity. It is used in moderate to severe Alzheimer's dementia. The initial dose is 5 mg/day, which is increased in 5-mg/day increments over 4 weeks to the final dose of 10 mg twice per day. Side effects include dizziness, headache, constipation, falls, and confusion. It may be effective in reducing caregiver distress, and it may help delay institutionalization.

Spar JE, La Rue A (eds): Clinical Manual of Geriatric Psychiatry, 1st ed. Washington, DC: American Psychiatric Publishing Inc; 2006. p. 213–214

Meeks TW, Lanouette N, Vahia I, Dawes S, Jeste DV, Lebowitz B. Psychiatric assessment and diagnosis in older adults. FOCUS. 2009 winter; 7(1):3–13

Which of the following genetic syndromes is caused by a 22q deletion and is clinically manifested by learning disabilities, palatal anomalies, cardiac defects and often schizophrenia?

  (A) Fragile X syndrome
  (B) Velocardiofacial syndrome
  (C) Down syndrome
  (D) Cri du chat syndrome
  (E) Angelman syndrome

The correct response is option **B**: Velocardiofacial (DiGeorge) syndrome

Velocardiofacial syndrome, also known as 2q11.2 deletion syndrome and DiGeorge syndrome, is caused by a large deletion from chromosome 22, produced by an error in recombination at meiosis. It is clinically manifested by learning disabilities, palatal anomalies, cardiac defects and often schizophrenia.

Jolin EM, Weller RA, Weller EB. Psychosis in children with velocardiofacial syndrome (22q11.2 deletion syndrome). Curr Psychiatry Rep. 2009 Apr;11(2):99–105.

DiGeorge Syndrome. http://ghr.nlm.nih.gov/condition=22q112deletionsyndrome

Smoller JW, Sheidley BR, Tsuang MT. Psychiatric Genetics: Applications in Clinical Practice. American Psychiatric Publishing, Inc.; 1st edition, 2008, pp. 200–212.

Which of the following refers to an ethical decision making approach that involves referring to similar, prior cases including legal precedents and applying reasoning from these cases to the case at hand?

  (A) Casuistry
  (B) Ethical principles
  (C) Expert opinion
  (D) General ethical theory
  (E) Tradition and current practice standards

The correct response is option **A**: Casuistry

Casuistry refers to an appeal to relevantly similar cases including legal precedents and the application of the reasoning about these cases to the case at hand. Ethical principles include respect for autonomy and beneficence. General ethical theory refers to consequentialism (the justification of a course of action is grounded on whether consequences of the right sort result from it) and deontological approaches (the justification of a course of action is grounded in considerations other than consequences). The quality of current practice standards in ethics are judged by the ethical analysis and argument that support them.

DeGrazia D, Beauchamp TL. Philosophy, in Methods in Medical Ethics. Edited by Sugarmen J, Sulmasy DP. Washington D.C., Georgetown University Press; 2001, pp 31–46.

Roberts LW, Dyer AR. Concise Guide to Ethics in Mental Health Care. American Psychiatric Publishing Inc., Washington D.C., 2004 p 11.

68

A 38-year-old woman with treatment resistant schizophrenia is prescribed clozapine. Two weeks after beginning the medication, the woman begins to experience episodes of tachycardia with a heart rate over 120 beats per minute. Electrocardiogram reveals sustained sinus tachycardia with non-specific ST-T wave changes and T-wave flattening while standing and supine. Which of the following medications is most likely to alleviate her tachycardia without increasing chances of a serious adverse effect?

(A) Atenolol
(B) Fludrocortisone
(C) Propranolol
(D) Verapamil

The correct response is option **A**: Atenolol

The cardiovascular side effects most frequently observed with clozapine are tachycardia and postural hypotension. The tachycardia is probably a direct effect of the vagolytic properties of the drug. It can present in the supine position and is thus not the result of orthostatic changes. Therefore, administration of fludrocortisone would not be beneficial. The patient would best benefit from a beta blocker. Propranolol should not be prescribed because it may increase the risk of agranulocytosis. Verapamil would be indicated for supraventricular tachycardia.

Sadock BJ, Sadock VA (eds): Kaplan and Sadock's Comprehensive Textbook of Psychiatry, 9th ed. Philadelphia, Lippincott Williams & Wilkins, 2009, pp. 3071, 3211

69

The course of dementia in individuals with 16 or more years of education differs from those with lower educational attainment in which way?

(A) Lower cognitive reserve
(B) Ability to maintain higher levels of cognitive functioning in early dementia
(C) Lower levels of cognitive function in early dementia
(D) Less disease burden when dementia is diagnosed
(E) Gentler slope of decline after dementia is diagnosed

The correct response is option **B**: Ability to maintain higher levels of cognitive functioning in early dementia

The most commonly used screening tool for measuring cognitive function is the Mini-Mental State Examination (MMSE). A score of ≤ 24 out of 30 is the usual cut point for detecting dementia. For highly educated individuals, defined as having 16 or more years of education, a score of ≤ 27 has been shown to have optimal sensitivity and specificity for pursuing a more extensive dementia workup. More highly educated individuals have a higher cognitive reserve and a greater ability to maintain cognitive function in the face of neurological insults. They function at a higher cognitive level early in dementia, show a greater disease burden before dementia is diagnosed, and show a steeper slope of cognitive decline and swifter mortality once dementia is finally diagnosed.

O'Bryant SE, Humphreys JD, Smith GE, Ivnik RJ, Graff-Radford NR, Petersen RC, Lucas JA. Detecting dementia with the Mini-Mental State Examination in highly educated individuals. Arch Neurol. 2008; 65:963–967

70

A 34-year-old woman with bipolar disorder has a body mass index of 31.2. To minimize the risk of aggravating this factor, which of the following medications would be most appropriate?

(A) Lithium
(B) Clozapine
(C) Lamotrigine
(D) Olanzapine
(E) Divalproex

The correct response is option **C**: Lamotrigine

Lamotrigine is a weight-neutral medication, while all of the others are associated with weight gain as a side effect. Weight neutrality does not exclude the possibility of weight gain in individual patients, but it reduces the likelihood considerably.

Bowden CL, Calabrese JR, Ketter TA, Sachs GS, White RL, Thompson TR: Impact of lamotrigine and lithium on weight in obese and nonobese patients with bipolar I disorder. Am J Psychiatry 2006; 163:1199–1201.

Merideth CH: A single-center, double-blind, placebo-controlled evaluation of lamotrigine in the treatment of obesity in adults. J Clin Psychiatry 2006; 258–262.

Taylor V, MacQueen G: Associations between bipolar disorder and metabolic syndrome: a review. J Clin Psychiatry 2006; 67:1034–1041.

71

According to the ethics primer of the American Psychiatric Association, which one of the following scenarios would most likely be considered a violation of the psychotherapeutic frame?

(A) A patient is late to his psychotherapy session due to an upcoming deadline at work, but the therapist still charges the full amount for the session.
(B) The therapist loses his office keys, but lives across the street. Rather than cancel his patients, he asks his wife and children to stay out for the day and sets up a temporary office in his living room.
(C) A patient does not bring his check book to his final session of the month, when payment is due. The therapist interprets this act as an expression of ambivalence about the treatment, and suggests this to the patient.
(D) The therapist is diagnosed with end-stage cancer, and informs his patient that due to serious illness, he will be terminating his practice over the next month.
(E) A grateful former patient wishes to donate money to the hospital with which his therapist is affiliated. Not wanting to handle the transaction himself, the therapist refers the patient to the hospital's development office.

The correct response is option **B**: The therapist loses his office keys, but lives across the street. Rather than cancel his patients, he asks his wife and children to stay out for the day and sets up a temporary office in his living room.

The Ethics Primer of the American Psychiatric Association states that psychotherapy necessarily takes place within a frame, which consists of mutually agreed upon constants of the relationship, as well as human elements of the therapeutic situation. Standard fees and billing practices are one of the mutually agreed upon constants, as is the location of the sessions. Changing the location from the office to the home would be a clear violation of this aspect of the frame, as well as many others including the therapist's relative anonymity. Efforts to understand all aspects of the therapist-patient relationship are included among the human elements that comprise the therapeutic situation. Finally, while accepting large gifts is typically viewed as exploiting of patients, the Ethics Primer specifically states that unsolicited institutional donations from former patients should be directed toward third parties uninvolved in the psychotherapy.

Gruenberg P: Boundary Violations, in Ethics Primer of the American Psychiatric Association. Washington DC, American Psychiatric Association, 2001. http://www.psych.org/Departments/EDU/residentmit/ethicsprimer.aspx

72

Genetic linkage analysis studies provide information about which one of the following aspects of a gene:

(A) Post-transitional processing
(B) Location
(C) Function
(D) Endophenotype
(E) Population frequency

The correct response is option **B**: Location

Linkage analysis is a method of positional cloning, and relies on the fact that when DNA segments or loci are near each other on a chromosome, they tend to be inherited together. Thus, it is an indirect method of tracking an unknown gene. It can be done without any knowledge of the nature of the gene itself, or of the mechanism by which the gene might influence a particular disorder.

Burmeister M. Genetics of psychiatric disorders: a primer. FOCUS 2006;4:317–326

73

A 17-year-old man is brought to the emergency department after fighting with his girlfriend and ingesting a bottle of alprazolam. En route to the hospital, the girlfriend lost control of the car causing the patient to hit his head against the windshield with loss of consciousness. Examination reveals the patient to be in stupor, with respiratory depression and coma. He has a 4 cm laceration over the right frontal area which is profusely bleeding. Which of the facts of the patient's presentation represents the greatest contraindication to the use of flumazenil?

(A) Age of patient
(B) CNS depression
(C) Benzodiazepine use
(D) Possible traumatic brain injury

The correct response is option **D**: Possible traumatic brain injury

The characteristic of the patient that represents the greatest contraindication to the use of flumazenil is the possible traumatic brain injury. Flumazenil can affect cerebral hemodynamics and is not recommended for situations in which intracranial pressure may already be increased, such as in head injury. Flumazenil should be administered carefully to benzodiazepine-dependent patients and patients who have ingested mixed substances to avoid the production of withdrawal seizures. None of the other characteristics of the patient represent contraindications.

Hales RE, Yudofsky SC: Substance use disorders in, The American Psychiatric Publishing Textbook of clinical psychiatry. Washington DC, American Psychiatric Publishing, 2003, pp 343–4.

74

A 42-year-old man is started on pharmacotherapy for treatment of major depressive disorder. Two weeks later he presents with complaints of dry mouth, impaired ability to focus at close range, constipation, urinary hesitation, tachycardia, and sexual dysfunction. Which of the following medications is most likely to have caused this presentation?

(A) Duloxetine
(B) Fluoxetine
(C) Imipramine
(D) Mirtazapine
(E) Venlafaxine

The correct response is option **C**: Imipramine

Imipramine is a tertiary amine tricyclic antidepressant. These medications block muscarinic receptors, producing anticholinergic effects such as the symptoms that the patient is describing. All tricyclic antidepressants have some degree of anticholinergic action. The other medications listed have much less anticholinergic activity and therefore are more widely used now. This difference in side effects improves patient compliance with taking the medicine.

Schatzberg AF, Nemeroff CB (eds). Essentials of Clinical Psychopharmacology, 2nd ed. Arlington, VA, American Psychiatric Publishing Inc., 2006. p 19

75

Which of the following medications has been the only one to demonstrate a decrease in suicide risk?

(A) Valproic acid
(B) Lithium
(C) Carbamazepine
(D) Lamotrigine
(E) Gabapentin

The correct response is option **B**: Lithium

Initial studies as well as a meta-analysis have demonstrated that lithium decreases suicide, and that abrupt discontinuation increases suicide. A meta-analysis of 31 studies of major affective disorders found a fivefold reduction in suicides and attempted suicides during lithium treatment compared to those not taking the drug. Other studies suggest that the antisuicidal effect of lithium extends beyond its mood stabilizing property.

Kessing LV et al: Suicide risk in patients treated with lithium. Arch Gen Psychiatry 2005; 62:860–866
Sadock BJ, Sadock VA: Kaplan & Sadock's Comprehensive Textbook of Psychiatry, 9th ed. Philadelphia, Lippincott Williams & Wilkins, 2009, p 3135
American Psychiatric Association: Practice Guideline for the Assessment and Treatment of Patients with Suicidal Behaviors. 2003. http://psychiatryonline.com/pracGuide/pracGuideHome.aspx

76

A 34 year-old woman, who has been treated with an antidepressant for the past month, complains that she no longer gets relief from her back pain when she takes codeine which has been prescribed by her orthopedist. Which one of the following antidepressants would be most likely to produce such an effect?

(A) Escitalopram
(B) Sertraline
(C) Paroxetine
(D) Mirtazapine
(E) Buproprion

The correct response is option **C**: Paroxetine

Paroxetine is a potent inhibitor of CYP2D6. The analgesic effect of codeine depends on it being metabolized by cytochrome P450 2D6 (CYP2D6) to its active metabolite morphine. The other antidepressant medications in this example are not potent inhibitors of the CYP2D6 system.

Sindrup SH, Brosen K: The pharmacogenetics of codeine hypoalgesia. Pharmacogenetics 1995; 5:335–346

Mannheimer B, Wettermark B, Lundberg M, Pettersson H, von Bahr C, Eliasson E: Nationwide drug-dispensing data reveal important differences in adherence to drug label recommendations on CYP2D6-dependent drug interactions. Br J Clin Pharmacol 2010 Apr; 69(4):411–7

77

Children of European descent with an early history of abuse have been found to be more likely to develop subsequent depression when they have a genetic polymorphism of which of the following neurotransmitter transporters?

(A) Norepinephrine
(B) Dopamine
(C) Serotonin
(D) Glutamate
(E) GABA

The correct response is option **C**: Serotonin

In studies replicated in children, adolescents and young adults with a history of abuse, those with a short allele of 5-HTTLPR, the serotonin transporter, exhibited more depression than those with a long allele.

Kendler KS, Kuhn JW, Vittum J, Prescott CA, Riley B. The interaction of stressful life events and a serotonin transporter polymorphism in the prediction of episodes of major depression: a replication. Arch Gen Psychiatry 2005;62:529–35.

78

A 45-year-old woman was a witness to a motor vehicle accident that resulted in a number of fatalities. The images and the sounds of the accident greatly distressed her. The day after the accident she was seen by her family physician. The most appropriate next treatment step is:

(A) education and support about possible reactions that may occur
(B) immediate referral to a mental health treatment program
(C) treatment with an antidepressant
(D) benzodiazepines as needed for sleep
(E) critical incident debriefing

The correct response is option **A**: Education and support about possible reactions that may occur

It is important not to pathologize all emotional responses to disaster. The initial response may represent what has been called "a normal response to an abnormal situation." Education about the normal course following a traumatic event and support are the most useful first step in addressing a patient's concerns after a trauma.

Disaster Psychiatry Handbook, American Psychiatric Association Committee on Psychiatric Dimensions of Disaster, 2004, pp. 21–22 http://www.psych.org/Resources/DisasterPsychiatry/APADisasterPsychiatryResources/DisasterPsychiatryHandbook.aspx

American Psychiatric Association Practice Guideline for the Treatment of Patients with Acute Stress Disorder and Posttraumatic Stress Disorder. Am J Psychiatry. 2004. p. 11 http://www.psychiatryonline.com/pracGuide/pracGuideTopic_11.aspx

79

A 48-year-old man with depression has been resistant to treatment with a variety of antidepressants. The decision is made to try him on a monoamine oxidase inhibitor. In order to avoid serotonin syndrome, a washout period of at least five weeks is MOST indicated if he has been taking which antidepressant?

(A) Bupropion
(B) Clomipramine
(C) Fluoxetine
(D) Paroxetine
(E) Venlafaxine

The correct response is option **C**: Fluoxetine

MAOIs must not be prescribed with serotoninergic medications to avoid serotonin syndrome. Because of the shorter half-life of clomipramine, paroxetine, and venlafaxine, a MAOI may be started two weeks after washout. The same applies to bupropion as it does not have serotonergic properties. However, due to the longer half-life of fluoxetine, MAOIs must not be administered for 5 weeks after discontinuation.

Pocket Handbook of Clinical Psychiatry, 4th ed, Sadock BA and Sadock VA, Lippinicott, Williams and Wilkins, 2005. p 161

80

Which of the following medications used to treat excessive daytime sleepiness associated with narcolepsy has also been abused as a "date-rape" drug?

(A) Sodium oxybate
(B) Modafinil
(C) Methylphenidate
(D) Selegiline
(E) Dextroamphetamine

The correct response is option **A**: Sodium oxybate

Sodium oxybate or gamma-hydroxybutyrate is FDA-approved for treating excessive daytime sleepiness and cataplexy in patients with narcolepsy. It had been banned in the U.S. in 1990 and listed as a Schedule I drug because of its abuse potential and use to facilitate sexual assaults. Because of its value in treating narcolepsy, it is now listed as a Schedule III drug when used medically, and its distribution is under strict control.

Robinson DM, Keating GM. Sodium oxybate: a review of its use in the management of narcolepsy. CNS Drugs. 2007; 21:350–352
Drasbek KR, Christensen J, Jensen K. Gamma-hydroxybutyrate – a drug of abuse. Acta Neurol Scand. 2006; 114:145

81

A patient recounts a story about getting angry with a store clerk. The therapist asks a factual question about the circumstance, inspiring rage in the patient, who finds him to be uncaring and seeking to blame her. The therapist says, "I wonder if what you're feeling right now is just like the feeling you had in the store, when you attributed the same uncaring attitude toward the clerk. These kinds of misreadings seem to make you very upset in many different settings." Which of the following most accurately describes this type of intervention?

(A) Genetic interpretation
(B) Transference interpretation
(C) Clarification
(D) Observation
(E) Empathic validation

The correct response is option **B**: Transference interpretation

This is a paraphrasing of a vignette example of a transference interpretation that appeared in an article by Gabbard and Horowitz in the American Journal of Psychiatry, March 2009. In a transference interpretation, the therapist points out how a patient's early relational pattern, which recurs in many domains of the patient's life, is repeating itself in the "here and now" between therapist and patient. Clarification refers to the process of helping a patient specify vague issues. In a genetic interpretation, the therapist draws a link between present occurrences and a patient's early family relationships. When a therapist strives to put himself in the patient's position and states how that must feel, he performs an empathic validation. Although the therapist is technically making an observation about the patient, "observation" in psychotherapy is different from interpretation in that it does not explain or link behaviors.

Gabbard GO, Horowitz MJ: Insight, transference interpretation, and therapeutic change in the dynamic psychotherapy of borderline personality disorder. Am J Psychiatry 2009; 166: p 517
Gabbard GO: Long-Term Psychodynamic Psychotherapy: A Basic Text. Washington DC, American Psychiatric Publishing Inc, 2004, pp 59–77

82

Consideration of genotyping for human leukocyte antigen allele HLA-B 1502 has been recommended by the FDA prior to starting carbamazepine on patients with which of the following ancestries?

(A) European
(B) African
(C) Asian
(D) Hispanic
(E) Native American

The correct response is option **C**: Asian.

According to the FDA, "the risk of Stevens Johnson syndrome (SJS)/toxic epidermal necrolysis (TEN) from carbamazepine is significantly increased in patients positive for the HLA-B*1502 allele. This allele is found almost exclusively in patients with ancestry across broad areas of Asia, including South Asian Indians. Due to wide variability in rates of HLA-B*1502 even within ethnic groups, the difficulty in ascertaining ethnic ancestry, and the likelihood of mixed ancestry, screening for HLA-B*1502 should be performed for most patients of Asian ancestry. Prevalence of HLA-B*1502 has not been studied in many regions of Asia. The following figures must therefore be considered no more than a rough guide in deciding which patients to screen:

- 10–15% or more of patients may carry the allele in parts of China, Thailand, Malaysia, Indonesia, the Philippines, and Taiwan.
- South Asians, including Indians, appear to have intermediate prevalence of HLA-B 1502, averaging 2 to 4%, but higher in some groups.
- HLA-B 1502 appears to be present at a low frequency, <1%, in Japan and Korea.

While testing negative for HLA-B*1502 allele is associated with a lower risk of such reactions, the risk is not reduced to zero."

FDA U.S. Food and Drug administration [Internet]:

http://www.fda.gov/Drugs/DrugSafety/PostmarketDrugSafetyInformationforPatientsandProviders/ucm124718.htm

Ferrel PB, Jr. and McLeod HL: Carbamazepine, *HLA-B*1502* and risk of Stevens-Johnson syndrome and toxic epidermal necrolysis: US FDA recommendations. Pharmacogenetics 2008; 9:1543–1546.

83

An 84-year-old woman with a history of Alzheimer's disease presents to an emergency department after a fall. She had been experiencing difficulty sleeping at night for several months and was increasingly combative and suspicious of her daughter, with whom she lived. In developing a plan of treatment for this patient, which of the following principles is most appropriate to incorporate?

(A) Adjust doses of medication slowly with long intervals between dose increments
(B) Prescribe small doses of several different medications rather than using one medication
(C) Use a long-acting injectable medication to aid adherence
(D) Use an initial loading dose of medication to speed response

The correct response is option **A**: Adjust doses of medication slowly with long intervals between dose increments

Individuals with dementia may be more sensitive to adverse effects such as anticholinergic effects, orthostasis, sedation and Parkinsonism because of alterations in absorption, distribution metabolism and/or elimination of medications. Consequently smaller initial doses, smaller increments in dose, and long periods of time between dose changes are recommended. The use of more than one medication, although sometimes unavoidable, may further influence the pharmacokinetics of many medications and obscure causes of adverse effects if they appear. Although long-acting injectable medications can aid adherence, the potential for long-lasting adverse effects would be problematic in an older patient with dementia.

American Psychiatric Association Practice Guideline for the Treatment of Patients with Alzheimer's disease and Other Dementias, 2nd ed. 2007 p. 12 http://www.psychiatryonline.com/pracGuide/pracGuideTopic_3.aspx

84

A 28-year-old woman with bipolar I disorder is pregnant for the first time. Throughout the pregnancy, she has been maintained on a mood stabilizer. At the time of birth, the baby is noted to have a cardiovascular defect consistent with Ebstein's anomaly. The mood stabilizer the woman was taking was most likely:

(A) Carbamazepine
(B) Haloperidol
(C) Lithium
(D) Lorazepam
(E) Valproate

The correct response is option **C**: Lithium

First-trimester exposure to lithium, valproate, or carbamazepine is associated with greater risk of birth defects. With lithium exposure, the relative risk for Ebstein's anomaly, a cardiovascular defect, is 10–20 times greater than the risk in the general population, although the absolute risk is low at about 1–2 per 1000 births. Exposure to carbamazepine and valproate during the first trimester is associated with neural tube defects and craniofacial abnormalities. High-potency antipsychotic medications are preferred in the treatment of psychotic symptoms during pregnancy because they are less likely to have associated anticholinergic, antihistaminergic, or hypotensive effects. In general, teratogenic effects with benzodiazepines are likely to be small.

American Psychiatric Association Practice Guideline for the Treatment of Patients with Bipolar Disorder, 2nd ed (2002). Reprinted in FOCUS: Bipolar Disorder, Winter 2003; 1:75.

85

According to simple Mendelian inheritance, if a disease gene is recessive, what is the likelihood of developing the disease if one parent has two dominant genes and the other two recessive genes?

(A) 0%
(B) 25%
(C) 50%
(D) 75%
(E) 100%

The correct response is option **A**: 0%

Because the disease will only occur in the absence of a dominant gene, two recessive genes will be necessary for the condition to appear. Therefore, the children will not be at risk for developing the disease, but they will be carriers.

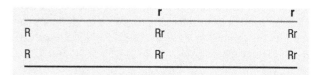

	r	r
R	Rr	Rr
R	Rr	Rr

Sadock BJ, Sadock VA (eds): Kaplan & Sadock's Comprehensive Textbook of Psychiatry, 9th ed. Philadelphia, Lippincott Williams & Wilkins, 2009, pp 301–302

Smoller JW, Sheidley BR, Tsuang MT. Psychiatric Genetics: Applications in Clinical Practice. American Psychiatric Publishing, Inc.; 1st edition, 2008, p. 196.

86

Which of the following is the medication most often associated with an increased risk of falls in persons age 80 or older?

(A) Antihypertensives
(B) Benzodiazepines
(C) Antidepressants
(D) Histamine H1 receptor antagonists
(E) Atypical antipsychotics

The correct response is option **B**: Benzodiazepines

In patients 80 years or older, it is estimated that at least one third of injurious falls (falls associated with hospitalization, fracture, head trauma or death) are related to the use of benzodiazepines. Approximately 10% of the falls in this age group are fatal.

Pariente A, Dartigues JF, Benichou J, Letenneur L, Moore N, Fourrier-Réglat A. Benzodiazepines and injurious falls in community dwelling elders. Drugs Aging. 2008; 25(1):61–70

Patients who are being treated with exposure therapy for anxiety disorders are:

(A) encouraged to think about non-threatening situations during the treatment.
(B) encouraged to focus on their fears and allow feelings of anxiety to occur.
(C) required to conduct the therapy in real life or fully realistic situations.
(D) required to develop a protocol and start with the most feared stimulus first.
(E) required to be on an appropriate type and dose of anti-anxiety medication.

The correct response is option **B**: encouraged to focus on their fears and allow feelings of anxiety to occur

For exposure therapy to be effective, the patient must pay attention fully to the details of the experience and allow the feelings of anxiety and arousal to occur. Exposure is designed to help the patient confront their fears while staying psychologically engaged, allowing the processes involved in fear reduction (habituation and extinction) to occur. Generally, patients start with the least feared situations. Exposure can occur using imagination, role-play, virtual reality or in real life situations. Thinking about other things can interfere with the process and medication is not a required component of the treatment.

Scheier FR, Luterek JA, Heimberg RG, Leonardo E: Social phobia, in Clinical Manual of Anxiety Disorders. Edited by DJ Stein. Washington, DC. American Psychiatric Publishing Inc, 2004, p 77.

What were the findings of the Treatment for Adolescents with Depression Study (TADS), with regard to efficacy of treatment?

(A) Fluoxetine alone was most effective.
(B) Cognitive behavioral therapy alone was most effective.
(C) Fluoxetine plus cognitive behavioral therapy was most effective.
(D) Interpersonal therapy alone was most effective.
(E) Fluoxetine plus interpersonal therapy was most effective.

The correct response is option **C**: Fluoxetine plus cognitive behavioral therapy was most effective.

The Treatment of Adolescents with Depression Study (TADS) evaluated and compared the efficacy of four treatment approaches: Combined CBT-fluoxetine, fluoxetine alone, CBT alone and placebo. The results of the study indicated that 71% of adolescents improved with the combined treatment, 60.6% improved with fluoxetine alone, 43.2% improved with CBT alone while 34.8% showed improvement with placebo. Interpersonal therapy was not evaluated in this study.

March JS, Silva S, Petrycki S, Curry J, Wells K, Fairbank J, Burns B, Domino M, McNulty S, Vitiello B, Severe J, Treatment for Adolescents with Depression Study (TADS) team. Fluoxetine, cognitive-behavioral therapy, and their combination for adolescents with depression: Treatment for Adolescents with Depression Study (TADS) randomized controlled trial. Journal of the American Medical Association. 2004 Aug 18; 292(7):807–820

AACAP practice parameter for the assessment and treatment of children and adolescents with depressive disorders. J Am Acad Child Adolesc Psychiatry. 2007. FOCUS: Child and Adolescent Psychiatry. Summer 2008; 6(3):387–8

Emslie GJ, Kennard BD, Mayes TL, Nightingale-Teresi J, Carmody T, Hughes CW, Rush AJ, Tao R, Rintelmann JW. Fluoxetine versus placebo in preventing relapse of major depression in children and adolescents. FOCUS: Child and Adolescent Psychiatry. Summer 2008; 6(3):356

A 76-year-old woman with a long history of generalized anxiety disorder presents to a psychiatrist. She is interested in the possibility of pharmacotherapy for this disorder. She has a history of hypertension, for which she takes amlodipine, but otherwise is in good health. The most accurate advice regarding the use of pharmacotherapy for this patient is that medications are:

(A) generally not effective in treating anxiety in elderly patients.
(B) contraindicated due to the increased side effects in older adults.
(C) less effective than psychotherapy for anxiety in older adults.
(D) not recommended due to the high potential for drug-drug interactions.
(E) a first line treatment for anxiety in the elderly.

The correct response is option **E**: A first line treatment for anxiety in the elderly

The same treatments that are effective for anxiety in younger persons are also effective in the elderly. Although both pharmacotherapy and behavioral interventions are reasonably effective, the weight of evidence suggests that there are higher average treatment effects with pharmacological interventions. Although side effects, drug interactions, and patient preferences should be taken into account, in most elderly patients pharmacotherapy is likely to be the first-line treatment recommendation for anxiety disorders. With regard to generalized anxiety disorder, the reference (Pinquart 2007) evaluated 6 medication studies and 8 behavioral studies.

Pinquart M, Duberstein PR. Treatment of anxiety disorders in older adults: a meta-analytic comparison of behavioral and pharmacological interventions. Am J Geriatr Psychiatry. 2007; 15(8):639–651

You are treating a 16-year-old patient for ADHD who has multiple café au lait spots visible on both arms and legs. A diagnosis of neurofibromatosis is made by a neurology consultant. Which one of the following modes of genetic transmission is seen in this illness?

(A) Autosomal dominant
(B) Autosomal recessive
(C) Non-Mendelian inheritance
(D) X-linked recessive
(E) X-linked dominant

The correct response is option **A**: Autosomal dominant

Neurofibromatosis type I is characterized by café au lait spots, neurofibromas, and Lisch nodules. It is also associated with ADHD and having an IQ 5-10 points below average. It is inherited on chromosome 17 in an autosomal dominant pattern.

Kaufman DM: Clinical Neurology for Psychiatrists, 5th ed. Philadelphia, WB Saunders Company, 2001, pp 329–333.
http://ghr.nlm.nih.gov/handbook/inheritance/inheritancepatterns
Smoller JW, Sheidley BR, Tsuang MT. Psychiatric Genetics: Applications in Clinical Practice. American Psychiatric Publishing, Inc.; 1st edition, 2008, p 202

91

Which of the following combination treatments has the best evidence for producing a short term benefit of more rapid stabilization for the acute symptom treatment of panic disorder?

(A) CBT and SSRI
(B) Benzodiazepine and SSRI
(C) CBT and benzodiazepine
(D) SSRI and buspirone

The correct response is option **B**: Benzodiazepine and SSRI

According to The American Psychiatric Association Practice Guideline for the Treatment of Patients with Panic Disorder benzodiazepines may be used along with antidepressants to help control symptoms until the antidepressant takes effect. Recent studies suggest that the benzodiazepine confers a short-tem benefit of stabilization of panic symptoms. However, the advantage of the combination does not continue and individuals receiving SSRI alone catch up to those receiving the combination after the first few weeks of treatment. The benefit of quicker stabilization should be weighed against the possibility of an increased side-effect burden. Studies of medication and psychosocial treatment have not shown a clear and lasting advantage for this combination.

Goddard AW, Brouette T, Almai A, Jetty P, Woods SW, Charney D. Early coadministration of clonazepam with sertraline for panic disorder. Arch Gen Psychiatry. 2001 Jul;58(7):681–6.

Pollack MH, Simon NM, Worthington JJ, Doyle AL, Peters P, Toshkov F, Otto MW. Combined paroxetine and clonazepam treatment strategies compared to paroxetine monotherapy for panic disorder. J Psychopharmacol. 2003 Sep;17(3):276–82.

92

A 22-year-old man presents repeatedly over a year with concerns that he is suffering from AIDS. He has never been found to be HIV positive, but is not convinced despite having negative tests. He does not meet the criteria for major depressive disorder, generalized anxiety disorder, or obsessive-compulsive disorder. Which of the following is the most likely diagnosis?

(A) Body dysmorphic disorder
(B) Hypochondriasis
(C) Conversion disorder
(D) Somatization disorder
(E) Undifferentiated somatoform disorder

The correct response is option **B**: Hypochondriasis

Hypochondriasis is characterized by 6 months or more of a general preoccupation with fears, or the idea of having a serious disease based on a misinterpretation of bodily symptoms. This preoccupation causes significant distress and impairment; it is not accounted for by another psychiatric or medical disorder. The emphasis in hypochondriasis is on fear of having a disease and emphasis in somatization disorder is the concern with symptoms. Hypochondriasis is equally distributed among men and women. Conversion disorder is acute and generally transient and usually involves a symptom rather than a particular disease.

Sadock BJ and Sadock VA (eds). Kaplan and Sadock's Synopsis of Psychiatry, 10th ed. Philadelphia: Lippincott Williams and Wilkins; 2007. p 643

93

Which of the following neurotransmitters has the largest body of evidence associating it with the reinforcing effects of various types of drugs of abuse?

(A) Acetylcholine
(B) Dopamine
(C) GABA
(D) Glutamate
(E) Serotonin

The correct response is option **B**: Dopamine

Although all of the answer choices have been associated in one way or another with the reinforcing effects of drugs, the most consistently associated neurotransmitter has been dopamine. The concentrations of dopamine are increased in the limbic regions by drugs of abuse. It is thought that the reinforcing effects of drugs of abuse are due to their ability to exceed the magnitude and duration of the increases in dopamine in the nucleus accumbens when compared to natural reinforcers like sleep and sex.

Kalivas PW, Volkow ND: The neural basis of addiction: a pathology of motivation and choice. Am J Psychiatry 2005; 162:1403–1413. Reprinted in FOCUS: Substance Abuse, Spring 2007; 2:208–219.

Pierce RC, Kumaresan V: The mesolimbic dopamine system: the final common pathway for the reinforcing effect of drugs of abuse? Neuroscience & Biobehavioral Reviews 2006; 30:215–38.

Volkow ND, Li TK: Drug addiction: the neurobiology of behaviour gone awry. Nature Reviews Neuroscience 2004; 5:963–70.

94

Which of the following is the preferred method to confirm a clinical diagnosis of narcolepsy?

(A) Functional magnetic resonance imaging (fMRI)
(B) Apnea monitoring
(C) Multiple sleep latency test (MSLT)
(D) Human leukocyte antigen (HLA) testing
(E) CSF hypocretin levels

The correct response is option **C**: Multiple sleep latency test (MSLT)

The MSLT, which involves measuring REM sleep latency, consists of 4 or 5 twenty-minute naps scheduled about two hours apart. It is usually performed after an overnight sleep study. HLA testing lacks diagnostic specificity, and CSF hypocretin levels require a lumbar puncture. Apnea monitoring is essential for diagnosing sleep apnea.

Dauvilliers Y, Arnulf I, Mignot E. Narcolepsy with cataplexy. Lancet. 2007; 369:499–511

Moore DP. Textbook of Clinical Neuropsychiatry, 2nd ed. London, Hodder Arnold, 2008. pp 575–577

95

Which of the following psychotherapeutic interventions represents the best approach for a patient with germ obsessions who washes his hands every time he touches something he considers dirty?

(A) Having the patient place his hands in a container of mud
(B) Having the patient snap his wrist with a rubber band when he washes his hands
(C) Pointing out to the patient that the germ phobia is an example of distorted thinking
(D) Having the patient touch a dirty object, then not allowing him to wash his hands
(E) Providing the patient with coping cards to remind him that the hand washing is unnecessary

The correct response is option **D**: Having the patient touch a dirty object, then not allowing him to wash his hands.

This is an example of exposure and response prevention (ERP). Wrist-snapping represents aversive conditioning. Placing the patient's hands in mud represents flooding. The coping cards and distorted thinking are tenets of CBT. While these may be helpful in some instances, ERP is the best form of therapy for OCD.

Sadock BJ, Sadock VA: Kaplan & Sadock's Synopsis of Psychiatry: Behavioral Sciences/Clinical Psychiatry, 10th ed. Philadelphia, Lippincott Williams & Wilkins, 2007, p 611

96

A military veteran is diagnosed with PTSD after his wife encourages him to seek treatment due to problems adjusting to civilian life. It is clear that survivor guilt is a major source of distress. Which of the following is the best intervention for this issue?

(A) Vocational counseling
(B) Couples therapy
(C) Individual psychotherapy
(D) Fluoxetine
(E) Risperidone

The correct response is option **C**: Individual psychotherapy

Individuals with PTSD often have multiple problems that require different interventions. Interpersonal withdrawal, survivor guilt, or shame may be more responsive to psychosocial interventions than medication. The other options may be helpful for other aspects of the patient's functioning.

American Psychiatric Association Practice Guideline for the Treatment of Patients with Acute Stress Disorder and Posttraumatic Stress Disorder. Am J Psychiatry. 2004; 161(11):37 http://psychiatryonline.com/pracGuide/pracGuideHome.aspx.

Gabbard GO (ed): Treatments of Psychiatric Disorders 4th ed. American Psychiatric Publishing, Inc., Washington, DC. 2007; pp. 520–525

97

Which of the following cultural groups is most likely to want to be informed of a terminal prognosis?

(A) Mexican Americans
(B) Korean Americans
(C) African Americans
(D) Japanese Americans
(E) Navajo Americans

The correct response is option **C**: African Americans

Blackhall et al (1995) studied cultural differences in attitudes toward disclosing information about terminal Illness. African Americans (and European Americans) were found to be more likely to want this disclosure than Mexican or Korean Americans. Japanese tend to expect little specific information from their physicians. On the other hand, Navajos believe that language can "shape reality and control events." Therefore being given a negative prognosis is felt to be dangerous physically and emotionally as well as disrespectful.

Breitbart W, Lintz K. Psychiatric Issues in the care of dying patients. Wise MG, Rundell JR (eds): Textbook of Consultation-Liaison Psychiatry, 2nd ed. Washington, DC, American Psychiatric Publishing, 2002, pp 775–776.

Blackhall LJ, Murphy ST, Frank G, et al: Ethnicity and attitudes toward patient autonomy. JAMA 1995, 278:820–825.

Levenson JL (ed): Textbook of Psychosomatic Medicine. Arlington, VA, American Psychiatric Publishing, 2005, p 996.

When diagnosing major depressive disorder in young children, which of the following signs or symptoms is MORE likely to be present than would be expected in an adolescent or adult?

(A) Diurnal variation in mood
(B) Hypersomnia
(C) Melancholia
(D) Poor self-esteem
(E) Somatic complaints

The correct response is option **E**: Somatic complaints

Although the essential features of major depressive disorder are similar in children, adolescents, and adults, there are noticeable differences in phenomenology. Younger children, unable to express emotions as adequately as adolescents and adults, tend to present with more somatic complaints, psychomotor agitation, and at times, mood-congruent hallucinations. The most common somatic complaints are headaches and abdominal pain/discomfort. With age, these symptoms begin to decrease, but self-esteem seems to worsen. By adolescence, somatic complaints and depressed appearance decrease in frequency and are commonly replaced by symptoms of anhedonia, diurnal variation, hopelessness, psychomotor retardation and delusions.

Dulcan MK and Wiener JM. Essentials of Child and Adolescent Psychiatry, Arlington VA, American Psychiatric Publishing, Inc., 2006. pp. 268–269.

A mutation on which of the following chromosomes has been associated with early-onset Alzheimer's dementia?

(A) Chromosome 2
(B) Chromosome 19
(C) Chromosome 21
(D) Y chromosome
(E) X chromosome

The correct response is option **C**: Chromosome 21

Many individuals with Down syndrome develop early-onset Alzheimer's dementia. Therefore, chromosome 21 has been linked to this illness. Other linked chromosomes are 1 and 14. Chromosome 19 is linked to late-onset Alzheimer's dementia. Alzheimer's is not sex-linked.

Alzheimer's Disease Genetics fact Sheet from U.S. National Institutes of Health National Institute on Aging [Retrieved 8/16/09] http://www.nia.nih.gov/Alzheimers/Publications/geneticsfs.htm
Smoller JW, Sheidley BR, Tsuang MT. Psychiatric Genetics: Applications in Clinical Practice. American Psychiatric Publishing, Inc.; 1st edition, 2008, p 181

A 16-year-old girl is brought by her parents for an evaluation as part of the admission process for a weight reduction program. The adolescent agrees that she is overweight and that she would like to lose weight. Which of the following would be MOST indicative that she will be successful in the program?

(A) BMI < 30
(B) No family history of eating disorders
(C) Mother successfully lost weight
(D) She is willing to take medication
(E) She is willing to change her eating habits

The correct response is option **E**: She is willing to change her eating habits.

To be able to participate successfully in a weight reduction and management program, adolescents must be willing to change their lifestyle habits.

Zametkin AJ, Zoon CK, Klein HW, Munson S. Psychiatric aspects of child and adolescent obesity: a review of the past 10 years. J Am Acad Child Adolesc Psychiatry 2004; Reprinted in FOCUS. Fall 2004; 2 (4):634

A 25-year-old woman complains about shortness of breath, chest pain and diaphoresis. She has had multiple attacks in the past 3 weeks. Her medical work-up is negative. Which of the following medications is the best choice considering efficacy and side-effect profile?

(A) Propranolol
(B) Desipramine
(C) Bupropion
(D) Sertraline
(E) Alprazolam

The correct response is option **D**: Sertraline

The APA Practice Guideline suggests the SSRIs as the most useful agents currently because of the data supporting their effectiveness and favorable side effect profile. The TCAs (desipramine) have been shown to be effective but the side effect profile makes them less well tolerated; e.g., anticholinergic, sleep disturbance, sweating, hypotension, weight gain, etc. There is no good evidence that either propranolol or bupropion are effective for panic disorder. Finally, alprazolam was a major choice for treatment some time ago but its side effect profile including tolerance, difficulty in discontinuing drug without rebounds, sedation and other common side effects of the benzodiazepines caused it to be replaced by other agents.

American Psychiatric Association Practice Guideline for the Treatment of Patients With Panic Disorder, 2nd ed (2008). (suppl; in press) http://www.psychiatryonline.com/pracGuide/pracGuideHome.aspx.

The "parent of origin" effect is defined as transmission of a risk for disease based on whether an autosome has been transmitted by the mother or father. As one example of this phenomenon in psychiatric genetics, duplications of chromosome 15q inherited from the mother, but not the father, have been found to account for a small but significant proportion of cases of which of the following disorders?

(A) Schizophrenia
(B) Bipolar disorder
(C) Obsessive-compulsive disorder
(D) Alcohol dependence
(E) Autism

The correct response is option **E**: Autism

Duplications of chromosome 15q inherited from the mother (but not from the father) have been associated with cases of autism. Duplicated genetic material may lead to normal development when originating with the father, but often leads to developmental abnormalities when originating with the mother. Each of the recent CNV studies of ASD has provided strong support for contribution of chromosome 15q11-13 duplication to ASD risk. The rate of chromosome 15q11-13 duplication is 1% in ASD.

Mason CE, State MW, Moldin SO. Genome, Transcriptome, and Proteome: Charting a New Course to Understanding the Molecular Neurobiology of Mental Disorders. Chapter 1.11. in Sadock BJ, Sadock VA. Ruiz P (eds): Kaplan and Sadock's Comprehensive Textbook of Psychiatry, 9th ed. Philadelphia, Lippincott Williams & Wilkins, 2009, pp 147–161.
Campbell DB. Advances and challenges in the genetics of autism. FOCUS Summer 2010;8(3):339–349

A 14-year-old girl presents with significant weight loss. She reports that about one year ago she became concerned that she was overweight and began self-inducing vomiting. Since then, she has continued to use purgatives in addition to misusing laxatives, diuretics and enemas as a means of weight control after binging. She is intensely afraid of becoming fat. She is in the 65th percentile for weight based on height, appears cachetic, but insists she is obese. She has not experienced menses for six months. Which of the following symptoms will MOST likely be elicited from the patient?

(A) A need for orderliness and control
(B) Competitiveness
(C) Obsessional thinking
(D) Perfectionism
(E) Co-morbid impulsivity

The correct response is option **E**: Co-morbid impulsivity

Anorexia nervosa typically has its onset in an adolescent female who perceives herself to be overweight. The four cardinal symptoms are refusal to maintain body weight at or above a minimally normal weight for age and height; intense fear of gaining weight; denial of the seriousness of the current low body weight; and amenorrhea. DSM-IV-TR distinguished between two subtypes—restricting and binge eating/purging. The binge eating/purging type is characterized by regularly engaging in binge-eating or purging behavior such as self-induced vomiting or the misuse of laxatives, diuretics, or enemas. When compared with patients with restricting anorexia, those with binge eating/purging type are more likely to have co-morbid impulsivity, including substance use disorder, personality disorders, mood lability, and suicidality.

Dulcan MK, Weiner JM. Essentials of Child and Adolescent Psychiatry. Arlington (VA): American Psychiatric Publishing, Inc., 2006. pp 527–528
Hales RE, Yudofsky SC, Gabbard GO (eds): The American Psychiatric Publishing Textbook of Psychiatry, 5th ed. Arlington, VA, American Psychiatric Publishing, Inc., 2008, p 974

Cognitive deficits in schizophrenia have been associated with a decrease in GABA$_A$ receptors in which of the following brain areas?

(A) Lateral amygdala
(B) Medial amygdala
(C) Dorsolateral prefrontal cortex
(D) Medial prefrontal cortex
(E) Nucleus accumbens

The correct response is option **C**: Dorsolateral prefrontal cortex

Several lines of evidence have linked cognitive impairments in schizophrenia with altered levels of GABA$_A$ receptors in the dorsolateral prefrontal cortex. While the prefrontal cortex in general has been associated with cognitive function, it is specifically the dorsolateral prefrontal cortex that has been associated with cognitive deficits in schizophrenia. The amygdala is primarily involved in regulating emotional behavior and the nucleus accumbens with reward.

Lewis DA, Moghaddam B. Cognitive dysfunction in schizophrenia: convergence of γ-aminobutyric acid and glutamate alterations. Arch Neurol 2006;63:1372–6.

A 19-year-old man presents for an outpatient evaluation of increasing concerns about germs and contamination that are now resulting in several hours per day of hand washing and cleaning rituals to relieve anxiety. He is started on sertraline, the dose of which is increased 50 mg every other day until reaching 200 mg daily. After one week of treatment at this dose, he has not experienced any relief of the symptoms. However, the medication is well tolerated without significant side effects. In developing further plan of treatment, which of the following is the appropriate total length of time to continue sertraline before changing to another pharmacologic agent?

(A) 2 weeks
(B) 4 weeks
(C) 6 weeks
(D) 8 weeks
(E) 10 weeks

The correct response is option **E**: 10 weeks

At least 10 and perhaps 12 weeks of pharmacological treatment is needed before one can conclude that an SSRI has failed in relieving symptoms of OCD. Equally important is an adequate dose, usually on the high end of the dosing spectrum. The SSRI chosen, as with other disorders, should be a good fit for a particular patient in terms of its side effect profile. Many SSRIs have FDA approval for OCD. The first challenge in treating with medication is working with the patient to maintain medication adherence.

Koran LM. Obsessive-compulsive disorder: an update for clinicians. FOCUS: OCD; Summer 2007; 3:299–313.
Stein DJ, Hollander E, Rothbaum BO (eds): Textbook of Anxiety Disorders, 2nd ed. Arlington, VA, American Psychiatric Publishing, 2010, p 314.

106

A psychiatric consult is requested for a patient who has burns over 60% of his body. The patient has begun refusing dressing changes despite pre-treatment with morphine. Pain control is adequate except during dressing changes. Upon examination, the patient reports that the pain is too severe to tolerate, and he does not feel that the morphine is adequately controlling his pain. The psychiatrist should recommend which of the following agents as an additional medication prior to dressing changes?

(A) Long-acting morphine
(B) Methadone
(C) Meperidine
(D) Fentanyl
(E) Codeine

The correct response is option **D**: Fentanyl

This patient is under-medicated during dressing changes and requires better analgesic control. Fentanyl is the recommended agent for managing the pain associated with dressing changes due to its rapid onset and short duration of action. The other medications have a less favorable onset/duration of action profile than fentanyl.

Wise MG, Rundell JR (eds): The American Psychiatric Publishing Textbook of Consultation-Liaison Psychiatry, 2nd ed. Washington, DC, American Psychiatric Publishing, Inc., 2002, p 612
American Psychiatric Publishing Textbook of Psychosomatic Medicine. Levenson JL (ed) 2005, p 660

107

A 36-year-old moderately obese man is seen for evaluation of depressed mood, difficulty falling asleep, poor appetite, and diminished concentration at work, all of which been worsening over the past few weeks. When treatment options are discussed, he reports particular concerns about sexual side effects. Considering the patient's concerns, which one of the following medications would be most appropriate to suggest as an initial treatment?

(A) Bupropion
(B) Fluoxetine
(C) Mirtazapine
(D) Nortriptyline
(E) Venlafaxine

The correct response is option **A**: Bupropion.

In direct comparative studies that specifically evaluated sexual functioning, bupropion was significantly less likely to be problematic than SSRIs, TCAs, or SNRIs. Mirtazapine does not cause significant problems with sexual side effects but may cause significant weight gain (as can nortriptyline). Thus bupropion would be the medication of choice.

Clayton AH, Croft HA, Horrigan JP, Wightman DS, Krishen A, Richard NE, Modell JG: Bupropion extended release compared with Escitalopram: effects on sexual functioning and antidepressant efficacy in 2 randomized, double-blind, placebo-controlled studies. J Clin Psychiatry 2006; 67:736–746
Jefferson JW: Bupropion extended-release for depressive disorders. Expert Rev Neurother 2008; 8:715–722

108

Which of the following disorders has the most evidence supporting familial aggregation of the disorder?

(A) Posttraumatic stress disorder
(B) Adjustment disorder, mixed features
(C) Panic disorder
(D) Social phobia
(E) Specific phobia

The correct response is option **C**: Panic disorder

Among anxiety disorders, the strongest aggregate evidence for familial aggregation is for panic disorder. Panic disorder, generalized anxiety disorder, phobias, and OCD all have significant familial aggregation. More research has been done on the genetics of panic disorder compared to other anxiety disorders.

Merikangas KR, Low NC. Genetic epidemiology of anxiety disorders. Handb Exp Pharmacol. 2005; (169):163–79.
Hettema JM, Neale MC & Kendler KS. A review and meta-analysis of the genetic epidemiology of anxiety disorders. Am J Psychiatry 2001; 158:1568–1578.

109

Which of the following medical complications is most likely to be seen in a patient with bulimia nervosa?

- (A) Decreased serum amylase
- (B) Hyperchloremia
- (C) Metabolic acidosis
- (D) Hypokalemia
- (E) Hyperthyroxinemia

The correct response is option **D**: Hypokalemia

Self-induced vomiting in patients with bulimia nervosa can result in metabolic alkalosis, hypochloremia, hypokalemia, increased serum amylase, and cardiac arrhythmias. Dangers of hypokalemia include weakness, lethargy, and possible cardiac arrhythmias.

Hales RE, Yudofsky SC, Gabbard GO (eds): The American Psychiatric Publishing Textbook of Psychiatry, 5th ed. Washington, DC, American Psychiatric Publishing, Inc., 2008. pp 983–985

Mehler PS. Bulimia nervosa. N Engl J Med 2003; 349:876–877

110

Evidence to date from OCD genetic studies indicate that its inheritance is best characterized by which pattern?

- (A) Automsomal dominant
- (B) Autosomal recessive
- (C) Sex-linked recessive
- (D) Complex
- (E) Mendelian

The correct response is option **D**: Complex

OCD is a complex genetic disorder that seems to also be strongly influenced by environmental and non-genetic biologic processes. There is emerging evidence that complex disorders may result from both rare genes of major effect and a combination of common genes of lesser effect. Studies of OCD report increased prevalence of this disorder among relatives. Twin studies have confirmed that a genetic component underlies the illness. Genome-wide significant findings have yet to be identified. Segration analyses have clarified that transmission does not occur in a simple mendelian fashion.

Stewart SE, Pauls DL: The genetics of obsessive-compulsive disorder. FOCUS Summer 2010;8(3):350–357

111

A 72-year-old woman is referred to a psychiatrist because the family has noticed increasing apathy. In evaluating the patient, which of the following would be the most useful first step for revealing the likely underlying pathology?

- (A) An empirical trial of an antidepressant
- (B) An MRI of the brain
- (C) History and a full mental status examination
- (D) Thyroid function testing
- (E) Neuropsychological evaluation

The correct response is option **C**: History and a full mental status examination

Apathy is common in the elderly, and recent research suggests that it is distinct from depression and should not be treated automatically as a variant of major depression. Both clinical and neurobiological research suggests that apathy in the elderly is most often associated with dementia and may be a harbinger of progressive cognitive decline. Laboratory tests such as an MRI, thyroid function and urine drug testing are most likely to play a confirmatory role when the history and examination suggest a specific pathology. MRI and similar neuroanatomical evaluations have shown that specific anatomical areas may underlie the pathology of apathy; however these findings represent relative differences seen in population comparisons, and are not sensitive enough to be considered a diagnostic tool.

Lyketsos C. Apathy and agitation: challenges and future directions. Am J Geriatr Psychiatry. 2007; 15(5):361–364

112

Which of the following is believed to be the chief factor in predicting outcome of psychodynamic psychotherapy?

(A) Transference
(B) Countertransference
(C) Therapeutic alliance
(D) Resistance
(E) On time payments

The correct response is option **C**: Therapeutic alliance.

While most of the above mentioned choices are significant aspects of psychotherapy, therapeutic alliance is a strong predictor of outcome in individual psychotherapy across diverse treatment orientations and modalities. The strength of the therapeutic relationship is correlated with outcome across schools of psychotherapy.

Sadock BJ, Sadock VA. Kaplan and Sadock's Synopsis of Psychiatry: Behavioral Sciences/Clinical Psychiatry. Lippincott Williams & Wilkins; 10th edition, 2007, p 495.
Gabbard GO (ed): Textbook of Psychotherapeutic Treatments. Arlington, VA: American Psychiatric Publishing, Inc., 2009, p 714

113

An adolescent girl becomes anxious and "panicky" at the thought of spiders. She cannot join her high school classmates for lunch outside due to the fear that she "will run into a spider." The most appropriate diagnosis is:

(A) agoraphobia.
(B) acute stress disorder.
(C) generalized anxiety disorder.
(D) specific phobia.
(E) social phobia.

The correct response is option **D**: Specific phobia

Specific phobias are marked and persistent fears that are excessive or unreasonable, cued by the presence of anticipation of a specific object (e.g. animals) or situation (e.g. heights, flying). Social phobias concern the avoidance of social situations, and agoraphobia is characterized by anxiety about being in places or situations from which escape might be difficult. In this case the anxiety is specifically related to a fear of spiders.

American Psychiatric Association: Diagnostic and Statistical Manual of Mental Disorders, 4th Edition. Text Revision (DSM-IVTR). Washington DC, American Psychiatric Association, 2000, pp 449–450.

114

A 31 year old female describes dramatic fluctuations in mood and self-esteem. Which one of the following features would be most helpful in distinguishing bipolar II disorder from borderline personality disorder during a period of elevated mood?

(A) Suicidal ideation with depressed mood
(B) Psychosis while mood is elevated or irritable
(C) Impulsivity while mood is elevated or irritable
(D) A history of continued functioning through mood fluctuations
(E) Mood fluctuations are observed by others

The correct response is option **B**: Psychosis while mood is elevated or irritable

In a hypomanic episode, psychosis is never present, whereas borderline patients may experience transient paranoia or dissociation when under stress.

American Psychiatric Association (2000) Diagnostic and Statistical Manual of Mental Disorders, 4th ed., Text Rev. APA, Washington DC. P 368 and 710.

115

Which of the following psychiatric conditions is most commonly associated with self neglect in the geriatric population?

(A) Depression
(B) Generalized anxiety disorder
(C) Panic disorder
(D) Schizophrenia
(E) Personality disorder

The correct response is option **A**: Depression

Depression is a predictor of self neglect. It has been shown to be as common as 62% in elders who self neglect in one case controlled study of older persons referred for self neglect (compared to 12% in those referred for other reasons). Elders who self neglect are frequently frail, live in squalor, have untreated medical conditions, and frequently refuse medical interventions. Dementia is also common in self neglectors.

Abrams RC, Lachs M, McAvay G, Keohane DJ, Bruce ML. Predictors of self-neglect in community-dwelling elders. Am J Psychiatry. 2002 Oct; 159(10):1724–30
Dyer CB, Pavlik VN, Murphy KP, Hyman DJ. The high prevalence of depression and dementia in elder abuse or neglect. J Am Geriatr Soc. 2000 Feb; 48(2):205–8

116

According to the AMA Code of Medical Ethics, which of the following educationally related gifts from a pharmaceutical company is ethically acceptable?

(A) Money to help defray hotel costs during a CME event
(B) Scholarships awarded to individual residents to attend educational conferences
(C) Reimbursement of travel for a guest faculty speaker
(D) Money to compensate a psychiatrist for time spent at a CME event

The correct response is option **C**: Reimbursement of travel for a guest faculty speaker

Scholarships awarded to students cannot be awarded to individuals, only to institutions. Gifts should serve an educational purpose and cannot be used to compensate a clinician for time or cost spent attending a CME event. Faculty speakers can be compensated financially by pharmaceutical companies.

Wahl DS, Milone RD et al: Ethics Primer of the American Psychiatric Association, Washington, DC, American Psychiatric Publishing, Inc, 2001; 48.

Jibson MD; Interactions between physicians and industry: FOCUS Fall 2007.

117

Which of the following statements best describes the association between PTSD and the subsequent emergence of drug use problems?

(A) Young adults with PTSD due to earlier life-time traumas, with no prior drug use disorders, are about five times more likely to develop drug related problems subsequently compared to traumatized young adults without PTSD.
(B) Experiencing significant trauma without the presence of PTSD is sufficient to subsequently increase the prevalence of drug use disorders substantially.
(C) After controlling for factors such as sex, age and ethnicity, PTSD confers no additional increased risk of subsequent drug use disorders.
(D) After controlling for factors such as childhood conduct problems and risk taking, PTSD confers no additional increased risk of subsequent drug use disorders.
(E) After controlling for factors such as family SES and years of education, PTSD confers no additional increased risk of subsequent drug use disorders.

The correct response is option **A**: Young adults with PTSD due to earlier life-time traumas, with no prior drug use disorders, are about five times more likely to develop drug related problems subsequently compared to traumatized young adults without PTSD.

A large, longitudinal prospective study has shown that in young adults who have no features of drug use disorder, the presence of PTSD following lifetime history of significant trauma increases the relative risk of subsequent drug use and abuse problems nearly 5 times (Relative Risk 4.9), and this increased risk remains substantial even after controlling for a host of early factors that in themselves also increase the risk for adult drug use including sex, age, ethnicity, childhood conduct problems, risk taking, family SES and years of education.

Reed PL, Anthony JC, Breslau N. Incidence of drug problems in young adults exposed to trauma and posttraumatic stress disorder: do early life experiences and predispositions matter? Arch Gen Psychiatry. 2007; 64(12):1435–1442

118

Borderline personality disorder is marked by pervasive instability of self-image, emotions and impulsivity. Which of the following is a DSM diagnostic criteria for this diagnosis?

(A) Consistent irresponsibility
(B) Lack of remorse after injuring others
(C) Requiring excessive admiration
(D) Sense of entitlement
(E) Unstable sense of self

The correct response is option **E**: Unstable sense of self

While patients with borderline personality disorder may display or possess any of the other features listed, unstable sense of self is the only one which is a diagnostic criterion for this diagnosis. Consistent irresponsibility as well as lack of remorse after injuring others are criteria for antisocial personality disorder; entitlement and requiring admiration are criteria for narcissistic personality disorder.

Diagnostic and Statistical Manual of Mental Disorders, 4th ed, Text Revi (DSM-IV-TR). Washington, DC, American Psychiatric Association, 2000, pp 701–717

119

Which of the following should be the initial treatment of hypochondriasis?

(A) Cognitive behavioral therapy
(B) Treatment of incidental physical exam findings
(C) Scheduling regular physical examinations
(D) Discussing the false nature of the illness
(E) Pharmacotherapy with SSRIs

The correct response is option **C**: Scheduling regular physical examinations

The first line treatment for hypochondriasis is reassurance to diminish the preoccupation with fear of having a disease. This can be accomplished by scheduling regular medical appointments with a clear goal. Cognitive therapy, as well as other forms of psychotherapy, may be helpful. Pharmacotherapy is helpful in treating any underlying drug-responsive conditions. Discussing the false nature of the illness is not helpful. Treatment of physical complaints should be done when objective evidence calls for it.

Hales RE, Yudofsky SC, Gabbard GO (eds): The American Psychiatric Publishing Textbook of Psychiatry, 5th ed. Washington, DC, American Psychiatric Publishing, 2008, p 632

120

A 33-year-old man with schizophrenia and alcohol dependence acknowledges that when he drinks beer the police tend to arrest him and bring him to the psychiatric hospital. He agrees to "take medicine to help [him] not drink so much." Due to issues of noncompliance, his current medication is a long-acting injectable antipsychotic. He lives on his own and keeps his clinic appointments, but has had difficulties adhering to oral medication regimens. The best medication to augment the treatment of his alcohol dependence would be:

(A) acamprosate.
(B) clozapine.
(C) disulfiram.
(D) naltrexone.
(E) ondansetron.

The correct response is option **D**: Naltrexone

Both acamprosate and disulfiram are available only as oral medications, so are not ideal for a patient with medication adherence problems. While there is some data suggesting that clozapine may be useful in treating symptoms of both schizophrenia and substance use disorders, it too is available as an oral medication only. Ondansetron has been insufficiently studied in this patient population to recommend its use here. Naltrexone is available as a long-acting injection (Vivitrol), so may be preferable in this situation.

Dermatis H, Galanter M. Clinical advances in pharmacological and integrated treatment approaches for alcohol and drug use disorders. FOCUS: Substance Abuse Spring 2007;2:142.
American Psychiatric Association Practice Guideline for the Treatment of Patients with Substance Use Disorders, 2nd Edition, (2006). http://psychiatryonline.com/pracGuide/pracGuideHome.aspx.

121

Avoidant personality disorder is marked by social inhibition, sense of inadequacy and hypersensitivity. Which of the following is a DSM criterion for this disorder?

(A) Requiring excessive admiration
(B) Difficulty making everyday decisions
(C) Excessive devotion to work to the exclusion of friendships
(D) Preoccupation with being socially criticized
(E) Reluctance to delegate tasks or to work with others

The correct response is option **D**: Preoccupation with being socially criticized

A patient with avoidant personality disorder may manifest any or all of the other features listed, but only [D] is a criterion for this diagnosis. Difficulty expressing disagreement and making everyday decisions is diagnostic for dependent personality disorder. Excessive devotion to work and reluctance to delegate is diagnostic criteria for obsessive compulsive personality disorder and requiring excessive admiration is a criteria for narcissistic personality disorder.

Diagnostic and Statistical Manual of Mental Disorders, 4ᵗʰ ed, Text Revi (DSM-IV-TR). Washington, DC, American Psychiatric Association, 2000, pp 718–729

122

Which of the following statements gives the most appropriate guidance for patients and their families regarding driving by patients with dementia?

(A) Families have no responsibility for getting involved in driving decisions of patients with mild cognitive impairment.
(B) All patients with mild cognitive impairment should be reported to their State Motor Vehicle Departments for mandatory tracking.
(C) Clinicians should advise all patients with mild cognitive impairment to stop driving and to turn in their driver's licenses.
(D) Mildly impaired patients should be advised to stop driving at night.
(E) Patients and families should be informed that even mild dementia increases the risk of vehicular accidents.

The correct response is option **E**: Patients and families should be informed that even mild dementia increases the risk of vehicular accidents.

The guidance from the APA's Practice Guideline for the Treatment of Patients with Alzheimer's Disease and Other Dementias points out that even mild dementia is associated with increased vehicular accidents. Accordingly, mildly impaired patients should be advised to limit their driving to safe situations or to stop driving (there is no imperative and no mandatory reporting law for mildly impaired patients). Families should be informed and involved, since the implementation of the recommendations often falls to them.

American Psychiatric Association Practice Guideline for the Treatment of Patients with Alzheimer's disease and Other Dementias, 2ⁿᵈ ed. 2007 p. 11, http://www.psychiatryonline.com/pracGuide/pracGuideTopic_3.aspx

123

An 8-year-old boy presents with a one-month history of stomachaches and headaches every morning just before going to school. When interviewed, he reports having persistent nightmares of being kidnapped and worries about his father having an accident. The most likely diagnosis is:

(A) normal childhood.
(B) agoraphobia.
(C) separation anxiety.
(D) generalized anxiety disorder.
(E) panic disorder.

The correct response is option **C**: Separation anxiety

Separation anxiety disorder is excessive anxiety concerning separation from the home or from those to whom the person is attached. When separated from major attachment figures, these individuals are often preoccupied with fears that accident or illnesses will befall them or their attachment figures. The disorder is rare in adults where the common diagnoses are agoraphobia or panic disorder with agoraphobia. It can be differentiated from generalized anxiety disorder by the fact that the anxiety is about separation and not generalized.

Diagnostic and Statistical Manual of Mental Disorders, 4th ed, Text Revision (DSM-IV-TR). Washington, DC, American Psychiatric Association, 2000, pp 121–124

Dulcan MK, Weiner JM. Essentials of Child and Adolescent Psychiatry. Arlington (VA): American Psychiatric Publishing, Inc., 2006. p 558

124

A 65-year-old man has metastatic head-and-neck cancer that leaves him with a ptosis, facial nerve palsy, and an inability to eat solid foods. He complains of feeling hopeless, that life has lost all meaning, and that he wants to die immediately. He does not meet criteria for major depression. The best descriptor for this triad of symptoms is:

(A) anticipatory grief.
(B) demoralization.
(C) mourning.
(D) denial.
(E) bargaining.

The correct response is option **B**: Demoralization

Anticipatory grief precedes death, and results from its expectation. Mourning is the process of adaptation to death. Kissane and colleagues described the triad of hopelessness, meaningless in life, and desire for death as the demoralization syndrome.

Breitbart W, Gibson C, Chochinov HM. Palliative care, in American Psychiatric Publishing Textbook of Psychosomatic Medicine, Edited by Levenson JA. Arlington, VA, 2005 pp 993–998.

Kissane DW. The contribution of demoralization to end of life decision-making. Hastings Cent Rep. 2004 Jul-Aug;34(4):21–31.

Clarke DM, Kissane DW. Demoralization: its phenomenology and importance. Australian & New Zealand Journal of Psychiatry 2002–12; 36:6 733(10) pp 733–742.

A 73-year-old woman was prescribed 10 mg of paroxetine for anxiety one week ago. She now presents to the physician's office with confusion. Lab work-up reveals low serum sodium and low plasma osmolarity. Her urine sodium and osmolarity are high. The physician should consider a diagnosis of:

(A) hypothyroidism.
(B) SIADH (Syndrome of Inappropriate Antidiuretic Hormone).
(C) hyperparathyroidism.
(D) renal failure.
(E) dehydration.

The correct response is option **B**: SIADH (Syndrome of Inappropriate Antidiuretic Hormone)

Hyponatremia and Syndrome of Inappropriate Antidiuretic Hormone (SIADH) have been associated with SSRI use in elderly patients. The incidence of SIADH does not appear to be dose-dependent. Most cases of SIADH occur within the first 2 weeks of SSRI treatment but could occur at any time. Risk factors for elderly patients could include low body mass index and lower baseline sodium (138 mEq/1).

Jacobson SA, Pies RW and Katz IR. Clinical Manual of Geriatric Psychopharmacology. Arlington, VA, American Psychiatric Publishing, Inc., 2007. pp 191–192.

A 37-year-old male software designer is brought to the psychiatrist's office by his brother, who reports that the patient has become increasingly suspicious over the last year. Last week, a shopping mall security guard observed him recording license plate numbers. The guard inquired, the patient explained that he was doing statistical research on license plates, and there was no further incident. He told his brother later that he thought he had noticed these cars parked in front of his home, and might be part of scoping the neighborhood in advance of a crime. The brother is now concerned that it is only a matter of time for the patient to get into his first legal skirmish as a result of this kind of behavior. The patient reports that since his teens, he has needed to be very observant of others to protect himself. He says he has never been a victim of assault or theft only because of his constant vigilance. He experienced several days of auditory hallucinations when he was about 20 years old; "voices" were making deprecatory comments, but he cannot recall further details . These symptoms remitted entirely, and he reports no other psychotic symptoms.

He has worked at the same software company for ten years and while he has been promoted several times, most recently 3 months ago, he thinks he was slighted by his supervisor who gave a better position to a colleague. He is satisfied with his single status. Which ONE of the following disorders is the most likely diagnosis?

(A) Paranoid personality disorder
(B) Delusional disorder
(C) Schizoid personality disorder
(D) Schizophrenia, paranoid type
(E) Schizotypal personality disorder

The correct response is option **A**: Paranoid personality disorder

The patient's suspiciousness and related behavior places paranoid personality disorder high on the differential diagnosis. The other Cluster A personality disorders are less likely but still on the differential diagnosis. His brief psychotic symptoms do not meet criteria for schizophrenia and thus rules out delusional disorder.

Diagnostic and Statistical Manual of Mental Disorders, Fourth Edition, Text Revision (DSM-IV-TR). Washington, DC, American Psychiatric Association, 2000, pp 297–313, 685–701

A 6-year-old girl is referred by her teacher because of "acting out" behaviors at school, including inappropriate touching of peers and insistence on sitting on adults' laps. During the session, she tells the psychiatrist that her father touches her "secret place." The father explains that he bathes the girl at night and is simply making sure she is clean everywhere. Which of the following is the most appropriate action for the psychiatrist?

(A) Advise the father not to give baths and see if the behavior resolves.
(B) Tell the teacher to call child protective services.
(C) Relay the findings to the teacher and tell her child protective services will not be necessary.
(D) Try to gather more history to see if this constitutes sexual abuse.
(E) Make a call to child protective services.

The correct response is option **E**: Make a call to child protective services.

The threshold for reporting is a *suspicion* of child abuse. The determination of abuse is not up to the individual doctor. Revealing findings to the teacher without consent from the parents is a confidentiality violation.

Wahl DS, Milone RD et al: Ethics Primer of the American Psychiatric Association, Washington, DC, American Psychiatric Publishing, Inc, 2001; 17–18.

Patients with acute stress disorder have been shown in controlled trials to be least likely to subsequently develop posttraumatic stress disorder when treated with:

(A) cognitive restructuring therapy.
(B) exposure therapy.
(C) systematic debriefing.
(D) couples therapy.
(E) internet-based CBT.

The correct response is option **B**: Exposure therapy

A controlled trial of 90 civilian patients with acute stress disorder following trauma treated with six 90-minute weekly sessions of imaginal and in-vivo exposure therapy, cognitive-restructuring therapy, or who were assigned to a waiting list control showed that exposure therapy was clearly superior to cognitive restructuring, which was in turn superior to wait-list control in preventing the subsequent appearance of PTSD. Whereas at six months 77% of those in the wait-list group developed PTSD, only 63% of those receiving cognitive restructuring and 33% of those receiving exposure therapy developed PTSD.

Bryant RA, Mastrodomenico J, Felmingham KL, Hopwood S, Kenny L, Kandris E, Cahill C, Creamer M. Treatment of acute stress disorder: a randomized controlled trial. Arch Gen Psychiatry. 2008; 65(6):659–667

129

According to the results of the Clinical Antipsychotic Trials of Intervention Effectiveness (CATIE) study, approximately what percentage of patients had continued on their initial antipsychotic medications by 18 months?

 (A) 10%
 (B) 25%
 (C) 50%
 (D) 75%
 (E) 90%

The correct response is option **B**: 25%

The most prominent finding of the CATIE study is the high all-cause discontinuation rate (74%) for all the antipsychotic medications. This implies that 74% of the patients discontinued the medication, before 18 months of being started on it. The causes for discontinuation included lack of tolerability, lack of efficacy, clinician decision (due to safety concerns) and patient decision (electing to terminate). Among the atypical antipsychotics, the time to discontinuation was significantly longer for patients treated with olanzapine when compared to patients on risperidone and quetiapine.

Lieberman JA, Stroup TS, McEvoy JP, Swartz MS, Rosenheck RA, Perkins DO, Keefe RS, Davis SM, Davis CE, Lebowitz BD, Severe J, Hsiao JK. Effectiveness of antipsychotic drugs in patients with chronic schizophrenia. N Engl J Med. 2005; 353(12):1209–23.
Nasrallah HA. The roles of efficacy, safety, and tolerability in antipsychotic effectiveness: practical implications of the CATIE schizophrenia trial. J Clin Psychiatry. 2007; 68 Suppl 1:5–11.

130

Temperament traits of Harm Avoidance, Novelty Seeking, Reward Dependence, and Persistence are defined as heritable differences underlying automatic responses to danger, novelty, social approval, and intermittent reward, respectively. Which of the following statements about the temperament traits in the general population is MOST accurate?

 (A) The phenotypic expression of these traits is primarily due to the experiences of the individual.
 (B) They are normally distributed quantitative traits.
 (C) They are modifiable based on the goodness of fit with the parent.
 (D) They are inconsistently manifested in different cultures.
 (E) They are similar to fluid intelligence in that they show demonstrable changes with aging.

The correct response is option **B**: They are normally distributed quantitative traits.

Each of the four major dimensions is normally distributed quantitative trait, moderately heritable, observable in early childhood, relatively stable in time, and moderately predictive of adolescent and adult behavior. The four dimensions have been repeatedly shown to be universal across different cultures, ethnic groups, and political systems.

Sadock BJ, Sadock VA (eds): Kaplan and Sadock's Comprehensive Textbook of Psychiatry, 9th ed. Philadelphia, Lippincott Williams & Wilkins, 2009, p. 2199.
Angres DH. The Temperament and Character Inventory in addiction treatment. Focus 2010 8: 192

131

A 37-year-old single man's sex life centers on donning women's lingerie before engaging in sexual activities with willing female partners. He considers himself heterosexual and has never had any interest in having sex with men. He is distressed about his sexual behavior and is now seeking treatment. Which of the following best describes his behavior?

 (A) Transvestic fetishism
 (B) Gender identity disorder
 (C) Frotteurism
 (D) Exhibitionism

The correct response is option **A**: Transvestic fetishism

The behaviors are consistent with transvestic fetishism. He is a heterosexual male who experiences intense sexual urges while cross-dressing. Furthermore, the behavior causes distress for him.

American Psychiatric Association: Diagnostic and Statistical Manual of Mental Disorders, 4th Edition, Text Revision (DSM-IV-TR). Washington DC, American Psychiatric Association. 2000. pp 5743–5575

A 28-year-old woman presents to the clinic concerned about having ADHD. She has noticed that for the last three days she has been "hyper." She stays up until 4 a.m. to rehearse her presentations and awakens easily at 7 a.m. She also now works as late as 9 p.m., whereas she would usually stop at 6 p.m. She finds herself easily distracted and strays from her routine presentation. She experiences these symptoms about three times a year. Talking with her husband reveals that these periods are always followed by a deep depression during which she will rarely get out of bed, does not eat, and will not see clients for about two weeks. Her presentation is most consistent with:

(A) cyclothymia.
(B) bipolar I disorder.
(C) bipolar II disorder.
(D) ADHD – inattentive type.
(E) ADHD – hyperactive/impulsive type.

The correct response is option **C**: Bipolar II disorder

The patient's hyperactivity and distractibility are confined to times in which she expresses the other manic symptoms, making ADHD unlikely. Her depressive phases are too severe to classify her as cyclothymic. The mania in bipolar I disorder is associated with *significant* social or occupational dysfunction or hospitalization. The patient in this scenario is impaired, but not significantly so.

Sadock BJ, Sadock VA, Ruiz P (eds): Kaplan & Sadock's Comprehensive Textbook of Psychiatry, 9th ed. Philadelphia, Lippincott Williams & Wilkins, 2009, pp 1719–20.

American Psychiatric Association Practice Guideline for the Treatment of Patients with Bipolar Disorder, 2nd Edition (2002), http://psychiatryonline.com/pracGuide/pracGuideHome.aspx.

A 19-year-old woman with anorexia presents with shortness of breath and symptoms consistent with heart failure. She admits to using large amounts of ipecac. Which of the following test results would be most consistent with ipecac-induced toxicity?

(A) Decrease in the serum CK value
(B) Decrease in lactate dehydrogenase
(C) Shortening of the QTC interval
(D) Enlarged heart
(E) Bradycardia

The correct response is option **D**: Enlarged heart

Ipecac abuse is associated most predominantly with a myopathy that involves "Z-band streaming." This can result in increased CPK and lactate dehydrogenase, and cardiac abnormalities including tachycardia, QTC prolongation, an enlarged heart on echocardiogram, and reduced ejection fraction. The cardiovascular changes usually reverse when the ipecac is stopped. Direct testing for ipecac alkaloids can be done in urine, serum, or tissue samples, and are present for several weeks after use.

Silber TJ: Ipecac syrup abuse, morbidity, and mortality: isn't it time to repeal its over-the-counter status? J Adolescent Health 2005; 37(3):256–260.

An assessment of a 25-year old woman as a candidate for psychotherapy reveals that she is able to delay gratification in order to attain personal goals but remains egocentric and defensive. She is noted to have frequent distress when attachments and desires are frustrated. She functions well under good conditions but frequently experiences problems under stress. Based upon the *stages in the development of self-awareness and well being* this woman is MOST likely at what stage?

(A) Stage 0: unaware
(B) Stage 1: average adult cognition
(C) Stage 2: metacognition
(D) Stage 3: contemplation

The correct response is option **B**: Stage 1: average adult cognition

A full assessment of personality requires consideration of a person's level of self-awareness and well-being. There are four stages of self-awareness along the path to well- being. Stage 0 (unaware) is characterized by immaturity; seeking immediate gratification and a "child-like" ego state. Stage 1 (average adult cognition) includes individuals who are purposeful but egocentric; they are able to delay gratification, but have frequent negative emotions such as anxiety, anger and disgust. In the Stage 2 (metacognition) individuals are mature and allocentric; they are aware of their own subconscious thinking; calm and patient; and so are able to supervise conflicts and relationships. Stage 3 (contemplation) is the highest stage. These people are calm; wise; demonstrate impartial awareness; creative and loving; able to access what was previously unconscious as needed without effort or distress.

Sadock BJ, Sadock VA (eds): Kaplan and Sadock's Comprehensive Textbook of Psychiatry, 9th ed. Philadelphia, Lippincott Williams & Wilkins, 2009, pp. 2233.

Which of the following techniques or therapies has been shown, in a randomized controlled trial, to be most helpful in the treatment of acute stress disorder?

(A) Cognitive restructuring
(B) Individual psychological debriefing
(C) Exposure-based therapy
(D) EMDR (Eye Movement Desensitization and Reprocessing)
(E) Group debriefing

The correct response is option **C**: Exposure-based therapy

The cognitive behavioral therapy technique of exposure-based therapy has been found to superior to cognitive restructuring. Debriefing, either individually or in group, has not been found to be effective. EMDR has not been tested for the treatment of acute stress disorder.

Gabbard, GO. Treatment of Psychiatric Disorders, 4th ed. Washington, DC, American Psychiatric Press, Inc. 2007; pp. 519-522

American Psychiatric Association Practice Guideline for the Treatment of Patients with Acute Stress Disorder and Posttraumatic Stress Disorder. 2004; pp 61–62 http://www.psychiatry-online.com/pracGuide/pracGuideTopic_11.aspx

Bryant RA, Mastrodomenico J, Felmingham KL, Hopwood S, Kenny L, Kandris E, Cahill C, Creamer M. Treatment of acute stress disorder: a randomized controlled trial. Arch Gen Psychiatry. 2008; 65(6):659–667

136

Which of the following medications should be the first line treatment for generalized anxiety disorder?

- (A) Diazepam
- (B) Lorazepam
- (C) Buspirone
- (D) Paroxetine
- (E) Hydroxyzine

The correct response is option **D**: Paroxetine

Efficacy and the favorable side effect profile make SSRIs (paroxetine) the current first line choice. Long acting benzodiazepines (diazepam) are also effective but concern about dependence and cognitive problems make them a second line choice. Short acting benzodiazepines (lorazepam) pose even greater risk for dependence. Buspirone has a longer wait until active. Although it has a favorable side effect profile, some consider it less effective than other drugs. Hydroxyzine, a histamine receptor antagonist, was found to be effective with no problem of dependence. Its major side effect is sedation. It does not appear to be very widely used.

Stein DJ, Hollander E, Rothbaum BO (eds): Textbook of Anxiety Disorders, 2nd ed. Arlington, VA, American Psychiatric Publishing, 2010, pp 193–213

Hales RE, Yudofsky SC, and Gabbard GO (eds). American Psychiatric Textbook of Psychiatry, 5th ed. Arlington, VA, American Psychiatric Publishing, Inc., 2008, pp 534–35

137

After performing a thorough history and physical, a psychiatrist suspects that the patient has bipolar I disorder, rapid-cycling. Which of the following tests should be ordered to rule out an underlying medical etiology?

- (A) CSF 5-HIAA
- (B) 24 hour urine
- (C) Thyroid function tests
- (D) Liver function tests
- (E) Dexamethasone suppression test

The correct response is option **C**: Thyroid function tests

The initial intervention in patients who experience rapid cycling is to identify and treat medical conditions such as hypothyroidism. Autoimmune thyroid disease as manifested in positive TPO antibodies, with or without frank hypothyroidism, may contribute to rapid cycling. Low levels of 5-HIAA are associated with increased impulsivity. 24 hour urine collections are most associated with pheochromocytomas. Liver function tests are often part of the monitoring requirements for mood stabilizers. Although a DST has had some studies linking it to bipolar disorder, it is rarely used.

Oomen HA, Schipperijn AJ, Drexhage HA. The prevalence of affective disorders and in particular rapid-cycling bipolar disorder in patients with abnormal thyroid function tests. Clin Endocrinol. 1996; 45:215–223.

American Psychiatric Association Practice Guideline for the Treatment of Patients with Bipolar Disorder, 2nd Edition (2002). Reprinted in FOCUS: Bipolar Disorder, 2003; 1:65.

138

The symptom domain most strongly correlated with functional impairment in schizophrenia is:

- (A) positive symptoms.
- (B) negative symptoms.
- (C) cognitive impairment.
- (D) mood disturbance.

The correct response is option **C**: Cognitive impairment

Among the four symptom domains of schizophrenia— positive symptoms (hallucinations, delusions); negative symptoms (blunted affect, alogia, anhedonia, social isolation, lack of motivation); cognitive impairment; and mood disturbance—cognitive dysfunction has the highest correlation with functional impairment. Improvements in cognition are highly correlated with better quality of life.

Marder SR. Neurocognition as a treatment target in schizophrenia. FOCUS: Schizophrenia. Spring 2008; 6(2):180–183

A 37-year-old woman, in dynamic psychotherapy for borderline personality disorder, has been expressing an unrealistic overvaluation of the therapist. After many months of this expressed high regard, she suddenly becomes enraged after the therapist fails to return her call, and now declares the therapist to be "the worst ever." Which of the following would be the most appropriate way to handle the patient's new reaction?

- (A) Avoid directly responding and instead encourage the patient to further express her emotions.
- (B) Apologize for the missed call and then suggest they move on with the current work.
- (C) Acknowledge the failing and then question how the patient's opinion could change so dramatically.
- (D) Propose that they clarify an appropriate call-back policy to avoid future mishaps.
- (E) Suggest to the patient that such inevitable mistakes are an important part of the therapy.

The correct response is option **C**: Acknowledge the failing but then question how the patient's opinion could change so dramatically.

One of the primary goals of dynamic psychotherapy is to increase a patient's insight into the workings of their own mind. Patients with borderline personality disorders have chaotic relationships with oscillations between idealization and devaluation. Although a therapist should honestly acknowledge mistakes, the patient's seeming overreaction to this mistake provides an opportunity to explore the patient's defensive style and help the patient see how these reactions likely affect other areas of the patient's life.

Cabaniss D. Personality disorders. FOCUS 2005;3:383–384

Which of the following is the most accurate information to give families regarding the risk of using antipsychotics to treat agitation in elderly patients with moderate dementia of the Alzheimer's type?

- (A) There is an increased risk of mortality, but only for the antipsychotics risperidone and olanzapine.
- (B) Increased mortality in the elderly has been associated with both atypical and conventional antipsychotics.
- (C) Although suggested by earlier studies, subsequent studies have not found a significant risk of mortality with atypical antipsychotics.
- (D) The risk is unknown, as inadequate data exists to make any conclusive statements.
- (E) Although newer antipsychotics may have a risk, typical antipsychotics appear to be safe.

The correct response is option **B**: Increased mortality in the elderly has been associated with both atypical and conventional antipsychotics.

Recently published studies suggest that both conventional and atypical antipsychotic medications are associated with increased risk of death in elderly patients, leading the FDA to require manufacturers to add a black box warning to this effect. In a prior FDA-conducted meta-analysis of 17 placebo controlled studies concerning atypical antipsychotics over the course of the 10 week trials, 4.5% of those taking active medications died compared to 2.6% of those taking placebo.

Gill SS, Bronskill SE, Normand SL, Anderson GM, Sykora K, Lam K, Bell CM, Lee PE, Fischer HD, Herrmann N, Gurwitz JH, Rochon PA. Antipsychotic drug use and mortality in older adults with dementia. Ann Intern Med. 2007; 146(11):777–786

Schneeweiss S, Setoguchi S, Brookhart A, Dormuth C, Wang PS. Risk of death associated with the use of conventional versus atypical antipsychotic drugs among elderly patients. CMAJ. 2007; 176(5):627–632

Kuehn BM. FDA: Antipsychotics risky for elderly. JAMA. 2008; 300(4):379–380

Cheong JA: Ask the expert: Geriatric Psychiatry. FOCUS. 2009; 7:36–37.

141

The use of stimulants to treat ADHD is relatively contraindicated if the child has which of the following co-morbid conditions?

(A) Tic disorder
(B) Pre-existing cardiovascular disease
(C) Seizure disorder
(D) Anxiety disorder
(E) Bipolar disorder

The correct response is option **B**: Pre-existing cardiovascular disease

The FDA indicates that stimulants should not be used when individuals have a number of co-morbid conditions. However, studies and the literature indicate that none of the options except B (pre-existing cardiovascular disease) appear to be significantly exacerbated by the use of stimulants. The American Heart Association has recommended that all children receiving stimulant medications receive an EKG prior to initiating treatment.

AACAP Practice parameter of the use of stimulant medications in the treatment of children, adolescents, and adults. J Am Acad Child Adolesc Psychiatry. 2007. Reprinted in FOCUS: Child and Adolescent Psychiatry. Fall 2004; 2(4):644–645.

Practice parameter for the assessment and treatment of children and adolescents with ADHD. J Am Acad Child Adolesc Psychiatry. 2007; 46:911–912. Reprinted in FOCUS: Child and Adolescent Psychiatry. Summer 2008; (3) pp 401–426.

Winterstein AG, Gerhard T, Shuster J, Johnson M, Zito JM, Saidi A. Cardiac safety of central nervous system stimulants in children and adolescents with attention-deficit/hyperactivity disorder. Pediatrics. Dec 2007; 120(6): e1494–501.

Cardiovascular monitoring of children and adolescents with heart disease receiving stimulant drugs: a scientific statement from the American Heart Association Council on Cardiovascular Disease in the Young Congenital Cardiac Defects Committee and the Council on Cardiovascular Nursing. Circulation. 2008 May 6; 117(18) pp 2407–23 Epub 2008 Apr 21.

142

A patient describes a dinner party at which he felt increasing anxiety and a sense that people were avoiding him. He discussed this with his wife and she became irritated with him, noting that it would help if he could look people in the eye and not wear the same worn-out suit jacket to every party. He tried to explain that this was his lucky jacket and it protected them both from car accidents, but she just shook her head. Based on this, which of the following personality disorders is most likely?

(A) Schizoid
(B) Schizotypal
(C) Antisocial
(D) Borderline
(E) Narcissistic

The correct response is option **B**: Schizotypal

Schizotypal personality disorder is a pervasive pattern of social and interpersonal deficits marked by acute discomfort with, and reduced capacity for, close relationships as well as cognitive distortions of behavior. This may include odd social behaviors, loose, vague or idiosyncratic speech, paranoia in social situations, and magical thinking.

Diagnostic and Statistical Manual of Mental Disorders, Fourth Edition, Text Revision (DSM-IV-TR). Washington, DC, American Psychiatric Association, 2000, pp 697–701.

143

What is the leading cause of disability in the world for persons 15–44 years of age?

(A) Bipolar disorder
(B) Schizophrenia
(C) Self-inflicted injuries
(D) Unipolar major depression
(E) Alcohol use

The correct response is option **D**: Unipolar major depression

When ranked according to the percent total disability–adjusted life year, the global burden of disease is greatest for major depression. All of the other listed mental illnesses are also ranked in the top ten leading causes of disability.

Murray CJL, Lopez AD: The Global Burden Of Disease: A Comprehensive Assessment Of Mortality And Disability From Diseases, Injuries, and Risk Factors in 1990 and Projected to 2020. Cambridge, MA, Harvard University Press, 1996 (Table 5.4)

Hales RE, Yudofsky SC, Gabbard GO (eds): The American Psychiatric Textbook of Psychiatry, 5th ed. Arlington, VA, American Psychiatric Publishing, Inc., 2008. pp 472

144

A busy 33-year-old female executive decides that she will end 10 years of smoking. She tried once before, but was unsuccessful. She travels several times a month, and agrees to use a nicotine inhaler, along with brief telephone counseling appointments. When is she most likely to relapse?

    (A) On the quit date
    (B) During the first few days of the quit date
    (C) One week after the quit date
    (D) Two weeks after the quit date

The correct response is option **B**: During the first few days of the quit date

Most patients relapse within a couple of days of stopping smoking. It's therefore important for the psychiatrist or the psychiatrist's staff to contact the patient right after the quit date for support.

American Psychiatric Association Practice Guideline for the Treatment of Patients with Substance Use Disorders, 2nd Edition (2006), p 362–364. http://psychiatryonline.com/pracGuide/pracGuideHome.aspx.

145

Clinical efficacy of typical (first generation) antipsychotic medications is highly correlated with binding to which of the following receptors?

    (A) Dopamine, D1
    (B) Dopamine, D2
    (C) Serotonin, 5-HT2a
    (D) Muscarinic, M4
    (E) Adrenoceptors, α_2

The correct response is option **B**: Dopamine, D2

Clinical efficacy of typical antipsychotic medications is highly correlated with binding to dopaminergic D2 receptors. The dose of a typical antipsychotic that is likely to be effective is the dose that occupies an appropriate number of D2 receptors. For dopamine receptor antagonists, this implies approximately 60–70% of receptors.

Kane JM, Stroup TS, Marder SR. Schizophrenia: Pharmacological Treatment, in Kaplan & Sadock's Comprehensive Textbook of Psychiatry, 9th ed. Edited by Sadock BJ, Sadock VA, Ruiz P. Philadelphia, Lippincott Williams & Wilkins, 2009, pp 1547–56
Miyamoto S, Duncan GE, Marx CE, Lieberman JA. Treatments for schizophrenia: a critical review of pharmacology and mechanisms of action of antipsychotic medications. Mol Psychiatry. 2005, Jan; 10(1):79–104

146

Which of the following is a single locus (monogenic) disorder?

    (A) Alzheimer's disease
    (B) Bipolar disorder
    (C) Autism
    (D) Huntington's disease
    (E) Obsessive-compulsive disorder

The correct response is option **D**: Huntington's disease

Huntington's disease is a neurodegenerative genetic disorder caused by a single gene mutation (the Huntingtin gene) producing a trinucleotide repeat on chromosome 4. Its transmission follows simple Mendelian inheritance. The other options are polygenic disorders with more complex inheritance patterns.

Smoller JW, Sheidley BR, Tsuang MT. Psychiatric Genetics: Applications in Clinical Practice. American Psychiatric Publishing, Inc.; 1st edition, 2008, p. 48
Sadock BJ, Sadock VA (eds): Kaplan & Sadock's Comprehensive Textbook of Psychiatry, 9th ed. Philadelphia, Lippincott Williams & Wilkins, 2009, pp 299–333.

147

Which of the following is considered the treatment of choice for the core deficit of children with Asperger's syndrome?

    (A) Speech and language therapy
    (B) Self-care assistance
    (C) Social skills training
    (D) Structured educational intervention
    (E) Vocational rehabilitation

The correct response is option **C**: Social skills training

Language, self-care and cognitive interventions are all treatments for autistic disorder. There are no significant delays in these areas in children with Asperger's syndrome, for which the hallmark is impairment and oddity of social interaction and restricted interests.

Sadock BJ and Sadock VA (eds): Kaplan & Sadock's Synopsis of Psychiatry, Tenth ed. Philadelphia, Lippincott Williams & Wilkins, 2007, pp 1201–2

148

Medications from which one of the following classes have the greatest potential for worsening symptoms of borderline personality disorder?

(A) Selective serotonin reuptake inhibitors
(B) Monoamine oxidase inhibitors
(C) Anticonvulsants
(D) Atypical antipsychotics
(E) Benzodiazepines

The correct response is option **E**: Benzodiazepines

Patients with borderline personality disorder may exhibit disinhibition with benzodiazepines. All of the other classes of drugs listed may be helpful in treating specific symptoms of this disorder.

Sadock BJ, Sadock VA: Kaplan and Sadock's Synopsis of Psychiatry, 10th ed. Philadelphia, Lippincott Williams & Wilkins, 2007, p. 801.

149

In order to be given the diagnosis of mild cognitive impairment (MCI), A patient must have:

(A) a memory impairment.
(B) a cognitive complaint in at least one domain.
(C) cognitive complaints in multiple domains.
(D) compromised general cognitive function.
(E) cognitive and memory complaints meeting criteria for mild dementia.

The correct response is option **B**: A cognitive complaint in at least one domain.

Core to the diagnosis of MCI is a cognitive complaint in at least one domain of the five cognitive domains of memory, attention, visuo spacial, language, executive function. By definition, MCI cannot meet criteria for dementia and cannot result in impaired general cognitive function. MCI is further characterized according to amnestic and non-amnestic subtypes and compromise in single or multiple domains. Subtypes can be helpful in predicting the type of dementia that is likely to develop eventually.

Petersen RC, Negash, S. Mild cognitive impairment: an overview. CNS Spectr 2008; 13:45–53

Palmer K, Bäckman L, Winblad B, Fratiglioni L. Mild cognitive impairment in the general population: occurrence and progression to Alzheimer disease. Am J Geriatr Psychiatry. 2008; 16(7):603–611

Chertkow H, Massoud F, Nasreddine Z, Belleville S, Joanette Y, Bocti C, Drolet V, Kirk J, Freedman M, Bergman H. Diagnosis and treatment of dementia:3. Mild cognitive impairment and cognitive impairment without dementia. CMAJ. 2008 May 6; 178(10):1273–85.

150

A 42-year-old patient requests treatment for anxiety and interpersonal difficulties. The patient reports feelings of social inadequacy and sensitivity to rejection for the past 20 years. The patient does not attend social events or interact with others as a result of this anxiety, worries excessively about being criticized by others, and feels inferior to others. This has caused occupational problems since the patient is only able to function in jobs that have virtually no social interaction. The patient is unhappy that he has no friends and has never been romantically involved. Which of the following is the most likely diagnosis?

(A) Schizoid personality disorder
(B) Generalized anxiety disorder
(C) Avoidant personality disorder
(D) Social anxiety disorder
(E) Obsessive-compulsive disorder

The correct response is option **C**: Avoidant personality disorder

This patient meets the DSM-IV-TR criteria for avoidant personality disorder. The differential diagnosis would include social anxiety disorder; however, avoidant personality disorder generally involves avoidance of situations and relationships with the potential for rejection or disappointment, whereas social anxiety disorder is characterized by specific fears related to social performance. The differential diagnosis also includes schizoid personality disorder. However, this patient is concerned about not having friends and romantic experiences, and a patient with schizoid personality disorder is likely not to desire these kinds of relationships.

Hales RE, Yudofsky SC, Gabbard GO (eds): The American Psychiatric Publishing Textbook of Psychiatry, 5th ed. American Psychiatric Publishing, Inc., Washington, DC. 2008. pp 846–847

The parents of a 10-year-old boy who has had both motor and vocal tics for over a year are wondering whether he will remain symptomatic as an adult. Which of the following statements MOST accurately describes the probable outcome of children with these symptoms?

(A) 50% of children are not symptomatic by age 18.
(B) Symptoms continue to increase in adolescence and adulthood.
(C) The motor tics resolve but the vocal tics persist.
(D) The tics decrease in adolescence but then increase again in adulthood.

The correct response is option **A**: 50% of children are not symptomatic by age 18

Tourette's disorder includes the presence of both vocal tics and multiple motor tics. Transient tic disorder also has both motor and verbal tics but if the symptoms last more than one 1 year the diagnosis is converted to Tourette's disorder. Therefore, this child meets the DSM-IV-TR criteria for the definition of Tourette's disorder. Although Tourette's disorder is described as a lifelong disease, prevalence is 10 times higher among children than adults, and longitudinal studies show that symptoms decrease or fully remit in 50% of affected individuals by age 18 years, demonstrating a more benign and less chronic outcome for many individuals.

Swain JE, Scahill L, Lombroso PL, King RA, Leckman JL. Tourette syndrome and tic disorders: a decade of progress. J Am Acad Child Adolesc Psychiatry. 2007; 46:948.

Bloch MH, Peterson BS, Scahill L, Otka J, Katsovich L, Zhang H, Leckman JF. Adulthood outcome of tic and obsessive-compulsive symptom severity in children with Tourette syndrome. Arch Pediatr Adolesc Med. 2006 Jan; 160(1):65–9.

Leckman JF, Zhang H, Vitale A, Lahnin F, Lynch K, Bondi C, Kim Y, Peterson BS. Course of tic severity in tourette syndrome:the first two decades. Pediatrics. 1998 July; 102(1):14–19.

Increased risk of developing diabetes mellitus and dyslipidemia have most commonly been linked to:

(A) perphenazine.
(B) quetiapine.
(C) risperidone.
(D) ziprasidone.
(E) olanzapine.

The correct response is option **E**: olanzapine.

Olanzapine and clozapine are associated with increased risks of developing diabetes mellitus and dyslipidemia. A recent comparative antipsychotic trial in schizophrenia suggested significantly greater weight gain for olanzapine than for the other antipsychotics—perphenazine, quetiapine, risperidone, and ziprasidone. Clozapine and olanzapine are associated with the most weight gain, risperidone and quetiapine with moderate weight gain, and ziprasidone and aripiprazole with minimal weight change.

Newcomer JW: Second-generation (atypical) antipsychotics and metabolic effects: a comprehensive literature review. CNS Drugs 2005; 19(suppl 1):1–93.

Lieberman JA, Stroup TS, McEvoy JP, Swartz MS, Rosenheck RA, Perkins DO, Keefe RS, Davis SM, Davis CE, Lebowitz BD, Severe J, Hsiao JK: Effectiveness of antipsychotic drugs in patients with chronic schizophrenia. N Engl J Med 2005; 353:1209–1223.

Hirschfeld RMA: "Guideline Watch: Practice Guideline for the Treatment of Patients with Bipolar Disorder, 2nd Edition" APA Practice Guidelines November 2005. Reprinted in FOCUS: Bipolar Disorder Winter 2007; 1:36.

153

Patients in a study were asked to exert behavioral inhibition when confronted with negative stimuli. fMRI investigations demonstrated decreased activation of the subgenual anterior cingulate cortex and the posterior medial orbitofrontal cortex, and increased activity in the left and right extended amygdala and ventral striatum relative to controls. These FMRI findings were associated with which of the following diagnoses?

(A) Narcissistic personality disorder
(B) Attention-deficit/hyperactivity disorder (ADHD)
(C) Paranoid personality disorder
(D) Borderline personality disorder
(E) Schizophrenia

The correct response is option **D**: Borderline personality disorder

Previous neuropsychological studies have suggested that impulsivity and negative affectivity may be related to orbitofrontal dysfunction. The study was organized to examine the hypothesis that patients with borderline personality disorder who are experiencing negative emotional states would show deficient inhibitory function of the prefrontal cortex. When confronted with negative stimuli and asked to exert behavioral inhibition, relative to controls, borderline personality disorder patients showed decreased activation of the subgenual anterior cingulate cortex and the posterior medial orbitofrontal cortex, and increased activity in the left and right extended amygdala and ventral striatum.

Silbersweig D, Clarkin JF, Goldstein M, Kernberg OF, Tuescher O, Levy KN, Brendel G, Pan H, Beutel M, Pavony MT, Epstein J, Lenzenweger MF, Thomas KM, Posner MI, Stern E. Failure of frontolimbic inhibitory function in the context of negative emotion in borderline personality disorder. Am J Psychiatry, December 2007; 164:1832–1841.

154

Binge eating disorder is characterized by:

(A) feelings of being unable to control one's intake of food.
(B) consumption of a large amount of food over a 24-hour period.
(C) purging after eating a large amount of food.
(D) increasing amounts of exercise.
(E) progressive weight loss.

The correct response is option **A**: Feelings of being unable to control one's intake of food.

Binge eating disorder occurs in patients without compensatory behaviors such as purging, fasting or excessive exercise. These patients consume a large quantity of food in a discrete period of time (e.g., within any 2-hour period) while feeling unable to control their intake. Comorbid psychopathology on both Axis I and II is common, including mood, anxiety, substance-use, and personality disorders.

American Psychiatric Association: Diagnostic and Statistical Manual of Mental Disorders, 4th Edition, Text Revision (DSM-IV-TR). Washington DC, American Psychiatric Association. 2000, pp 785–787

155

A patient who has been diagnosed with PTSD reports nightmares and sleep disruption. Which one of the following medications has been shown to be effective for the treatment of trauma-related nightmares and sleep disruption in patients with PTSD?

(A) Topiramate
(B) Sertraline
(C) Prazosin
(D) Gabapentin
(E) Propranolol

The correct response is option **C**: Prazosin

According to the March 2009 Guideline Watch of the APA, prazosin is the pharmacotherapy for sleep problems related to PTSD that is supported by the greatest number of peer-reviewed studies. SSRIs are not effective in treating PTSD-related nightmares. Anticonvulsants have not been shown to be efficacious for PTSD symptoms. Although propranolol has some efficacy in reducing symptoms of post-traumatic physiologic arousal, recent studies failed to demonstrate a significant separation from placebo for PTSD symptoms in general.

Benedek DM, Friedman MJ, Zatzick D, Ursano RJ: Guideline Watch (March 2009): Practice Guideline for the Treatment of Patients With Acute Stress Disorder and Posttraumatic Stress Disorder; Focus 2009; 7:204–213.

A 3-day-postpartum mother with no prior psychiatric diagnosis is concerned about feeling depressed. She endorses a decrease in energy, difficulty sleeping despite being tired, decreased appetite, and frequent mood swings saying, "One minute I'm fine, the next minute I'm crying." Which of the following is the most appropriate treatment?

(A) Psychoeducation
(B) Cognitive behavioral therapy
(C) Pharmacotherapy
(D) Hospitalization
(E) Psychodynamic psychotherapy

The correct response is option **A**: Psychoeducation

The mother is most likely experiencing postpartum blues or baby blues. The symptoms of postpartum blues mimic depression and usually peak by day five and resolve by day 10 postpartum. By definition, postpartum blues is transient. In addition to psychoeducation and validation of her experience, she should also be monitored for signs and symptoms of a progression into a full postpartum depression or anxiety disorder.

Sadock BJ, Sadock VA, Ruiz P (eds): Kaplan & Sadock's Comprehensive Textbook of Psychiatry, 9th ed. Philadelphia, Lippincott Williams & Wilkins, 2009, p 2553
Payne JL. Antidepressant use in the postpartum period: practical considerations Am J Psychiatry. 2007 Sep; 164(9):1329–32

A 44-year-old woman presents with a general history of alcohol abuse and significant depressive and anxiety symptoms over 20 years. It is unclear whether the substance use was in response to the affective symptoms or if the affective symptoms were substance-induced. Which of the following procedures would help make this determination?

(A) Administer the MacAndrew Alcoholism Scale—Revised (MAC-R).
(B) Conduct a detailed mental status exam, focusing on form of thought.
(C) Draw a timeline of all substances used and all psychiatric symptoms.
(D) Measure the percent carbohydrate-deficient transferrin.
(E) Obtain serial urine toxicology tests.

The correct response is option **C**: Draw a timeline of all substances used and all psychiatric symptoms.

Plotting a life timeline of both substance use and psychiatric symptoms can help delineate the respective courses of substance-related and psychiatric symptomatology and any relationships between the two. The MacAndrew scale may help distinguish patients with substance abuse problems from those without, but is less reliable among psychiatric populations. The other options would provide information about more recent use or psychiatric status and so are unlikely to provide the desired historical clarification.

Practice Guideline for the Treatment of Patients with Substance Use Disorders, 2nd Edition in American Psychiatric Association Practice Guidelines for the Treatment of Psychiatric Disorders, Compendium 2006, Arlington VA, APA, 2006Section II.B., General Treatment Principles, Assessment http://www.psych.org/psych_pract/treatg/pg/SUD2ePG_04-28-06.pdf.

A depressed 62-year-old man being treated with an SSRI is admitted to the hospital with motoric immobility, posturing, grimacing, echolalia and echopraxia. Intravenous administration of lorazepam and amobarbital leads to no relief. Which of the following treatments should be considered?

(A) Add a second antidepressant.
(B) Begin a mood stabilizer.
(C) Initiate electroconvulsive therapy.
(D) Add dantrolene.
(E) Administer intravenous haloperidol.

The correct response is option **C**: Initiate electroconvulsive therapy.

Catatonic features may occur in the context of mood disorders and are characterized by at least two of the following manifestations: motoric immobility, as evidence by catalepsy or stupor; extreme agitation; extreme negativism; peculiarities of voluntary movement, as evidenced by posturing, stereotyped movements, mannerisms, or grimacing; and echolalia or echopraxia. When catatonia dominates the presentation, urgent biological treatment is indicated. Immediate relief may be obtained by intravenous benzodiazepines. Concurrent antidepressant mediation treatment should be considered. However, when relief is not immediately obtained, the urgent provision of electroconvulsive therapy is indicated.

American Psychiatric Association Practice Guideline for the Treatment of Patients with Major Depressive Disorder, 3rd ed (2010), http://www.psychiatryonline.com/pracGuide/pracGuideHome.aspx

Which of the following antidepressants is the best choice for a patient who wants to avoid orgasm dysfunction as a side effect?

(A) Bupropion
(B) Sertraline
(C) Venlafaxine
(D) Escitalopram
(E) Fluoxetine

The correct response is option **A**: Bupropion

In double-blind studies that specifically assessed sexual function, bupropion has been shown to have a more favorable sexual side effect profile than any of the other options.

Clayton AH, Croft HA, Horrigan JP, Wightman DS, Krishen A, Richard NE, Modell JH. Bupropion extended release compared with escitalopram: effects on sexual functioning and antidepressant efficacy in 2 randomized, double-blind, placebo- controlled studies. J Clin Psychiatry. 2006; 67:736–746

Modell JG, Katholi CR, Modell JD, DePalma RL. Comparative sexual side effects of bupropion, fluoxetine, paroxetine, and sertraline. Clin Pharmacol Ther. 1997; 61:476–487

Thase ME, Clayton AH, Haight BR, Thompson AH, Modell JG, Johnston JA. A double-blind comparison between bupropion XL and venlafaxine XR. J Clin Psychopharmacol. 2006; 26:482–488

A 20-year-old female college student presents to the counseling center with concerns about her alcohol use. She describes two occasions in the past year when she attended parties and had "way too much to drink." Following these occasions she feels "lousy," postpones studying, and then must stay up late to study for tests. When she's gone to most other parties she's had four or five drinks with no ill effects. There are no other substance-related symptoms. She expresses some concern about her drinking and asks for recommendations. The best intervention at this point would be to:

(A) provide a brief intervention.
(B) prescribe disulfiram.
(C) recommend attending Alcoholics Anonymous.
(D) prescribe naltrexone.
(E) prescribe acamprosate.

The correct response is option **A**: Provide a brief intervention.

Brief Intervention is the term used to describe a therapy delivered over one to three sessions, sometimes with telephone follow-up, that provides assessment of substance use, advice on reducing or stopping use and motivational feedback. Its efficacy has been demonstrated in a variety of treatment settings, including the primary care physician's office.

Prescribing medication or recommending attending Alcoholics Anonymous would be more appropriate for someone with a diagnosis of alcohol dependence rather than misuse. The patient is a heavy drinker and is at risk for developing a substance use disorder as well as other complications related to heavy alcohol use, so intervention is indicated.

American Psychiatric Association Practice Guideline for the Treatment of Patients with Substance Use Disorders, 2nd Edition (2006), http://psychiatryonline.com/pracGuide/pracGuideHome.aspx

Which of the following medications has the greatest body of evidence supporting its use as a monotherapy for acute bipolar depression?

(A) Bupropion
(B) Lamotrigine
(C) Valproate
(D) Olanzapine
(E) Quetiapine

The correct response is option **E**: Quetiapine

Quetiapine is FDA-approved as monotherapy for acute bipolar depression (both bipolar I and II). Olanzapine's effectiveness has been established only when combined with fluoxetine. None of the conventional antidepressants have been approved for this indication, and their usefulness remains a matter of debate. While lamotrigine is often rated high for this indication, most placebo-controlled studies have been negative. There have been no studies of adequate size to establish the value of valproate.

Thase ME, Macfadden W, Weisler RH, Chang W, Paulsson B, Khan A, Calabrese JR: Efficacy of quetiapine monotherapy in bipolar I and II depression: a double-blind, placebo-controlled study (The Bolder II Study). J Clin Psychopharmacol 2006; 26:600–609

Fountoulakis KN, Grunze H, Panagiotidis P, Kaprinis G: Treatment of bipolar depression: an update. J Affect Disord 2008; 109:21–34

Calabrese JR, Huffman RF, White RL, Edwards S, Thompson TR, Ascher JA, Monaghan ET, Leadbetter RA: Lamotrigine in the acute treatment of bipolar depression: results of five double-blind, placebo-controlled clinical trials. Bipolar Disord 2008; 10: 323–333

162

A patient reports feeling that he has always had to please others, and that, if he is not liked by everyone, he will never be successful. Which of the following statements would be characteristic of a cognitive behavioral approach to the patient's problem?

(A) "Let's draw out your circle of friends and examine which ones you feel you must please."
(B) "Feeling you must please others is acting more out of an emotional mind than a rational mind."
(C) "Tell me about your experience that you can only be successful by pleasing others."
(D) "Is it possible that feeling you're not being liked by everyone is a way to ease the pressure of having to be successful?"

The correct response is option **C**: "Tell me about your experience that you can only be successful by pleasing others?"

Option C attempts to elucidate maladaptive cognitions. Option A demonstrates one of the first techniques in interpersonal therapy. Emotional and rational mind are concepts of dialectical behavioral therapy. Option D starts to examine defense mechanisms, which is part of psychodynamic psychotherapy.

Hales RE, Yudofsky SC, Gabbard GO (eds): The American Psychiatric Publishing Textbook of Psychiatry, 5th ed, Arlington, VA, American Psychiatric Publishing Inc, 2008, pp 1176–1177, 1194, 1227

163

A 32-year-old woman presents with a history of frequent, unanticipated panic attacks. Which of the following medications is most likely to be of benefit for treating her disorder?

(A) Bupropion
(B) Aripiprazole
(C) Gabapentin
(D) Clonazepam
(E) Buspirone

The correct response is option **D**: Clonazepam

According to the APA Practice Guideline for the Treatment of Patients with Panic Disorder, "SSRIs, SNRIs, TCAs, and benzodiazepines appear roughly comparable in their efficacy. . ." Bupropion, gabapentin, and buspirone have not been found to be effective, and aripiprazole has not been studied adequately.

American Psychiatric Association Practice Guideline for the Treatment of Patients with Panic Disorder, 2nd ed., 2009, p11 http://psychiatryonline.com/pracGuide/PracGuideHome.aspx

164

Which of the following is the best established psychosocial intervention for the treatment of panic disorder?

(A) Dialectical behavioral therapy
(B) Interpersonal psychotherapy
(C) Psychodynamic psychotherapy
(D) Marital and family therapy
(E) Cognitive-behavioral therapy

The correct response is option **E**: Cognitive-behavioral therapy

Cognitive-behavioral therapy is the most widely studied and best validated psychosocial treatment for panic disorder. According to Roy-Byrne, et al., "two large meta-analyses reported large effect sizes of 1.55 (response of 63%) and 0.90." Unfortunately, as they point out, "Although the nature of the evidence is robust, such approaches are underused in the USA, compared with drug treatment." There are limited data suggesting that psychodynamic psychotherapy may be useful and less data supporting the use of family and marital therapy. Although exercise and psychoeducation may be of value for patients, there are slight data investigating the efficacy of either of these as a monotherapy.

Mitte K. A meta-analysis of the efficacy of psycho- and pharmacotherapy in panic disorder with and without agoraphobia. J Affect Disord 2005; 88:22–45

Roy-Byrne PP, Craske MG, Stein MG. Panic disorder. Lancet 2006; 368:1023–1032

American Psychiatric Association Practice Guideline for the Treatment of Patients With Panic Disorder, 2nd ed (2008). http://psychiatryonline.com/pracGuide/pracGuideHome.aspx

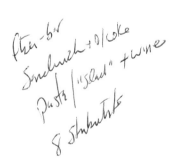

165

A patient with a history of substance dependence and depression treated with tranylcypromine presents to the emergency room with hypertension, tachycardia, chest pain and severe occipital headache. The patient says he had a relapse of his drug use. Which of the following substances is the most likely contributor to his clinical presentation at this time?

- (A) Vodka
- (B) Methamphetamine
- (C) PCP
- (D) Marijuana
- (E) Inhalants

The correct response is option **B**: Methamphetamine

While aged foods are commonly known to potentially cause hypertensive crisis with MAOI's, there are also several drugs which will also do this. These include ephedrine, pseudoephedrine, amphetamine, cocaine, guanethidine, methyldopa, reserpine, meperidine, and dextromethorphan.

Rapaport MH: Dietary restrictions and drug interactions with monoamine oxidase inhibitors: the state of the art. Journal of Clinical Psychiatry 2007; 68 Suppl 8:42–6

166

Trazodone exerts its hypnotic effects by interaction with which of the following neurotransmitter receptors?

- (A) Dopamine
- (B) GABA
- (C) Histamine
- (D) Alpha$_2$
- (E) Acetylcholine

The correct response is option **C**: Histamine

The sedation caused by trazodone is thought to be due to histamine$_1$ and alpha$_1$ receptors antagonism. Muscarinic cholinergic blockade can also lead to drowsiness, but trazodone does not have significant direct cholinergic effects. Dopamine interaction is not associated with sedation.

Stahl SM: Stahl's Essential Psychopharmacology, 3rd ed. New York, Cambridge University Press, 2008, pp 338–341, 845

167

Based on the results of Phase 1 of the Clinical Antipsychotic Trials of Intervention Effectiveness (CATIE) study, which of the following antipsychotic medications is most likely to be associated with the development of metabolic complications?

- (A) Olanzapine
- (B) Quetiapine
- (C) Risperidone
- (D) Ziprasidone
- (E) Perphenazine

The correct answer is option **A**: Olanzapine

During the CATIE study, olanzapine was associated with greater weight gain and increases in measures of glucose and lipid metabolism. Patients in the olanzapine group gained more weight than patients in any other group, with an average weight gain of 2 lb (0.9 kg) per month. Furthermore, 30% of patients in the olanzapine group gained 7% or more of their baseline body weight. Olanzapine use also was associated with greater increases in glycosylated hemoglobin, total cholesterol, and triglycerides even after adjustment for the duration of treatment in the study.

Buckley PF, Foster A, Miller B. Schizophrenia host vulnerability and risk of metabolic disturbance during treatment with antipsychotics. FOCUS: Schizophrenia. Spring 2008; 6(2):172–179.

Lieberman JA, Stroup TS, McEvoy JP, Swartz MS, Rosenheck RA, Perkins DO, Keefe RS, Davis SM, Davis CE, Lebowitz BD, Severe J, Hsiao JK. Clinical Antipsychotic Trials of Intervention Effectiveness (CATIE) Investigators. Effectiveness of antipsychotic drugs in patients with chronic schizophrenia. N Engl J Med. 2005; 353(12):1209–23.

Nasrallah HA. The roles of efficacy, safety, and tolerability in antipsychotic effectiveness: practical implications of the CATIE schizophrenia trial. J Clin Psychiatry. 2007; 68 Suppl 1:5–11.

168

Which of the following SSRIs is designated as FDA pregnancy category D?

(A) Fluoxetine
(B) Paroxetine
(C) Sertraline
(D) Citalopram
(E) Escitalopram

The correct response is option **B**: Paroxetine

All SSRIs are pregnancy category C with the exception of paroxetine, which has been associated with increased risk of fetal cardiovascular malformations, primarily VSDs and ASDs, when given during the first trimester.

Current Categories for Drug Use in Pregnancy

Category	Description
A	Adequate, well-controlled studies in pregnant women have not shown an increased risk of fetal abnormalities.
B	Animal studies have revealed no evidence of harm to the fetus, however, there are no adequate and well-controlled studies in pregnant women. or Animal studies have shown an adverse effect, but adequate and well-controlled studies in pregnant women have failed to demonstrate a risk to the fetus.
C	Animal studies have shown an adverse effect and there are no adequate and well-controlled studies in pregnant women. or No animal studies have been conducted and there are no adequate and well-controlled studies in pregnant women.
D	Studies, adequate well-controlled or observational, in pregnant women have demonstrated a risk to the fetus. However, the benefits of therapy may outweigh the potential risk.
X	Studies, adequate well-controlled or observational, in animals or pregnant women have demonstrated positive evidence of fetal abnormalities. The use of the product is contraindicated in women who are or may become pregnant.

U.S. Food and Drug Administration (FDA). FDA Advising of Risk of Birth Defects with Paxil. http://www.fda.gov/bbs/topics/NEWS/2005/NEW01270.html.

U.S. Food and Drug Administration (FDA), Pregnancy and Lactation Labeling http://www.fda.gov/cder/regulatory/pregnancy_labeling/default.htm

169

According to the National Comorbidity Survey (NCS), which of the following experiences is most frequently associated with PTSD in women in the U.S.?

(A) Being in a life-threatening accident
(B) Combat exposure
(C) Being involved in a natural disaster
(D) Sexual assault
(E) Witnessing someone being badly injured or killed

The correct response is option **D**: Sexual assault

In the NCS, which was carried out in the early 1990s, the most common stressor precipitants for women were sexual assault with physical attack, being threatened with a weapon, and childhood physical abuse, respectively. Combat exposure was the most common stressor for men. A recent review points out that PTSD lifetime prevalence in the NCS was twice as high in women as men and that combat exposure accounts for a significant proportion of PTSD in U.S. men. It also emphasizes that the main PTSD burden in the U.S. stems not from war but from criminal victimization, motor vehicle accidents, intimate partner violence, and childhood maltreatment. Women are more likely to have experienced sexual abuse, and men are more likely to have encountered physical violence, whether in the U.S. or while at war.

Hales RE, Yudofsky SC, Gabbard GO (eds): The American Psychiatric Publishing Textbook of Psychiatry, 5th ed. Washington, DC, American Psychiatric Publishing, Inc., 2008. pp 565–567

Kessler RC, Sonnega A, Bromet E, Hughes M, Nelson CB: Posttraumatic stress disorder in the National Comorbidity Survey. Arch Gen Psychiatry 1995; 52:1048–1060

Nemeroff CB, Bremner JD, Foa EB, Mayberg HS, North CS, Stein MB. Posttraumatic stress disorder: a state-of-the-science review. J Psychiatr Res. 2006; 40(1):1–21. Reprinted in FOCUS 2009; 7(2):254–273

170

The core techniques of open-ended questions, affirmation, reflective statements, and summary statements (OARS) are central to which one of the following therapies?

(A) Cognitive behavioral
(B) Interpersonal
(C) Motivational interviewing
(D) Twelve-step facilitation
(E) Prolonged exposure

The correct response is option **C**: Motivational interviewing

While some of these techniques may be used in a variety of psychotherapeutic modalities, together they represent the four core techniques, or "microskills," of motivational interviewing.

Galanter M, Kleber HD (eds): The American Psychiatric Publishing Textbook of Substance Abuse Treatment, 3rd ed. Washington DC, American Psychiatric Publishing Inc, 2004, pp 371–2

171

Which of the following is the most common sleep problem in persons with major depressive disorder?

(A) Vivid mood congruent dreams
(B) Hypersomnia
(C) Restless leg syndrome
(D) Insomnia
(E) Sleep phase disorder

The correct response is option **D**: Insomnia

The most common type of sleep disorder associated with depression is insomnia of some type – usually middle or late insomnia. Eighty percent of patients complain of insomnia while roughly 10 percent of depressed patients describe hypersomnia. Less frequently individuals will have initial insomnia, hypersomnia in the form of prolonged sleep episodes, or increased daytime sleepiness. Sleep studies in major depression have shown prolonged sleep latency, shortened total sleep, and increased arousals during the night. Slow wave sleep is usually reduced. Restless leg syndrome is usually associated with increased age and may be related to metabolic, vascular, and neurological causes.

American Psychiatric Association: Diagnostic and Statistical Manual of Mental Disorders, 4th Edition. Text Revision (DSM-IV-TR). Washington DC, American Psychiatric Association, 2000. p 350
Sadock BJ, Sadock VA, Ruiz P (eds): Kaplan & Sadock's Comprehensive Textbook of Psychiatry, 9th ed. Philadelphia, Lippincott Williams & Wilkins, 2009, pp 2152–53, 4047.

172

Which of the following psychotherapeutic techniques has the greatest body of evidence supporting it as a first line treatment for PTSD?

(A) Hypnosis
(B) EMDR (Eye Movement Desensitization and Reprocessing)
(C) Prolonged exposure therapy
(D) Stress inoculation training
(E) Systematic desensitization

The correct response is option **C**: Prolonged exposure therapy

Prolonged exposure therapy involves repeated exposure to the same traumatic memory over a series of sessions, and is considered a first-line treatment for PTSD. EMDR remains controversial, but has been shown in some studies to have benefits. Hypnosis has been used to induce relaxation to help with autonomic arousal symptoms. Stress inoculation training involves the combination of relaxation, elements of distraction, thought-stopping, and self-guided dialogue. Systematic desensitization is effective for a phobic anxiety associated with PTSD. Cognitive processing/restructuring, has been shown to have comparative effectiveness to prolonged exposure.

Hales RE, Yudofsky SC, Gabbard GO (eds): The American Psychiatric Textbook of Psychiatry, 5th ed. Washington, DC, American Psychiatric Publishing, Inc., 2008. pp 579-580
Nemeroff CB, Bremner JD, Foa EB, Mayberg HS, North CS, Stein MB. Posttraumatic stress disorder: a state-of-the-science review. J Psychiatr Res. 2006; 40(1):1–21. Reprinted in FOCUS 2009; 2:254–273
Foa EB. Psychosocial therapy for posttraumatic stress disorder. J Clin Psychiatry 2006; 67 Suppl 2:40–45

173

Which of the following is most characteristic of symptoms of PTSD?

(A) Persist long after the precipitating event is over
(B) Exist only while the trauma is present
(C) Directly proportional to the magnitude of the trauma
(D) Occur only in response to certain types of trauma
(E) Develop immediately upon experiencing the trauma

The correct response is option **A**: Persist long after the precipitating event is over

Posttraumatic stress disorder may persist for years after the stressful event. PTSD can develop in anyone exposed to a traumatic event and is not limited to veterans or certain types of trauma.

American Psychiatric Association: Diagnostic and Statistical Manual of Mental Disorders, 4th Edition. Text Revision (DSM-IVTR). Washington DC, American Psychiatric Association, 2000. pp 463–467.

174

A 38-year-old woman with a history of estrogen receptor-positive breast cancer is currently taking tamoxifen to reduce the risk of recurrence. However, she has become increasingly tearful, withdrawn, and anergic over the past month. She also notes difficulty with sleep and concentration as well as distressing hot flashes since initiating tamoxifen. Which one of the following medications is most appropriate to treat her symptoms?

  (A) Venlafaxine
  (B) Paroxetine
  (C) Gabapentin
  (D) Fluoxetine
  (E) Duloxetine

The correct response is option **A**: Venlafaxine

Potent CYP2D6 inhibitors should be avoided in women taking tamoxifen. Of the antidepressants listed, only venlafaxine does not inhibit CYP2D6. Gabapentin is not an appropriate treatment for depression.

Henry NL, Stearns V, Flockhart DA, Hayes DF, Riba M: Drug interactions and pharmacogenomics in the treatment of breast cancer and depression. Am J Psychiatry 2008; 165:1251–1255

175

In addition to time course, which of the following symptoms is more prominent in ASD compared to PTSD?

  (A) Impairment in functioning
  (B) Dissociative symptoms
  (C) Fear or helplessness response
  (D) Reexperiencing

The correct response is option **B**: Dissociative symptoms

Acute stress disorder is time limited up to one month after the precipitating event and features prominent dissociative symptoms. Both acute stress disorder and PTSD cause impairment in functioning and require a response of intense fear, helplessness or horror. Neither features psychotic symptoms. At least one of the symptoms from each of the cardinal symptom clusters of PTSD (reexperiencing, avoidance and hyperarousal) must be present in acute stress disorder. According to the APA practice guideline, to meet the diagnostic criteria for ASD, a patient must exhibit dissociative symptoms either during or immediately after the traumatic event. In PTSD, dissociative symptoms (e.g., inability to recall important aspects of the trauma) are not necessary to the diagnosis but are often observed.

American Psychiatric Association: Diagnostic and Statistical Manual of Mental Disorders, 4th Edition. Text Revision (DSM-IV TR). Washington DC, American Psychiatric Association, 2000. pp 469–471

Hales RE, Yudofsky SC, Gabbard GO (eds): The American Psychiatric Textbook of Psychiatry, 5th ed. Washington, DC. American Psychiatric Publishing, Inc., 2008. pp 565–567

176

Presence of which of the following symptoms is sufficient to meet DSM-IV-TR criteria for alcohol abuse?

    (A) A need to drink increasing amounts to become intoxicated
    (B) Continued use despite recurrent liver dysfunction
    (C) Repeatedly driving while intoxicated
    (D) Unsuccessful attempts to quit drinking
    (E) Consuming a greater amount of alcohol than planned

The correct response is option **C**: Repeatedly driving while intoxicated

A diagnosis of alcohol abuse requires presence of a maladaptive pattern of substance use leading to impairment plus at least one of the following within a 12 month period: failure to fulfill major role obligations due to substance use, use in physically hazardous situations (e.g., driving while intoxicated), recurrent substance-related legal problems, or substance use despite social or interpersonal problems. The remaining choices are symptoms of alcohol dependence.

Levine BH, Albucher RC. Patient management exercise for substance abuse. FOCUS: Substance Abuse, Spring 2007, p 180–181.

Diagnostic and Statistical Manual of Mental Disorders, Fourth Edition, Text Revision (DSM-IV-TR). Washington, DC, American Psychiatric Association, 2000, pp 197–9.

177

A psychiatrist is asked by the local school to consult on a 13-year-old boy who has exhibited problems with compulsive eating and failure to make academic progress. The boy's parents report that he has always eaten "everything in sight" and has been delayed in his development. Medical history is remarkable for poor muscle tone and failure to thrive as an infant. Physical examination reveals hypotonia, obesity, hypogonadism, a narrow-appearing forehead, downslanting palpebral fissures, small-appearing hands and feet and downturning of the corners of the mouth. Intelligence testing is consistent with mental retardation. What is the MOST LIKELY cause of the patient's signs and symptoms?

    (A) Childhood degenerative disorder
    (B) Congenital rubella infection
    (C) Homocystinuria
    (D) Prader-Willi syndrome
    (E) Tuberous sclerosis

The correct response is option **D**: Prader-Willi syndrome

Prader-Willi Syndrome is characterized by hypotonia, obesity, developmental and behavioral problems (including mental retardation), hyperphagia (typically after the first year of life), hypogonadism in males, and dysmorphic features, including a narrow-appearing forehead, downslanting palpebral fissures, small-appearing hands and feet, and downturning of the corners of the mouth. Children often present in the neonatal period with low muscle tone and failure to thrive. DNA analysis enables molecular confirmation of the diagnosis in most cases.

Essentials of Child and Adolescent Psychiatry, Dulcan MK, Wiener JM American Psychiatric Publishing, Inc., 2006, pp 129–130

Which of the following psychosocial treatments for social phobia has the most evidence supporting effectiveness?

(A) Cognitive-behavioral therapy
(B) Interpersonal psychotherapy
(C) Psychodynamic psychotherapy
(D) Family focused therapy
(E) Group psychoeducation

The correct response is option **A**: Cognitive-behavioral therapy

Several controlled studies have demonstrated the effectiveness of cognitive-behavioral therapy (CBT) for treatment social phobia. These have involved both individual and group CBT. A central feature of such treatments involves exposure to feared situations. There have been several small studies suggesting that IPT may be an effective treatment for social phobia. At this time there are no evidence supporting the efficacy of psychodynamic, family focused or group psychoeducation.

Foa EB. Social anxiety disorder treatments: psychosocial therapies. J Clin Psychiatry 2006; 67(suppl 12):27–30

Van Ameringen M, Allgulander C, Bandelow B, Greist JH, Hollander E, Montgomery SA, Nutt DJ, Okasha A, Pollack MH, Stein DJ, Swinson RP. WCA recommendations for the long-term treatment of social phobia. CNS Spectrums 2003; 8:40–52

Hales RE, Yudofsky SC, Gabbard GO (eds): The American Psychiatric Publishing Textbook of Psychiatry, 5th ed. Arlington, VA, American Psychiatric Publishing, Inc., 2008. p 544–5

A 62-year-old woman presents for assessment and treatment of a three year history of mild but persistent depressive symptoms. One year ago she was named board chairman of her association and also began a new relationship with a very wealthy individual. The relationship is going well emotionally and sexually, but she sometimes feels inadequate in her new social circles. She misses her former partner particularly when she feels socially awkward. After a discussion of treatment options for improving her overall level of functioning and self satisfaction, she and her psychiatrist decide upon a structured, time-limited course of interpersonal psychotherapy (IPT). Which ONE of the following would be the most appropriate focus of the IPT?

(A) Analysis of transference
(B) Delayed grief
(C) Interpersonal deficits
(D) Role dispute
(E) Role transition

The correct response is option **E**: Role transition

IPT focuses on the interpersonal rather than primarily on one's own psychology. Therefore, focusing on transference is not the vehicle of IPT. The remaining four options can be the focus in IPT; in this case role transition is the best answer because it aligns well with her main goal of treatment: functioning in her new role as board chairman, and in her new romantic relationship. Delayed grief might be a focus if that is what the patient were experiencing. She does not present with interpersonal deficits in the IPT sense.

Weissman, MM, Markowitz, JC, & Klerman, GL: Clinician's Quick Guide to Interpersonal Psychotherapy. New York, Oxford University Press, 2007. http://www.interpersonalpsychotherapy.org/

Markowitz JC: The clinical conduct of interpersonal psychotherapy. Focus 2006; 4(2): 179–84

Which of the following congenital abnormalities is associated with maternal use of carbamazepine in the first trimester of pregnancy?

(A) An increased risk of Ebstein's anomaly, the downward displacement of the tricuspid valve into the right ventricle and variable levels of right ventricular hyperplasia
(B) Craniofacial defects, fingernail hypoplasia, and developmental delay
(C) Fetal development of skin rash in a neonate who has antigen characteristics different from those of the mother
(D) Impaired temperature regulation and apnea

The correct response is option **B**: Craniofacial defects, fingernail hypoplasia, and developmental delay

In the first trimester of pregnancy carbamazepine is associated with craniofacial defects, fingernail hypoplasia, and developmental delay; lithium is associated with an increased risk of Ebstein's anomaly; valproate is associated with neural tube defects secondary to the failure of the neural tube to close, and lamotrigine is associated with fetal development of skin rash in a neonate who has antigen characteristics different from those of the mother. Benzodiazepines are only rarely associated with organ dysgenisis but have been associated with impaired temperature regulation, apnea, hypotonia, and lower Apgar scores at birth.

Yonkers KA, Wisner KL, Stowe Z, Leibenluft E, Cohen L, Miller L, Manber R, Viguera A, Suppes T, Altshuler L: Management of bipolar disorder during pregnancy and the postpartum period. Am J Psychiatry 2004; 161:608–20.
American Psychiatric Association Practice Guideline for the Treatment of Patients with Bipolar Disorder, 2nd ed (2002). Reprinted in FOCUS: Bipolar Disorder, Winter 2003; 1:75.

When initiating treatment with long-acting injectable haloperidol every 4 weeks, what period of time is required to reach steady-state?

(A) 4 weeks
(B) 8 weeks
(C) 12 weeks
(D) 16 weeks
(E) 20 weeks

The correct response is option **E**: 20 weeks

Five injection intervals are required to reach steady-state. Haloperidol is typically dosed every 4 weeks; it therefore takes 20 weeks to reach steady-state. Five half lives are required to reach steady state.

Hales RE, Yudofsky SC, Gabbard GO (eds): The American Psychiatric Publishing Textbook of Psychiatry, 5th ed. Washington DC; American Psychiatric Publishing Inc., 2008. p 1104

In addition to pharmacotherapy, psychotherapy plays an important role in treating bipolar disorder. Which ONE of the following circumstances best describes when cognitive behavioral therapy (CBT) is most effective in the adjunctive treatment of bipolar disorder?

(A) Acutely ill, depressed
(B) Acutely ill, manic
(C) After four or more episodes
(D) Moderately or acutely ill states
(E) Recovered from acute episode

The correct response is option **E**: Recovered from acute episode

Miklowitz (2008) reports on when and which types of psychotherapy are most useful in the adjunctive treatment of bipolar disorder. He reviewed 18 trials of individual and group psychoeducation, systematic care, family therapy, interpersonal therapy, and cognitive-behavioral therapy. Amongst his findings are that family therapy, interpersonal therapy, and systematic care were most effective in preventing recurrences when initiated after an acute episode; while cognitive behavioral therapy and group psychoeducation were most effective when initiated during a period of recovery. Psychotherapies that emphasize medication adherence and early recognition of mood symptoms have stronger effects on mania, while treatments that emphasize cognitive and interpersonal coping strategies have stronger effects on depression. He also cited a five-site U.K. study that showed CBT was effective in delaying recurrences among patients with fewer than 12 prior episodes.

Miklowitz DJ: Adjunctive psychotherapy for bipolar disorder: state of the evidence. Am J Psychiatry 2008; 165:1408–1419

Behavioral approaches such as the Semans pause maneuver, the start-stop method of Kaplan, and the pause-squeeze technique of Masters and Johnson have been employed to treat which of the following?

(A) Male erectile disorder
(B) Female sexual arousal disorder
(C) Premature ejaculation
(D) Hypoactive sexual desire disorder
(E) Female orgasmic disorder

The correct response is option **C**: Premature ejaculation

These behavioral techniques were developed to treat premature ejaculation, a condition considered to be the most prevalent sexual dysfunction in men. They would not be appropriate treatments for the other options.

Gabbard GO (ed), Gabbard's Treatment of Psychiatric Disorders, 4th ed., Washington, DC, American Psychiatric Press. 2007, pp 641–655

184

A 25-year-old man with no past history of abnormal involuntary movements is being treated with haloperidol. He should be evaluated for abnormal involuntary movements every

(A) 1 month
(B) 3 months
(C) 6 months
(D) 12 months
(E) 18 months

The correct response is option **C**: 6 months

Individuals taking first-generation (typical) neuroleptics are at increased risk for developing tardive dyskinesia. The APA Practice Guideline for Schizophrenia recommends: "Clinical assessment of abnormal involuntary movements every 6 months in patients taking first-generation antipsychotics and every 12 months in those taking second generation antipsychotics." In patients at increased risk, assessment should be done every 3 months and every 6 months with treatment using first- and second-generation antipsychotics, respectively. Patients at increased risk for developing abnormal involuntary movements include elderly patients and patients who experience acute dystonic reactions, other clinically significant extrapyramidal side effects, or akathisias."

American Psychiatric Association Practice Guideline for the Treatment of Patients with Schizophrenia, 2nd ed (2004), pp 586–7. http://www.psychiatryonline.com/pracGuide/pracGuideHome.aspx

185

A 19-year old private in the U.S. Army loses his left leg after his vehicle drives over an improvised explosive device. Two months later he reports ongoing recurrent and intrusive recollections of the event, nightmares and flashbacks to the explosion, avoidance of any activities that remind him of the event, irritability and disturbed sleep. Which of the following psychotherapeutic interventions is MOST likely to be effective in alleviating his symptoms?

(A) Biofeedback
(B) Eye movement desensitization and reprocessing
(C) Exposure-based cognitive-behavior therapy
(D) Guided imagery therapy
(E) Hypnotherapy

The correct response is option **C**: Exposure-based cognitive-behavior therapy

In response to increased attention on U.S. military veterans returning from combat in Iraq and Afghanistan, the Institute of Medicine reviewed and summarized the evidence supporting treatment for PTSD. The 2007 report recognizes that there is evidence for the pharmacological treatment of combat-related PTSD but states that this evidence is not as strong as the evidence for treatment of other trauma-related PTSD. In particular, the report states that large randomized controlled trials, considered a standard of evidence in other areas of medicine, are lacking from the evidence base. The report concludes that existing evidence is sufficient only to establish the efficacy of exposure-based psychotherapies in the treatment of PTSD.

Institute of Medicine (2007). Treatment of posttraumatic stress disorder: An assessment of the evidence. Washington DC: National Academy of Sciences. Available online at http://books.nap.edu/catalog.php?record_id=11955#toc

186

A 40-year-old patient is taking clozapine for treatment-resistant schizophrenia. Assuming no abnormal laboratory results, after what period of time could complete blood count monitoring be reduced to every four weeks?

(A) 3 months
(B) 6 months
(C) 12 months
(D) 18 months
(E) 24 months

The correct response is option **C**: 12 months

After initiating clozapine, weekly complete blood count (CBC) monitoring is required. If the WBC remains $3500/mm^3$ and the ANC $2000/mm^3$ during the first 6 months of therapy, then the monitoring frequency may be decreased to every 2 weeks. If the WBC remains $3500/mm^3$ and the ANC $2000/mm^3$ for another 6 months, then the monitoring frequency may be decreased to every 4 weeks.

According to the APA Practice Guideline for the Treatment of Patients with Schizophrenia, the risk of agranulocytosis (absolute neutrophil count $500/mm^3$) has been estimated at 1.3% of patients per year of treatment with clozapine. The risk is highest in the first 6 months of treatment. Weekly WBC and neutrophil monitoring is required. After 6 months, monitoring may occur every 2 weeks, as the risk of agranulocytosis appears to diminish. WBC counts must remain above $3000/mm^3$ during clozapine treatment, and absolute neutrophil counts must remain above $1500/mm^3$.

Clozaril® package insert, Novartis Pharmaceuticals Corporation, East Hanover, NJ, 2005 http://www.pharma.us.novartis.com/product/pi/pdf/Clozaril.pdf.

American Psychiatric Association Practice Guideline for the Treatment of Patients with Schizophrenia, 2nd ed (2004). pp 636 http://www.psychiatryonline.com/pracGuide/pracGuideHome.aspx.

187

For patients with functional gastrointestinal disorders, which of the following medications would be most likely to alleviate the visceral pain associated with irritable bowel syndrome?

(A) Bupropion
(B) Clonazepam
(C) Fluoxetine
(D) Quetiapine
(E) Amitriptyline

The correct response is option **E**: Amitriptyline

Patients with functional gastrointestinal disorders are frequently disabled by visceral pain. Antidepressants have been commonly used for this, and the analgesic properties appear to be independent of the antidepressant effect. Among the antidepressants, the ones that have dual actions on both serotonin and norepinephrine, such as the tricyclic antidepressants, appear to be the most effective in relieving the pain associated with functional gastrointestinal disorders. Amitriptyline is the best studied among them, however several others such as trimipramine and doxepin have also shown positive results. Desipramine has shown more equivocal results; this may be due to the drug's somewhat more selective affinity for norepinephrine reuptake. Studies with selective serotonin reuptake inhibitors have not been as positive (although some more recent data showed positive results for paroxetine), and bupropion generally has not been used in this context.

Jones MP, Crowell MD, Olden KW, Creed F. Functional gastrointestinal disorders: an update for the psychiatrist. Psychosomatics. 2007; 48(2):93–102

188

A 56-year old man with major depression is prescribed paroxetine. One month later, he complains of significant nausea. His dose is lowered from 20 to 10 mg, however he continues to feel nauseated. He is motivated to remain on the medication if possible since he feels it has been enormously helpful for his depression. A genotyping of the cytochrome P450 2D6 gene reveals that he has one inactive copy, and one partially inactive copy. Which of the following would be the most appropriate step to take?

(A) Discontinue paroxetine immediately and wait one month.
(B) Attempt even lower doses of paroxetine.
(C) Discontinue paroxetine and begin fluoxetine.
(D) Discontinue paroxetine and begin citalopram.
(E) Continue paroxetine but add ondansetron.

The correct response is option **B**: Attempt even lower doses of paroxetine.

Although not currently clinical standard practice to conduct genetic analysis, the CYP450 2D6 has particular clinical relevance; it is involved in the primary metabolism of more than 70 medications. The 2D6 gene, which codes for this enzyme, has a high degree of allelic variability, with more than 100 variations of the gene having been recorded. It is also unique in that multiple copies of the gene can occur on the same chromosome. Alleles are classified by their degree of activity, and the number of active alleles directly affects the enzymes' ability to metabolize substances. Individuals with at least 2 active copies are able to tolerate those medications metabolized by the enzyme at regular doses, those with 3 or more active copies are considered "ultra-rapid metabolizers" and may need higher doses of medication. Those with two inactive copies are considered to be poor metabolizers and may not be able to tolerate medications metabolized by this enzyme. However, there is an intermediate group of slow metabolizers who have one inactive copy of the allele and one partially inactive copy. These individuals may be able to tolerate 2D6 substrate medications but in lower than average doses; often the doses would be considered subtherapeutic in those with normal metabolism. In the case above, given the robust response to the medication, an attempt to continue the patient on paroxetine is indicated. Although ondansetron is effective for nausea, it would not be indicated here as it is also metabolized by 2D6. Should the patient fail a trial of paroxetine, duloxetine (which can be metabolized by other pathways if 2D6 is not available) and citalopram (which is not metabolized by this enzyme) would be reasonable alternatives.

Mrazek DA. Psychiatric pharmacogenomics. FOCUS 2006;4:339–343

de Leon J. AmpliChip CYP450 Test: personalized medicine has arrived in psychiatry. Expert Rev. Mol. Diagn 2006; 6:277–286.

189

Which symptom is characteristically seen in patients with Münchausen syndrome?

(A) Thoughts of death
(B) Pathological lying
(C) Fear of pain
(D) Perceptual disturbances
(E) Feelings of inadequacy

The correct response is option **B**: Pathological lying

Patients with Münchausen syndrome usually have a history of multiple hospitalizations, wandering from hospital to hospital (peregrination), and pathological lying (pseudologia fantastica, the telling of dramatic tales that merge truth and falsehood).

Hales RE, Yudofsky SC, Gabbard GO (eds): The American Psychiatric Publishing Textbook of Psychiatry, 5th ed. Washington, DC, American Psychiatric Publishing, Inc., 2008, p 429

190

A patient with bipolar disorder is receiving maintenance treatment with extended-release divalproex. How many hours should elapse between his last dose and drawing of the trough level of valproic acid?

(A) 4
(B) 8
(C) 12
(D) 18

The correct response is option **D**: 18.

A trough level of valproate occurs 21 to 24 hours after the last dose of the extended-release preparation. Blood drawn 12 to 15 hours later will have a concentration 18% to 25% higher than trough. It appears that samples drawn 18 to 21 hours later will deviate from trough by only 3% to 13%, which is felt to be clinically acceptable. In practice, giving this preparation as a single daily dose in the morning and having blood drawn prior to the next morning dose will result in consistent trough levels.

Reed RC, Dutta S: Does it really matter when a blood sample for valproic acid concentration is taken following once-daily administration of divalproex-ER? Ther Drug Monit 2006; 28:413–418

191

A woman presents for help in coping with stress. During the assessment, it becomes clear that she is excessively preoccupied with her appearance, particularly her face. She spends hours a day examining and caring for her face. She is convinced that her cheekbones are uneven and make her look like a freak. Her appearance is unremarkable. After the assessment is complete, the psychiatrist's best initial approach is to:

(A) reassure the patient about her appearance.
(B) agree that the situation is quite distressing.
(C) point out that her thinking is quite distorted.
(D) agree that her appearance is a problem.
(E) explain the benefits of medication.

The correct response is option **B**: Agree that the situation is quite distressing

Patients with body dysmorphic disorder tend to have difficulty acknowledging that they have a psychiatric disorder that needs treatment. The recommended initial steps in treatment are to empathize with the patient and engage them in treatment. At the same time it is important not to agree with the patient's view of her appearance.

Phillips KA, Hollander E. Treating body dysmorphic disorder with medication: evidence, misconceptions, and a suggested approach. Body Image. 2008; 5:16

Hales RE, Yudofsky SC, Gabbard GO (eds): The American Psychiatric Publishing Textbook of Psychiatry, 5th ed. Washington, DC, American Psychiatric Publishing, 2008, p 634

Phillips KA. Clinical features and treatment of body dysmorphic disorder. FOCUS. 2005; 2:179–183

192

Which of the following is a common symptom of seasonal affective disorder?

(A) Light sensitivity
(B) Somatic complaints
(C) Insomnia
(D) Overeating
(E) Impulsiveness

The correct response is option **D**: Overeating

The syndrome of seasonal affective disorder frequently has several atypical symptoms in common with atypical affective disorder; viz., hypersomnia, overeating, prominent anergy, weight gain, and a craving for carbohydrates.

American Psychiatric Association: Diagnostic and Statistical Manual of Mental Disorders. Text Revision (DSM-IV–TR), 4th Edition. Washington, DC; American Psychiatric Association, 2000. pp. 425–26

193

Which of the following techniques is commonly used in motivational interviewing?

(A) Confrontation
(B) Interpretation of transference
(C) Identification of cognitive distortions
(D) Decision balance
(E) Relaxation training

The correct response is option **D**: Decision balance

During the process of motivational interviewing, decision balance is used to help the patient increase self-awareness, self-efficacy, and the intention to change. Confrontation is to be avoided in motivational interviewing. Interpretation of transference is a technique of psychoanalysis, identification of cognitive distortions is a technique of cognitive therapy, and relaxation training is a technique used in behavior therapy.

Hales RE, Yudofsky SC, Gabbard GO (eds): The American Psychiatric Publishing Textbook of Psychiatry, 5th ed. Arlington VA, American Psychiatric Publishing Inc, 2003, pp 1267–8, 1160, 1230

Galanter M, Kleber HD (eds): The American Psychiatric Publishing Textbook of Substance Abuse Treatment, 4th ed. Arlington VA, American Psychiatric Publishing Inc, 2008, pp 353–4

194

Which of the following factors best differentiates acute stress disorder from PTSD?

(A) Chronicity
(B) Traumatic event severity
(C) Presence of nightmares
(D) Level of functional impairment
(E) Severity of subjective response to the event

The correct response is option **A**: Chronicity

DSM-IV-TR criteria require that the symptoms of PTSD must be present for more than one month. Acute stress disorder is distinguished from posttraumatic stress disorder because the symptom pattern in acute stress disorder must occur within four weeks of the traumatic event and resolve within that four-week period. If the symptoms persist for more than one month and meet criteria for posttraumatic stress disorder, the diagnosis is changed from acute stress disorder to posttraumatic stress disorder.

Diagnostic and Statistical Manual of Mental Disorders, Fourth Edition, Text Revision (DSM-IV-TR). Washington, DC, American Psychiatric Association, 2000, pp 467–8.

195

Which of the following best describes the mechanism of action of flumazenil in the treatment of benzodiazepine overdose?

(A) Flumazenil blocks benzodiazepines from crossing the blood-brain barrier.
(B) Flumazenil competes with benzodiazepines at central synaptic GABA receptor sites.
(C) Flumazenil decreases the influx of chloride ions into GABAergic neurons preventing hyperpolarization.
(D) Flumazenil increases the influx of sodium ions into GABAergic neurons causing depolarization.
(E) Flumazenil increases the rate of oxidative metabolism of benzodiazepines.

The correct response is option **B**: Flumazenil competes with benzodiazepines at central synaptic GABA receptor sites.

Flumazenil is a potent benzodiazepine-specific antagonist that competes at central synaptic GABA receptor sites in a dose-dependent manner.

Hales RE, Yudofsky SC: Substance use disorders in, The American Psychiatric Publishing Textbook of Clinical Psychiatry. Washington DC, American Psychiatric Publishing, 2003, pp 343–4.

196

A 22-year-old woman was involved in a severe motor vehicle accident in which several people were significantly injured. She had difficulty recalling portions of the accident, nightmares and difficulty falling asleep. She refused to drive her car, had difficulty concentrating and felt emotionally numb. She was unable to attend work. Her symptoms spontaneously resolved after a month and she was able to return to work. The most likely diagnosis is:

(A) acute stress disorder.
(B) adjustment disorder.
(C) posttraumatic stress disorder.
(D) panic disorder.
(E) brief psychotic disorder.

The correct response is option **A**: Acute stress disorder

The symptoms of acute stress disorder include marked symptoms of anxiety or increased arousal, difficulty sleeping, irritability, poor concentration, hypervigilance, exaggerated startle response and motor restlessness. Acute stress disorder occurs within four weeks of the traumatic event and resolves within four weeks.

American Psychiatric Association: Diagnostic and Statistical Manual of Mental Disorders, 4th Edition. Text Revision (DSM-IVTR). Washington DC, American Psychiatric Association, 2000. p 468.

197

Which of the following is the most common form of affective illness in families of patients with bipolar disorder?

(A) Bipolar disorder
(B) Unipolar depression
(C) Dysthymia
(D) Premenstrual dysphoric disorder
(E) Cyclothymia

The correct response is option **B**: Unipolar depression

Mood disorders have a strong genetic component, with the greater the presence in families, the greater the risk to the child. Bipolar disorder has a particularly high degree of familial association. Although a family history of bipolar disorder confers a greater risk of mood disorders on the child, it is unipolar, and not bipolar disorder (or any of the others listed), that is the most common mood disorder in families of bipolar patients.

Sadock BJ, Sadock VA (eds): Kaplan & Sadock's Synopsis of Psychiatry: Behavioral Sciences/Clinical Psychiatry, 10th ed. Philadelphia, Lippincott Williams & Wilkins, 2007, p 532.
Fanous AH, Kendler KS. Genetic heterogeneity, modifier genes, and quantitative phenotypes in psychiatric illness: Searching for a framework. Molecular Psychiatry 2005;10:6–13. Reprinted with permission in FOCUS 2006;4:423–430

198

The use of bright light treatment has been shown to be efficacious and safe for the treatment of:

(A) dysthymia.
(B) nonseasonal depression.
(C) bipolar disorder.
(D) PTSD.

The correct response is option **B**: Nonseasonal depression

A meta-analysis by Golden et al. found that bright light treatment and dawn simulation was efficacious for seasonal affective disorder and for non-seasonal depression, with effect sizes equivalent to those in most antidepressant pharmacotherapy trials. Bright light therapy has caused some patients with bipolar disorder to switch into mania, and is therefore contraindicated.

Golden RN, Bradley N, Gaynes R, Ekstrom D, Hamer RM, Jacobsen FM, Suppes T, Wisner KL, and Nemeroff CB. The efficacy of light therapy in the treatment of mood disorder: A review and meta-analysis of the evidence. Am J Psychiatry. Apr 2005; 162(4):656–662.

A 42-year-old woman is referred for a polysomnogram to evaluate her complaint of insomnia. During the polysomnogram, she seems to fall asleep within 15 minutes, and her EEG reflects normal sleep throughout the night. When she wakes in the morning in the sleep lab, she reports that she was awake most of the night. Which type of primary insomnia is this patient most likely to have?

- (A) Psychophysiological insomnia
- (B) Sleep state misperception
- (C) Idiopathic insomnia
- (D) Obstructive sleep apnea
- (E) Delayed sleep-phase syndrome

The correct response is option **B**: Sleep state misperception

Sleep state misperception involves dissociation between the subjective experience of sleep and the objective measure of sleep. Obstructive sleep apnea and delayed sleep-phase syndrome are not types of primary insomnia. Psychophysiological insomnia involves difficulty falling asleep, and idiopathic insomnia frequently involves sleep latency, decreased total sleep, or increased arousals.

Sadock BJ, Sadock VA (eds). Kaplan and Sadock's Comprehensive Textbook of Psychiatry, 8th ed. Philadelphia, Lippincott Williams & Wilkins, 2005, pp 2023–2024, 2027–2028

Which of the following is one of the standards used to determine mental capacity in decision making?

- (A) Absence of psychosis
- (B) Agreement with the medical recommendations
- (C) Severity of psychiatric illness
- (D) Rational decision making
- (E) Presence of abstract thought

The correct response is option **D**: Rational decision making

Case law and the literature generally describe four standards for determining mental capacity in decision making: communication of choice, understanding of relevant information provided, appreciation of available options and consequences, and rational decision making.

Simon RI. The law and psychiatry. FOCUS: Forensic and Ethical Issues; Fall 2003; 4:363–367.

Which of the following treatments has the best body of evidence in preventing post-stroke depression in older populations?

- (A) Escitalopram
- (B) Mianserin
- (C) Sertraline
- (D) Problem solving therapy
- (E) Cognitive behavioral therapy

The correct response is option **A**: Escitalopram

In a 2008 published double-blind placebo controlled trial of non-depressed patients in their 60s with recent stroke, escitalopram or problem-solving therapy administered for a year were less likely to develop depression than patients receiving placebo, however using an intention-to-treat conservative method of analyzing the data, problem-solving therapy was not significantly better than placebo whereas escitalopram continued to be superior to placebo. Studies using mianserin (not available in the U.S.) and sertraline to prevent post-stroke depression have been unsuccessful, as have studies with cognitive behavioral therapy.

Robinson RG, Jorge RE, Moser DJ, Acion L, Solodkin A, Small SL, Fonzetti P, Hegel M, Arndt S. Escitalopram and problem-solving therapy for prevention of poststroke depression: a randomized controlled trial. JAMA. 2008; 299(20): 2391–2400

Robinson RG, Jorge RE, Arndt S. Escitalopram, problem-solving therapy, and poststroke depression—reply. *JAMA.* 2008;300(15): 1758–1759.

A single mother reports that her 12-year-old child has become increasingly defiant with parental requests, at times becoming physically aggressive by kicking doors and hitting walls. She notes that the child does not exhibit these problems with the father. Which of the following is the most appropriate treatment?

(A) Inoculation techniques, such as boot camp
(B) Contingency management
(C) Medication management
(D) Send the child to live with the father temporarily
(E) Brief hospitalization

The correct response is option **B**: Contingency management

The child is displaying signs of oppositional defiant disorder (ODD). One of the most effective approaches to managing disruptive behavior associated with ODD is training parents to use contingency management techniques. Inoculation techniques, such as boot camp, have no evidence of efficacy and have been shown to be harmful in some cases. Medication management should not be used as the primary treatment for ODD. Sending the child to live with his father would provide no therapeutic benefit for the interactions between the child and his mother. Hospitalization at this time is unwarranted.

Steiner H, Remsing L (2007). Practice Parameter for the Assessment and Treatment of Children and Adolescents with Oppositional Defiant Disorder. J Am Acad Child Adolesc Psychiatry 46; 1:126–41

A 22-year-old man with chronic schizophrenia developed gynecomastia after being treated with risperidone for many months. His prolactin level is markedly elevated and you want to switch him to the antipsychotic drug that is less likely to cause this problem. Which one of the following would be the most appropriate choice?

(A) Aripiprazole
(B) Olanzapine
(C) Perphenazine
(D) Haloperidol
(E) Paliperidone

The correct response is option **A**: Aripiprazole

Dopamine release from the hypothalamus stimulates dopamine D_2 receptors in the anterior pituitary gland and has an inhibiting effect on prolactin secretion. Antipsychotic drug-induced hyperprolactinemia is due to blockade of D_2 receptors. Unlike the other options which block D_2 receptors, aripiprazole is a partial D_2 receptor agonist and it does not elevate serum prolactin levels.

Haddad PM, Wieck A: Antipsychotic-induced hyperprolactinaemia: mechanisms, clinical features and management. Drugs 2004; 64:2291–2314

Wood M, Reavill C: Aripiprazole acts as a selective dopamine D_2 receptor partial agonist. Expert Opin Investig Drugs 2007; 16: 771–775

204

A 70-year-old man presents to a clinic with progressive memory loss. Which of the following findings is most representative of cortical dementia in this patient?

(A) Apathy
(B) Aphasia
(C) Decreased attention
(D) Bradyphrenia
(E) Mood lability

The correct response is option **B**: Aphasia

Cortical dementias arise from disorders that affect the cerebral cortex (Alzheimer's, Creutzfeldt-Jakob). Cortical dementia is characterized by impairment in recall and recognition, language deficits including aphasia, apraxia, agnosia, and visuospatial deficits. In general, cortical dementias are not associated with prominent motor signs. Subcortical dementias are associated with greater impairment in recall memory, a decrease in verbal fluency without anomia, bradyphrenia (slowed thinking), depressed mood, affective lability, apathy, and decreased attention/concentration.

Sadock BJ, Sadock VA (eds): Kaplan and Sadock's Synopsis of Psychiatry: Behavioral Sciences/Clinical Psychiatry (Synopsis of Psychiatry), 10th ed. Philadelphia, Lippincott Williams and Wilkins, 2007. pp 1353

205

A psychiatrist is asked to determine if a very ill, delirious and possibly senile patient has the capacity to make a new will. Which of the following features must be present to determine that the patient has the capacity?

(A) Orientation to time and place
(B) Unimpaired attention span
(C) Awareness that she is making a will
(D) Choice of beneficiary that is not frivolous
(E) Ability to recognize family

The correct response is option **C**: Awareness that she is making a will

The capacity to make a will has the fewest cognitive requirements of any legal document. All that is needed is awareness that a will is being made, knowledge of who the rightful heirs should be and some idea of the value of the estate. Knowing who the rightful heirs should be does not mean that they must be named as the beneficiary. The patient could in fact choose a beneficiary that others might consider frivolous. Neither unimpaired orientation nor attention span is necessary if the patient can cooperate to the extent needed for the cognitive requirements. Even if the patient is delusional or hallucinating the will can be written, as long as the symptoms do not interfere with decision making as regards the will.

Rosner R, (Ed) Principles and Practice of Forensic Psychiatry, 2nd ed, London, Arnold, 2003 p 309.

206

Which of the following types of therapy used to treat schizophrenia is based on the premise that attempting to suppress or control mental events is NOT helpful?

(A) Traditional cognitive-behavioral therapy (CBT)
(B) Compliance therapy
(C) Acceptance and commitment therapy (ACT)
(D) Supportive psychotherapy
(E) Illness education

The correct response is option **C**: Acceptance and commitment therapy (ACT)

Acceptance and commitment therapy (ACT) is a variation of CBT originally developed for the treatment of nonpsychotic conditions. In contrast with traditional CBT, which aims to change the individual's cognitions and to facilitate the development of a more rational perspective, the goal in ACT is to modify the individual's relationship to his or her thinking more broadly. ACT is based on the premise that attempting to suppress or control mental events is not helpful and rather encourages persons to accept and to experience thoughts and feelings nonjudgmentally, or mindfully.

Dickerson FB, Lehman AF: Evidence-based psychotherapy for schizophrenia. J of Nervous & Mental Disease. 2006; 194:3–9

207

A 45-year-old patient requests a medication to treat symptoms consistent with generalized anxiety disorder. The patient has a history of heavy drinking. Which of the following medications would be most appropriate to prescribe?

(A) Clonazepam
(B) Bupropion
(C) Quetiapine
(D) Diazepam
(E) Venlafaxine

The correct response is option **E**: Venlafaxine

The most appropriate option is venlafaxine, which is an efficacious treatment for GAD. While benzodiazepines, such as clonazepam, alprazolam, and diazepam, are effective in treating generalized anxiety disorder (GAD), the risk of benzodiazepine abuse or dependence among alcohol abusers limits their utility. Bupropion is not generally considered to be a first-line treatment for GAD. Quetiapine is not an approved treatment for GAD.

Schatzberg AF, Nemeroff CB (eds): Essentials of Clinical Psychopharmacology, 2nd ed, Washington, DC, American Psychiatric Publishing, 2006, pp 141–4, 189, 542–5.

Tyrer T, Baldwin D. Generalized anxiety disorder. Lancet 2006; 368: 2156–2166.

Hoge EA, Oppenheimer JE, Simon NM: Generalized anxiety disorder. FOCUS: Anxiety Disorders, Summer 2004; 3:353–354.

208

A bus driver calls in sick whenever there is inclement weather such as rain or light snow. He has never had an accident while driving, nor does he know anyone personally who had an accident due to inclement weather. He also avoids driving his own car in poor weather and attempts to convince his family members to do the same. He admits he is very cautious about many things, which interferes with his sleep, causes fatigue, and makes him irritable. Which of the following is the most likely diagnosis?

    (A) Panic disorder
    (B) Social phobia: situational
    (C) Posttraumatic stress disorder
    (D) OCD
    (E) Generalized anxiety disorder

The correct response is option **E**: Generalized anxiety disorder

The bus driver's excessive concern about driving in inclement weather, as well as his worry over others driving under those conditions, plus his report that he is very cautious suggests that generalized anxiety disorder is the most likely choice. In addition, the report that he is cautious suggests there are other areas of his life in which he worries excessively. Insomnia, fatigue and irritability are also part of the diagnostic picture. Panic disorder with agoraphobia is unlikely because his worries are so generalized (a cautious man) with no history of panic attacks or evidence of typical agoraphobia. Similarly, social phobia is unlikely because his driving avoidance relates to weather and not meeting bus passengers. There is no evidence of a trauma that could explain his avoidance (PTSD). Finally, he reports no rituals and his worries, unlike many obsessions, are reasonable but excessive.

American Psychiatric Association: Diagnostic and Statistical Manual of Mental Disorders, 4th Edition. Text Revision (DSM-IVTR). Washington DC, American Psychiatric Association, 2000, pp 472–6.

209

A 20-year-old woman was brought to the emergency department by police after disrupting one of her university classes. She was agitated and demanded that her intellectual abilities be acknowledged. She had pressured speech and her affect alternated between periods of euphoria and irritability. Her roommate told the emergency staff that the patient had been very energetic, unable to sleep for several days and had previously been admitted to hospital for similar behavior. Which of the following diagnoses is most likely?

    (A) Delirium
    (B) Cyclothymia
    (C) Bipolar disorder, manic
    (D) Bipolar disorder, mixed state
    (E) Schizophrenia

The correct response is option **C**: Bipolar disorder, manic

Inflated self-esteem, grandiosity, decreased need for sleep, pressure of speech, flight of ideas, mood elevation, mood lability, irritability, and disinhibition are characteristic symptoms of acute mania. According to DSM-IV-TR, a mixed episode is defined by diagnostic criteria being met for both a manic episode and a major depressive episode nearly every day for at least a week.

American Psychiatric Association: Diagnostic and Statistical Manual of Mental Disorders, 4th Edition. Text Revision (DSM-IVTR). Washington DC, American Psychiatric Association, 2000.

210

Children and adolescents are considered a vulnerable population in the conduct of research because they:

    (A) cannot consent.
    (B) suffer more adverse effects.
    (C) are in riskier studies.
    (D) cannot assent.
    (E) do not benefit.

The correct response is option **A**: Cannot consent.

Children and adolescents are considered a vulnerable population in terms of research due to their inability to consent and the risk that they will be exploited. Children and adolescents are expected to give assent depending on their age and capabilities. Studies involving children and adolescents are not necessarily more risky and subjects do not necessarily suffer more adverse effects. Subjects may directly benefit depending on the study.

Levine RJ. Respect for children as research subjects, in Lewis' Comprehensive Textbook of Child and Adolescent Psychiatry. Martin A, Volkmar FR, eds. Philadelphia, Lippincott Williams & Wilkins, 2007. p 143.

A 53-year-old man presents asking for help with drinking. He reports frequent swelling of his ankles and says that when he goes to the corner store, he has to walk slowly or he'll get too short of breath. He says he's supposed to be taking "some heart pills," but hasn't had any for a number of months and can't remember their names. He has attempted to quit drinking on two prior occasions and was treated with diazepam for "the shakes." He has been drinking one to two pints of rum daily for the past 10 months. His last drink was several hours ago. What would be the most appropriate initial referral?

(A) Medical hospitalization
(B) Partial hospitalization program
(C) Intensive outpatient program
(D) Office-based program
(E) Therapeutic community

The correct response is option **A**: Medical hospitalization

The patient's physical symptoms and history are strongly suggestive of significant untreated cardiac disease. His history also suggests that with continued abstinence he will go through alcohol withdrawal. His initial treatment should be in a setting where he can be closely medically monitored and his heart disease treated as needed.

Mee-Lee D, Shulman G, Fishman M, et al. (eds): ASAM Patient Placement Criteria for the Treatment of Substance-Related Disorders, 2nd ed, revised. Chevy Chase, MD, American Society of Addiction Medicine, 2001.

A 46-year-old man is begun on citalopram 20 mg daily for a major depressive episode. After four weeks he returns to his psychiatrist citing little if any change in his symptoms. Which of the following would be the most appropriate next step in the patient's treatment?

(A) Increase the patient to 40 mg of citalopram.
(B) Discontinue citalopram and begin venlafaxine.
(C) Continue citalopram but add lithium.
(D) Begin vagal nerve stimulation.
(E) Continue citalopram and begin aripiprazole.

The correct response is option **A**: Increase the patient to 40 mg of citalopram.

The management of "difficult to treat" depression remains a challenge, with various strategies suggested, including switching to different antidepressants, augmenting with various medications, and non-pharmacological treatments such as electroconvulsive therapy and vagal nerve stimulation. Before such approaches are considered, however, one wants to make sure that the patient has had an adequate trial of their initial antidepressant, defined as a sufficient dose for a sufficient duration. In the STAR*D trial, the mean dose of citalopram needed for remission was 40 mg. Similarly, of the patients in STAR*D who remitted while taking citalopram, only 30% responded within 4 weeks and another 30% who remitted did not do so until 10 weeks or more. In general, if no improvement in depressive symptoms is seen on an SSRI after 4 weeks, a trial of a higher dose may be warranted. However, higher doses tend not to be more effective than standard doses.

Zisook S: Ask the Expert: Psychopharmacology: major depressive disorder. FOCUS 2006;4:484–486
Yudofsky SC, Hales RE (eds): The American Psychiatric Publishing Textbook of Neuropsychiatry and Behavioral Sciences, 5th ed. Arlington VA, American Psychiatric Publishing Inc, 2008, pp 1058–1061

213

Which of the following features would be most predictive of a favorable response to lithium maintenance in bipolar disorder?

(A) Euthymic intervals
(B) Rapid cycling
(C) Mixed episodes
(D) Substance abuse
(E) Psychosis

The correct response is option **A**: Euthymic intervals

Features predictive of a good response to lithium include euphoric mania, full interepisode remission (euthymia), the absence of comorbidity, few lifetime episodes, the absence of rapid cycling, and a mania-depression-euthymia sequence of clinical course.

Jefferson JW, Greist JH: Lithium, in Kaplan & Sadock's Comprehensive Textbook of Psychiatry, 9th ed. Edited by Sadock BJ, Sadock VA, Ruiz P. Philadelphia, Lippincott Williams & Wilkins, 2009, pp 3132–45.

Grof P: Responders to long-term lithium treatment, in Lithium in Neuropsychiatry: The Comprehensive Guide. Edited by Bauer M, Grof P, Müller-Oerlinghausen B Abingdon, UK, Informa Healthcare, 2006, pp 157–178.

214

Which of the following medications has shown the most evidence for reducing suicide risk in the long-term treatment of bipolar disorder?

(A) Carbamazepine
(B) Divalproex
(C) Gabapentin
(D) Lithium
(E) Olanzapine

The correct response is option **D**: Lithium

Lithium has more research evidence than any other anitmanic agent regarding its effect on reducing suicide and suicidal acts during long-term treatment of bipolar disorder. Lithium has been shown to be more effective than any other antimanic agent in reducing suicide risk. Patients treated with other antimanic agents likely have lower suicide risk than bipolar persons not medicated at all.

Tondo L, Isacsson G, Baldessarini RJ: Suicidal behavior in bipolar disorder: risk and prevention. CNS Drugs 2003; 17:491–511.

Goodwin FK, Fireman B, Simon GE, Hunkeler EM, Lee J, Revicki D: Suicide risk in bipolar disorder during treatment with lithium and divalproex. JAMA 2003; 290:1467–1473.

Cipriani A, Pretty H, Hawton K, Geddes JR. Lithium in the prevention of suicidal behavior and all-cause mortality in patients with mood disorders: A systematic review of randomized trials. Am J Psychiatry, Oct 2005; 162:1805–1819.

215

A 56-year-old man with a history of cancer presents with confusion, pure amnestic syndrome, and affective symptoms. Diagnostic studies are consistent with paraneoplastic limbic encephalitis. Which of the following cancers is the most common cause of this paraneoplastic syndrome?

(A) Pancreatic cancer
(B) Prostate cancer
(C) Renal cancer
(D) Small cell lung cancer
(E) Testicular cancer

The correct response is option **D**: Small cell lung cancer

Paraneoplastic "limbic encephalitis" results from an immunological cross-reaction between tumor antigens and antigens within the CNS. It can cause a range of psychiatric presentations including cognitive deficits, confusional states, a pure amnestic syndrome, and affective symptoms. Small cell carcinoma of the lung is the most common cause of paraneoplastic syndrome.

Levenson JL (ed): Essentials of Psychosomatic Medicine. American Psychiatric Publishing, Inc., Washington, DC, 2007. p 323

216

A 24-year-old man on lithium maintenance therapy develops severe, persistent polyuria and polydipsia. Which of the following medications is most likely to be effective in treating these side effects without requiring administration of supplemental electrolytes?

(A) Amiloride
(B) Furosemide
(C) Hydrochlorothiazide
(D) Metolazone
(E) Torsemide

The correct response is option **A**: Amiloride

The most common renal effect of lithium is impaired concentrating capacity caused by reduced renal response to ADH, manifested as polyuria, polydipsia, or both. Although the polyuria associated with early lithium treatment may resolve, persistent polyuria may occur. Concurrent administration of a thiazide diuretic such as hydrochlorothiazide may be helpful. However, potassium levels must be monitored, and potassium replacement may be necessary. Amiloride, a potassium-sparing diuretic, is reported to be effective in treating lithium-induced polyuria and polydipsia. Its advantages are that it does not alter lithium levels and does not require administration of supplemental potassium.

American Psychiatric Association Practice Guideline for the Treatment of Patients with Bipolar Disorder, 2nd Edition (2002). Reprinted in FOCUS: Bipolar Disorder, 2003; 1:81–82. http://psychiatryonline.com/pracGuide/pracGuideHome.aspx.

217

A 17-year-old patient diagnosed with anorexia nervosa at age 14 is brought to a psychiatrist by her parents. They are concerned because she is 65% of her expected body weight. The most appropriate intervention is to:

    (A) suggest a group therapy program.
    (B) initiate treatment with an antidepressant.
    (C) restore the patient's nutritional state.
    (D) refer the patient and family for counseling.
    (E) provide cognitive therapy.

The correct response is option **C**: Restore the patient's nutritional state.

The immediate aim of treatment should be to restore the patient's nutritional state to normal. Emaciation can cause irritability, depression, preoccupation with food, and sleep disturbance. It is exceedingly difficult to achieve behavioral change with psychotherapy in a patient who is experiencing the psychological effects of emaciation.

Hales RE, Yudofsky SC, Gabbard GO (eds): The American Psychiatric Publishing Textbook of Psychiatry, 5th ed. Washington, DC, American Psychiatric Publishing, Inc., 2008. p 980

218

According to the results of the Clinical Antipsychotic Trials of Intervention Effectiveness (CATIE) study, which antipsychotic medication had the lowest all-cause discontinuation rate?

    (A) Olanzapine
    (B) Quetiapine
    (C) Risperidone
    (D) Ziprasidone
    (E) Perphanazine

The correct response is option **A**: Olanzapine

The most prominent finding of the CATIE study was the 74% all-cause discontinuation rate before 18 months. The causes for discontinuation included lack of tolerability, lack of efficacy, clinician decision (due to safety concerns) and patient decision (electing to terminate). Among the atypical antipsychotics, the time to discontinuation was significantly longer for patients treated with olanzapine compared to those on risperidone and quetiapine, but not compared to those on perphanazine or ziprasidone. In addition, completion rates for the 18 month study were olanzapine 36%, perphanazine 25%, quetiapine 18%, risperidone 26%, ziprasidone 21%.

Lieberman JA, Stroup TS, McEvoy JP, Swartz MS, Rosenheck RA, Perkins DO, Keefe RSE, Davis SM, Davis CD, Lebowitz BD, Severe J, Hsiao JK. Effectiveness of antipsychotic drugs in patients with chronic schizophrenia. N Engl J Med. 2005; 353:1209–23.

219

Which of the following medication combinations for individuals with OCD comorbid with tic disorder is supported best by evidence?

    (A) Fluoxetine plus clonazepam
    (B) Sertraline plus buspirone
    (C) Nefazodone plus naltrexone
    (D) Fluvoxamine plus haloperidol

The correct response is option **D**: Fluvoxamine plus haloperidol

Evidence indicates that individuals with OCD and comorbid tic disorder respond better to fluvoxamine plus haloperidol. While SSRI's are typical first-line treatments for OCD, clonazepam has not consistently demonstrated effectiveness for OCD, nor for OCD with a tic disorder. The combination of clomipramine and risperidone can be helpful in treating difficult cases of OCD, but it is not as effective as an SSRI plus haloperidol for OCD comorbid with a tic disorder.

Fineberg NA, Gale TM, Sivakumaran T. A review of antipsychotics in the treatment of obsessive compulsive disorder. J Psychopharmacology 2006; 20:97–103. Reprinted in FOCUS: OCD summer 2007 3:

Hales RE, Yudofsky SC, Gabbard GO (eds): The American Psychiatric Publishing Textbook of Psychiatry, 5th ed. Arlington, VA, American Psychiatric Publishing, 2008, pp 558–63.

Schatzberg AF, Nemeroff CB (eds): Essentials of Clinical Psychopharmacology, 2nd ed, Washington, DC, American Psychiatric Publishing, 2006, p 536.

Geller DA, Biederman J, Stewart SE, et al. Which SSRI? A meta-analysis of pharmacotherapy trials in pediatric obsessivecompulsive disorder. Am J Psychiatry 2003; 160:1919–1928.

220

Studies of the neurobiological correlates of borderline personality disorder have revealed hyperactivity in which one of the following?

(A) Amygdala
(B) Prefrontal cortex
(C) Tegmental area
(D) Cingulate
(E) Accumbens

The correct response is option **A**: Amygdala

The amygdala, prefrontal and preorbital cortex, and the anterior cingulate have all been implicated in the neurobiology of borderline personality disorder. Specifically, the prefrontal cortex and anterior cingulate are hypoactive, whereas the amygdala is hyperactive, in borderline personality disorder. The ventral tegmental area and the nucleus accumbens have not been clearly linked to borderline personality disorder.

Kernberg OF, Michels R: Borderline personality disorder. Am J Psychiatry. 2009; 166:505–8.

221

A 38-year-old patient with major depressive disorder has had a partial response to 80 mgs of citalopram. He states this is the best drug that he has been on, but continues to experience symptoms despite being on the medication for 7 weeks. He continues to occasionally have suicidal thoughts which frighten him because he made a suicide attempt 4 years ago. The best intervention at this time is to augment with:

(A) fluoxetine.
(B) lamotrigine.
(C) lithium.
(D) thyroid.
(E) buspirone.

The correct response is option **C**: Lithium

The choice of lithium is best for 2 reasons; it has the best data as being an effective augmentation drug and it lowers the risk of suicide. Lamotrigine and thyroid are used for augmentation, but the data supporting this use is not as strong as that for lithium and there is no data on their impact on suicide. Buspirone is a possibility, but lithium is a better choice for the reasons listed above. There is no reason to augment with a second SSRI (fluoxetine) because the serotonin transporters are already inhibited by citalopram.

American Psychiatric Association Practice Guideline for the Treatment of Patients with Major Depressive Disorder, 3rd ed (2010), http://psychiatryonline.com/pracGuide/pracGuideHome.aspx
American Psychiatric Association Practice Guideline for the Treatment of Patients with Suicidal Behaviors, 2nd ed (2000), pp 1375 http://www.psychiatryonline.com/pracGuide/pracGuideHome.aspx

Which of the following medications for bipolar disorder has been associated with polycystic ovarian syndrome (PCOS)?

(A) Topiramate
(B) Divalproex
(C) Carbamazepine
(D) Lamotrigine
(E) Lithium

The correct response is option **B**: Divalproex

In the Systematic Treatment Enhancement Program for Bipolar Disorder (STEP-BD), 230 women ages 18–45 were evaluated for PCOS. Oligoamenorrhea with hyperandrogenism developed in 10.5% of women on valproate compared to 1.4% of women on lithium or a non-valproate anticonvulsant. Oligoamenorrhea always had its onset during the first year of valproate therapy. While not all studies have found such an association, divalproex (valproate) is the only drug of those listed above that has been linked to PCOS.

Joffe H, Cohen LS, Suppes T, McLaughlin WL, Lavori P, Adams JM, Hwang CH, Hall JE, Sachs GS: Valproate is associated with new-onset oligoamenorrhea with hyperandrogenism in women with bipolar disorder. Biol Psychiatry 2006; 59:1078–1086.

Rasgon N: The relationship between polycystic ovary syndrome and antiepileptic drugs: a review of the evidence. J Clin Psychopharmacol 2004; 24:322–334.

The parents of a 4-year-old boy report that a few hours after he goes to sleep, their son will suddenly get up in the bed and look extremely frightened. His heart races; he is diaphoretic and cries out. He is difficult to awaken and has no recall for the event the next morning. Which of the following is the most appropriate next step in the management of this patient?

(A) Administer a short-acting hypnotic for two weeks.
(B) Have the child go to bed at a later time.
(C) Obtain an electroencephalogram to rule out temporal lobe epilepsy.
(D) Reassure the parents that their son will outgrow the disorder.
(E) Suggest to the parents that they allow their son to sleep with them for a temporary period.

The correct response is option **D**: Reassure the parents that their son will outgrow the disorder.

The patient presents with classic symptoms of night terror. These occur during stage 3 and 4 of non-REM sleep, so are not associated with nightmares. Because the child is in deep sleep, he will be difficult to arouse and have no recall of a bad dream. The episodes tend to occur during the first third of the night when individuals are most likely to be in stage 3 or 4 of non-REM sleep. Occurrence usually is in childhood. If onset is later, such as adolescence, it may be prudent to obtain an electroencephalogram to rule out temporal lobe epilepsy. This is usually a self-limiting disorder which children outgrow. So, the next best step is to reassure the parents. Rarely is there a need to administer a hypnotic.

Saddock BJ, Saddock VA. Pocket Handbook of Clinical Psychiatry. 4th ed. Philadelphia, PA. Lippincott Williams and Wilkins, 2005. pp 243–244

224

A 68-year-old woman being treated for bipolar disorder became semi-comatose and incontinent of urine. Her serum sodium concentration was 110 mmol/L. Which of the following medications is the most likely cause?

(A) Lithium
(B) Divalproex
(C) Oxcarbazepine
(D) Lamotrigine
(E) Olanzapine

The correct response is option **C**: Oxcarbazepine

Dong and colleagues found that the frequency of hyponatremia (NA≤134) was 29.9% among 97 oxcarbazepine-treated patients having severe (NA≤128) hyponatremia. Hyponatremia was much more likely in patients over 40 years of age and in patients treated simultaneously with levetiracetam. Patients whose sodium levels were low at their initial visit after starting oxcarbazepine were much more likely than patients with normal sodium at the initial visit to have persistent hyponatremia.

Dong X, Leppik IE, White J, Rarick J: Hyponatremia from oxcarbazepine and carbamazepine. Neurology 2005; 65:1976–1978.

Sachdeo RC, Wasserstein A, Mesenbrink PJ, D'Souza J: Effects of oxcarbazepine on sodium concentration and water handling. Ann Neurol 2002; 51:613–620.

225

In bipolar disorder, which of the following characteristics BEST differentiates adultonset bipolar disorder from childhood-onset?

(A) Presence of psychotic features
(B) Prolonged early course
(C) Mixed episodes
(D) Recurrent depression
(E) Treatment resistance

The correct response is option **D**: Recurrent depression

Patients with childhood-onset bipolar disorder are more likely to have psychotic features; have a more severe course of illness; be male; have a co-morbid substance abuse disorder; experience fewer remissions; have manic and mixed episodes; have a more prolonged early course; and be treatment resistant. Patients with adult-onset bipolar disorder are more likely to experience recurrent episodes of depression.

Dulcan MK, Weiner JM. Essentials of Child and Adolescent Psychiatry. Arlington (VA): American Psychiatric Publishing, Inc., 2006. pp 273–274

226

A psychiatrist's neighbor tells her that he is having trouble sleeping due to work related stresses. He asks for recommendations and some medication until he can get an appointment with his internist. What ethical problem results if the psychiatrist gives the neighbor the medication?

(A) Prescribing medication creates a doctor-patient relationship.
(B) The assistance may be ineffective, straining the relationship.
(C) Providing free care can foster resentment.
(D) Assisting this neighbor creates an expectation that the psychiatrist will treat other neighbors.

The correct response is option **A**: Prescribing medication creates a doctor patient relationship.

Giving advice and medication may create a doctor patient relationship with an associated expectation of duty of care.

Simon RI. Quick reference for forensic and ethical issues in psychiatry, FOCUS: Forensic and Ethical Issues; Fall 2003; 4:345.

227

A local radio talk show host comes to see you for psychotherapy because you were described as "the best doctor at the clinic" by one of his friends. He spends most of the hour talking about problems he is having with a workmate who he feels is treating him rudely. At the end of the session he asks to be seen at a special time to accommodate his work schedule. When you tell him you will be unavailable at that time, he becomes dismissive and angry. These traits are suggestive of which ONE of the following:

(A) Schizoid
(B) Antisocial
(C) Obsessive-compulsive
(D) Narcissistic
(E) Borderline

The correct response is option **D**: Narcissistic

Criteria for narcissistic personality disorder can include having a grandiose sense of self-importance, believing that one is special and can only be understood by other special people, and a sense of entitlement including unreasonable expectations of favorable treatment.

Diagnostic and Statistical Manual of Mental Disorders, Fourth Edition, Text Revision (DSM-IV-TR). Washington, DC, American Psychiatric Association, 2000, pp 714–717.

228

A 14-year-old patient with anorexia nervosa has achieved a stable weight and nutritional status. Which of the following interventions has the MOST evidence demonstrating effectiveness in the treatment of this disorder?

(A) Family based therapies
(B) Fluoxetine
(C) Individual cognitive behavioral therapy
(D) Individual interpersonal psychotherapy
(E) Olanzapine

The correct response is option **A**: Family based therapies

Family based interventions have demonstrated effectiveness in treating adolescents with anorexia nervosa and bulimia nervosa. The other interventions may be helpful in individual cases but have not demonstrated systematic effectiveness in adolescents. Controlled trials suggest that family treatment is the most effective intervention. For patients who initially lack motivation, awareness and desire for recovery may be increased by psychotherapeutic techniques based on motivational enhancement, although solid evidence for this is lacking.

American Psychiatric Association Practice Guideline for the Treatment of Patients with Eating Disorders, 3rd ed. (2005), p 1110 http://www.psychiatryonline.com/pracGuide/pracGuideHome.aspx
Bulik CM, Berkman ND, Brownley KA, Sedway JA, Lohr KN. Anorexia nervosa treatment: a systematic review of randomized controlled trials. International Journal of Eating Disorders. 40(4): 310–20, 2007 May 40:310–20

229

Which of the following traumatic events is MOST likely to induce PTSD in exposed individuals?

(A) Unexpected death
(B) Natural disasters
(C) Motor vehicle accidents
(D) Witness to violence
(E) Sexual assault

The correct response is option **E**: Sexual assault

Individuals exposed to interpersonal violence tend to have higher rates of PTSD. While PTSD can occur after any type of trauma, some types of trauma are more likely to be problematic.

American Psychiatric Association Practice Guideline for the Treatment of Patients with Acute Stress Disorder and Posttraumatic Stress Disorder. Am J Psychiatry. 2004; 161(11):48 http://www.psychiatryonline.com/pracGuide/pracGuideTopic_11.aspx

230

A 9-year-old boy is brought by his mother at the insistence of the school for the assessment of behavior problems. The diagnosis of attention-deficit/hyperactivity disorder is made, along with the recommendation to start stimulant medication. The mother is concerned that stimulant medication might put her son at risk for developing substance use problems. Regarding the risk of developing substance use problems, what is known about stimulant treatment for ADHD?

(A) Increased risk of drug dependence only
(B) Increased risk of both alcohol and drug dependence
(C) Decreased risk of drug dependence only
(D) Decreased risk of both alcohol and drug dependence
(E) Unchanged risk for both alcohol and drug dependence

The correct response is option **D**: Decreased risk of both alcohol and drug dependence

Treatment of childhood ADHD with psychostimulant medication reduces the risk of both alcohol and drug use disorders during adolescence and adulthood. Individuals with untreated ADHD are at greater risk for developing substance use disorders.

Wilens TE, Faraone SV, Biederman J, et al.: Does stimulant therapy of attention-deficit/hyperactivity disorder beget later substance abuse? A meta-analytic review of the literature. Pediatrics 2003; 111:179–85.
Biederman J, Wilens T, Mick E, et al.: Is ADHD a risk factor for psychoactive substance use disorders? Findings from a four-year prospective follow-up study. J Am Acad Child Adolesc Psychiatry 1997; 36:21–29. Reprinted in FOCUS: Substance Related Disorders; Spring 2003.; 2:96–204.

231

Which of the following disorders must be considered in the differential diagnosis of individuals with late onset obsessive-compulsive disorder (after the age of 45 years)?

(A) Huntington's disease
(B) Asperger's syndrome
(C) Delusional disorder
(D) Body dysmorphic disorder
(E) Schizophrenia

The correct response is option **A**: Huntington's disease

Individuals diagnosed with OCD after the age of 45 years (late onset) should specifically be evaluated for neurodegenerative illnesses (e.g., Huntington's disease), traumatic injury or neoplastic and vascular causes. The other answers should be considered at any age at onset.

Martis B, Keuthen NJ, Wilson KA, Jenike M. Obsessive-compulsive disorder, in Clinical Manual of Anxiety Disorders. Edited by Stein DJ. American Psychiatric Publishing Inc, Washington DC, 2004, p 94.

232

A psychiatrist has been seeing a terminally ill woman in psychotherapy. The patient has become too ill to come to the office so the psychiatrist elects to make a house call. In committing this boundary crossing, he should:

(A) act in a more social manner.
(B) discuss this variation from usual practice with a lawyer before going.
(C) discuss the implications of this change of venue with the patient.
(D) never go to the patient's home.

The correct response is option **C**: Discuss the implications of this change of venue with the patient.

The psychiatrist should act professionally, discuss the situation with his patient, and document the discussion.

Gutheil TG. Boundary issues in: American Psychiatric Publishing Textbook of Personality Disorders, edited by Oldham J, Skodol AE, Bender DS. American Psychiatric Publishing, 2005, p 428.

233

Which of the following is the most common psychiatric symptom found in patients with fibromyalgia?

(A) Anorexia
(B) Psychosis
(C) Hypersomnia
(D) Mania
(E) Depression

The correct response is option **E**: Depression

Patients with fibromyalgia commonly have depression, anxiety and insomnia. Individuals with this disorder also tend to have a family or prior history of depression and antidepressant use.

Arnold LM. Management of fibromyalgia and comorbid psychiatric disorders. J Clin Psychiatry. 2008; 69(supplement 2):14

234

Which type of treatment program has the best short-term outcomes for cocaine dependence?

(A) Voucher-based contingency management
(B) Psychodynamic group psychotherapy
(C) Interpersonal psychotherapy
(D) Twelve-step groups (without other counseling)
(E) Cue exposure therapy

The correct response is option **A**: Voucher-based contingency management

Voucher-based contingency management has yielded good outcomes in a number of studies with diverse populations. The psychodynamically-based psychotherapies, group and interpersonal psychotherapy, have shown good outcomes predominantly in case series, so they do not have a sufficient evidence base to recommend them in this situation. Attendance at 12-step groups alone has not been shown to be an acceptable alternative to more formal treatment. Twelve-step Facilitation Therapy and individual drug counseling both use 12-step principles and encourage group participation; these modalities have been shown to have good outcomes. Cue exposure therapy, while not extensively studied, has been shown to be not effective.

American Psychiatric Association Practice Guideline for the Treatment of Patients with Substance Use Disorders, 2nd Edition (2006), p 449–451. http://psychiatryonline.com/pracGuide/pracGuideHome.aspx

Pechnick RN, Glasner-Edwards S, Hrymoc M, Wilkins, JN. Preclinical development and clinical implementation of treatments for substance abuse disorders. FOCUS: Substance Abuse: Spring 2007; 2:158–159.

235

A patient in therapy has recently been told that his psychiatrist may change jobs and will be transferring his care to another psychiatrist. He has always needed a great deal of reassurance but now calls almost daily asking for opinions on decisions he is trying to make in his life. He often worries his ill wife will die before he does. Each time he is advised to attend day treatment to get further support, he often agrees to do so but does not follow through. Based on this vignette, which of the following personality disorders is most likely?

    (A) Dependent
    (B) Antisocial
    (C) Paranoid
    (D) Borderline
    (E) Narcissistic

The correct response is option **A**: Dependent

Criteria for dependent personality disorder include unrealistic fears of abandonment, urgently seeking another relationship as a source of support when a close relationship ends, difficulty in expressing disagreements with others, and difficulty initiating projects on one's own.

Diagnostic and Statistical Manual of Mental Disorders, Fourth Edition, Text Revision (DSM-IV-TR). Washington, DC, American Psychiatric Association, 2000, pp 721–725.

236

During an initial evaluation, a patient complains of multiple episodes of having palpitations, sweating and intense anxiety. Information that would be most supportive of panic disorder is that the episodes occur when the patient:

    (A) is reminded of a past assault.
    (B) must use a public bathroom.
    (C) attends a large party.
    (D) is in essentially any setting.
    (E) must use an elevator.

The correct response is option **D**: Is in essentially any setting

Panic episodes can occur in multiple types of settings and panic disorder should not be diagnosed if these episodes occur within the context of another anxiety disorder. Panic episodes also can occur due to medical causes or substances. Answer A is suggestive of posttraumatic stress disorder. Answer B may indicate OCD. Answer C may be social phobia. Answer D is most indicative of panic disorder. Answer E may be a simple phobia or agoraphobia.

Kinrys G, Pollack MH. Panic disorder and agoraphobia, in Clinical Manual of Anxiety Disorders. Edited by Stein DJ. American Psychiatric Publishing Inc, Washington DC, 2004, 13–16.

237

Which of the following statements most accurately describes the benefits of SSRIs in the treatment of PTSD? SSRIs have been shown to:

    (A) ameliorate core PTSD and other associated symptoms.
    (B) treat primarily the comorbid psychiatric disorders.
    (C) improve primarily hyperarousal symptoms.
    (D) improve the effectiveness of alpha 2 adrenergic agonists.
    (E) act only to augment psychotherapy in PTSD.

The correct response is option **A**: Ameliorate core PTSD and other associated symptoms

SSRIs have been demonstrated in randomized, double blind controlled studies to be effective in the treatment of PTSD due to their effectiveness in treating the core symptoms of PTSD, the disorders typically comorbid with PTSD, the associated problematic behavioral symptoms and their side effect profile. SSRIs are considered the first line medication treatment for PTSD.

American Psychiatric Association Practice Guideline for the Treatment of Patients with Acute Stress Disorder and Posttraumatic Stress Disorder. Am J Psychiatry. 2004; 161(11):17 http://www.psychiatryonline.com/pracGuide/pracGuideTopic_11.aspx

238

Which of the following factors will increase the potential for toxicity with lithium?

(A) Cigarette smoking
(B) Concomitant administration of mirtazapine (Remeron)
(C) Drinking a lot of water
(D) Exercising outdoors on a hot day

The correct response is option **D**: Exercising outdoors on a hot day

Exercise leads to dehydration and reduced volume of distribution (and therefore lithium toxicity). A first response to lithium toxicity is to encourage drinking water. Lithium is excreted through the kidney and not the liver. Antidepressants are generally safely administered with lithium. Cigarette smoking has known effects on cytochrome P450 enzymes in liver, but lithium is renally secreted without hepatic involvement.

Sadock BJ, Sadock VA, Ruiz P (eds): Kaplan & Sadock's Comprehensive Textbook of Psychiatry, 9th ed. Philadelphia, Lippincott Williams & Wilkins, 2009, pp 1353–59.

239

An individual with a history of opiate dependence admits to daily use of opiates, but a confirmatory urine toxicology screen is negative. Which of the following opiates is the patient most likely using?

(A) Hydrocodone
(B) Morphine
(C) Codeine
(D) Heroin
(E) Opium

The correct response is option **A**: Hydrocodone

In testing for opioids, urine toxicology screens primarily test for drugs derived from opium, such as morphine, codeine, and heroin. Synthetic opioids such as hydrocodone, methadone, and oxycodone may not be detected by standard tests.

Center for Substance Abuse Treatment. Detoxification and Substance Abuse Treatment. Treatment Improvement Protocol (TIP) Series 45. DHHS Publication No. (SMA) 06-4131. Rockville, MD: Substance Abuse and Mental Health Services Administration, 2006, pp 50–1. Also available at https://ncadistore.samhsa.gov/catalog/productDetails.aspx? ProductID_17398.

240

A 72-year-old man with severe chronic obstructive airway disease complains of anxiety, muscle tension and a general feeling of uneasiness. The most appropriate psychotropic medication for this patient's condition would be:

(A) clonazepam.
(B) diazepam.
(C) alprazolam.
(D) sorazepam.
(E) buspirone.

The correct response is option **E**: Buspirone

In treating anxiety disorders in patients with significant respiratory problems, it is often important to consider respiratory function. Anxiolytics may depress respiratory drive and further aggravate the patient's condition. Since buspirone produces no respiratory depression, it is an option to be considered in treating anxiety in these patients.

Schatzberg AF, Nemeroff CB (eds): Textbook of Psychopharmacology, 4th ed. Arlington, VA, American Psychiatric Publishing, 2009, pp 491–94.

241

Which of the following statements best describes the mechanism of action of acamprosate, thought to occur in the treatment of alcohol dependence?

(A) Acamprosate blocks the reuptake of chloride ions in central GABAergic neurons.
(B) Acamprosate competes with alcohol for central GABAergic neurons in a dose-dependent fashion.
(C) Acamprosate affects mu opiate receptors blocking the centrally mediated reinforcing effects of alcohol.
(D) Acamprosate inhibits aldehyde dehydrogenase, resulting in the accumulation of toxic levels of acetaldehyde.
(E) Acamposate reduces neuronal hyperactivity during early alcohol recovery.

The correct response is option **E**: Acamprosate reduces neuronal hyperactivity during early alcohol recovery.

Acamprosate is a small, flexible molecule that resembles GABA and decreases glutamatergic neurotransmission, perhaps by acting as an N-methyl-D-aspartate antagonist. It has been proposed that this medication helps sustain abstinence in detoxified alcohol-dependent individuals by reducing neuronal hyperactivity during early recovery.

American Psychiatric Association Practice Guideline for the Treatment of Patients with Substance Use Disorders, Second Edition, (2006). p 383–384. http://psychiatryonline.com/pracGuide/pracGuideHome.aspx.
Mason B. Acamprosate for alcohol dependence: an update for the clinician. FOCUS: Psychopharmacology Fall 2006; 4:505–506.
Dermatis H, Galanter M. Clinical advances in pharmacological and integrated treatment approaches for alcohol and drug use disorders. FOCUS: Substance Abuse Spring 2007:2:142.

242

In a recent study, which of the following substances was associated with an increase in the long term risk of developing psychotic disorder?

(A) Alcohol
(B) Cannabis
(C) Nicotine
(D) Opiates
(E) Inhalants

The correct response is option **B**: Cannabis

A recent large meta-analysis demonstrated that cannabis use increases the risk of psychotic outcomes independent of transient intoxication. While other substances may cause psychotic symptoms during periods of intoxication, no evidence exists to support an independent risk for psychosis as a result of using these other substances.

Moore THM, Zammit S, Lingford-Hughes A, Barnes TRE, Jones PB, Burke M, Lewis G. Cannabis use and risk of psychotic or affective mental health outcomes: a systematic review. Lancet 2007; 370:319–28
Veen ND, Selten J, Van der Tweel I, Feller WG, Hoek HW and Kahn RS. Cannabis Use and Age at Onset of Schizophrenia. Am J Psychiatry. 2004;161:501–506

243

A psychiatrist may terminate care of a patient in which of the following circumstances?

(A) Patient has not paid a bill
(B) Patient has failed to be cooperative in treatment
(C) Patient has consultation with another psychiatrist
(D) Patient misses two appointments and does not return the psychiatrist's calls
(E) Patient is hospitalized on an inpatient unit and care is permanently transferred

The correct response is option **E**: The patient is hospitalized on an inpatient unit and care is permanently transferred.

If a patient is hospitalized and his/her care is permanently transferred to another physician, then termination is legal and ethical. However, unless the patient is being permanently transferred to the care of the hospitalizing psychiatrist, failure to attend to a patient during hospitalization may be considered abandonment. Mere nonpayment of a bill, failure to be cooperative, consultation with another mental health professional, or failure to keep an appointment are not appropriate causes for termination if the patient continues to need treatment.

Simon RI, Shuman DW. Clinical Manual of Psychiatry and Law. Arlington, VA, American Psychiatric Publishing, 2007, pp 28–34.

244

Which of the following medications, commonly used in alcohol treatment to decrease craving, has been shown to be more effective if given after a period of sobriety?

- (A) Acamprosate
- (B) Disulfiram
- (C) Gabapentin
- (D) Naltrexone
- (E) Topiramate

The correct response is option **A**: Acamprosate

The goal of using acamprosate is to decrease the relapse rate after an initial abstinence period has been achieved. In European clinical trials, acamprosate has been shown to be most effective in those who have achieved a period of abstinence from alcohol (usually 7–10 days). U.S. studies have not replicated this finding. However it is suspected that this is because of a difference in the psychotherapies provided. The European studies tended to use more formalized counseling as opposed to the medication management visit approach used in the U.S. studies.

American Psychiatric Association Practice Guideline for the Treatment of Patients with Substance Use Disorders, 2nd Edition 2006, pp 383–384. http://psychiatryonline.com/pracGuide/pracGuideHome. aspx.

Connery HS, Kleber HD: Guideline Watch: Practice Guideline for the Treatment of Patients with Substance Use Disorders, 2nd ed April 2007. http://psychiatryonline.com/pracGuide/pracGuideHome. aspx

Mason B. Acamprosate for alcohol dependence: an update for the clinician. FOCUS: Psychopharmacology Fall 2006; 4:507–508.

245

Which of the following is characteristic of social phobia?

- (A) Spontaneous uncued panic attacks
- (B) Avoiding public speaking because of trembling
- (C) Fear of humiliation when speaking in a group setting
- (D) Fainting while having blood drawn
- (E) Avoiding parties because of fear of contamination

The correct response is option **C**: Fear of humiliation when speaking in a group setting

According to DSM-IV-TR, "the essential feature of social phobia is a marked and persistent fear of social or performance situations in which embarrassment may occur." While panic attacks can be associated with social phobia, they tend to be cued by the social situation and not spontaneous or uncued as seen in panic disorder. Social avoidance because of concern about a potentially embarrassing manifestation of a medical disorder (e.g., tremor of Parkinson's disease) is more appropriately diagnosed as anxiety disorder, not otherwise specified. Fainting during a blood draw would be diagnosed as specific phobia, blood-injection-injury type. Avoidance due to fear of contamination would be characteristic of obsessive-compulsive disorder.

Diagnostic and Statistical Manual of Mental Disorders, 4th ed, Text Revision (DSM-IV-TR). Washington, DC, American Psychiatric Association, 2000, pp 450–451

246

A patient with OCD and fears of contamination insists that his family remove their shoes when they enter his living space. Which of the following concepts best describes this behavior?

(A) Repetition compulsion
(B) Displacement
(C) Ritual by proxy
(D) Projection
(E) Reaction formation

The correct response is option **C**: Ritual by proxy

As rituals become an essential act to control anxiety, patients may attempt to get family members to partake in the behavior. Called "ritual by proxy," the patient's demands may extend to insisting the family have "outside" and "inside" clothes. Sometimes the patient insists the family reassure him that he has completed a task that will avoid a "dangerous" outcome; e.g., "Did I turn off the gas?" The family must tell him that he did, numerous times. The treatment for such behavior is "ritual prevention" in which the family reminds the patient that the psychiatrist has told the family not to comply. The other choices are defense mechanisms that are not specific to OCD.

Stein DJ, Hollander E, Rothbaum BO (eds): Textbook of Anxiety Disorders, 2nd ed. Arlington, VA, American Psychiatric Publishing, 2010, p 343.

247

A 48-year-old woman is brought to the emergency department after being found unconscious. Examination reveals respiratory depression, extreme miosis, stupor, coma and pulmonary edema. The patient's presentation is MOST consistent with an overdose of:

(A) alcohol.
(B) cannabis.
(C) inhalants.
(D) opioids.
(E) sedative-hypnotics.

The correct response is option **D**: Opioids

The syndrome of acute opioid overdose is recognized by extreme miosis or in severe cases by mydriasis (due to anoxia), drowsiness, slurred speech and impairment in attention and memory and sometimes pulmonary edema. Overdose is a medical emergency and can result in coma, shock and death. Naloxone is an opioid receptor antagonist that can be used to reverse the effects of opiates used in overdose.

Hales RE, Yudofsky SC: Substance use disorders, in The American Psychiatric Publishing Textbook of Psychiatry, 5th ed. Arlington, VA, American Psychiatric Publishing, 2008, pp 384–87.

248

Patients with obsessive-compulsive disorder are most likely to respond to which of the following therapy modalities?

(A) Psychoanalysis
(B) Dynamic psychotherapy
(C) Dialectical behavior therapy
(D) Motivational enhancement therapy
(E) Exposure and response prevention

The correct response is option **E**: Exposure and response prevention

Behavioral treatment, in particular exposure therapy, to decrease anxiety associated with obsessions and response prevention to decrease the frequency of rituals or obsessions, has been demonstrated to be very effective in the treatment of OCD. There are no controlled studies that demonstrate effectiveness of dynamic psychotherapy or psychoanalysis in dealing with the core symptoms of OCD. Dialectical behavior therapy is a specialized form of therapy developed for the treatment of borderline personality disorder, and motivational enhancement therapy is a type of therapy developed for the treatment of substance use disorders.

American Psychiatric Association Practice Guideline for the Treatment of Patients with Obsessive-Compulsive Disorder 2007. http://psychiatryonline.com/pracGuide/pracGuideHome.aspx
Hales RE, Yudofsky SC, Gabbard GO (eds): The American Psychiatric Publishing Textbook of Psychiatry, 5th ed. Arlington, VA, American Psychiatric Publishing, 2008, pp 374, 564–65, 842, 1235.

Which of following is the most common fear during the dying process?

(A) Loneliness
(B) Abandonment
(C) Pain
(D) Uncertainty

The correct response is option **C**: Pain

All of the above choices are important to the dying patient, but fear of physical suffering appears to be the most common. It is the issue most often mentioned in the definition of a "good death." There is increased attention paid to pain relief currently; hospital staff members are required to ask patients to rate their pain on a scale of 1 (least) to 10 (unbearable). Staff should make efforts to keep the pain level at 5 or below.

Roberts LW, Dyer AR: A Concise Guide to Ethics in Mental Health Care, Washington, DC, American Psychiatric Publishing, 2004, pp 187–188.
Wise MG, Rundell JR (eds): Textbook of Consultation-Liaison Psychiatry., 2nd ed. Washington, DC, American Psychiatric Publishing, 2002, pp 772–773.
Levenson JL (ed): Textbook of Psychosomatic Medicine. Arlington, VA, American Psychiatric Publishing, 2005, pp 981–82.

A 38-year-old woman is admitted to the hospital with a severe manic episode. On examination, she is noted to have motor excitement, mutism and stereotypic movements. Which of the following medications would be the most appropriate in treating this patient?

(A) Carbamazepine
(B) Haloperidol
(C) Lamotrigine
(D) Lorazepam
(E) Olanzapine

The correct response is option **D**: Lorazepam

Motor excitement, mutism and stereotypic movements are consistent with catatonia. Catatonic features may develop in up to one-third of patients during a manic episode. In treating catatonia, neuroleptics have generally exhibited poor efficacy and may be associated with an increased likelihood of neuroleptic malignant syndrome. In contrast, prospective studies have demonstrated the efficacy of lorazepam in the treatment of catatonic syndromes, including those associated with mania.

American Psychiatric Association Practice Guideline for the Treatment of Patients with Bipolar Disorder, 2nd ed (2002). Reprinted in FOCUS: Bipolar Disorder, Winter 2003; 1:73.
Taylor MA, Fink M. Catatonia in psychiatric classification: a home of its own. Am J Psychiatry. 2003 Jul;160(7):1233–41.
Bush G, Fink M, Petrides G, Dowling F, Francis A. Catatonia. II. Treatment with lorazepam and electroconvulsive therapy. Acta Psychiatr Scand. 1996 Feb;93(2):137–43.

A 35-year-old man with a history of opiate dependence is brought to the emergency department after being found unconscious. Examination reveals respiratory depression, extreme miosis, stupor, coma and pulmonary edema. The emergency department physician administers naloxone 1.0 mg intravenously every three minutes until a maximum dosage of 10 mg has been given. However, the patient remains unresponsive. What would be the most appropriate next step?

(A) Double the next intravenous dose of naloxone.
(B) Increase the frequency with which the naloxone is administered.
(C) Reconsider the diagnosis of an opioid overdose.
(D) Start a continuous infusion of naloxone.
(E) Switch from intravenous naloxone to nasogastric administration of naltrexone.

The correct response is option **C**: Reconsider the diagnosis of an opioid overdose.

The recommendations for the administration of naloxone are repeated doses every 3 minutes until respiratory or CNS depression is completely reversed or until a maximum dose of 10 mg i.v. has been given. Because of the poor bioavailability from significant hepatic first-pass effects, naloxone for acute intoxication is typically administered intravenously rather than nasogastrically. After the patient has received 10 mg of naloxone and remains unresponsive, it is very unlikely that the symptoms are due to an opioid overdose and other diagnoses should be considered.

American Psychiatric Association Practice Guideline for the Treatment of Patients with Substance Use Disorders, 2nd Edition (2006), p 35, http://psychiatryonline.com/pracGuide/pracGuideHome.aspx.
Hales RE, Yudofsky SC: Substance use disorders, in The American Psychiatric Publishing Textbook of Psychiatry, 5th ed. Arlington, VA, American Psychiatric Publishing, 2008, pp 384–87.

The concept that directs child psychiatrists and health care providers to involve children in decisions about their care commensurate with their developmental capacity is referred to as:

(A) cognitive incapacity.
(B) pediatric assent.
(C) pediatric consent.
(D) remaining autonomy.

The correct response is option **B**: Pediatric assent

Informed consent applies to patients who have reached adulthood, except when the patient has been determined to lack capacity. As argued by the American Academy of Pediatrics Committee on Bioethics, decision making involving the healthcare of older children and adolescents should include, to the greatest extent possible, the assent of the patient as well as the participation of the parents and the physician. Pediatricians should not necessarily treat children as rational autonomous decision makers (pediatric consent) but should give serious consideration to each patient's developing capacities (vs. incapacities) for participating in decision making, including rationality and autonomy. "Remaining autonomy" refers to geriatric patients who are becoming increasingly impaired in cognition.

American Academy of Pediatrics, Committee on Bioethics. Informed consent, parental permission, and assent in pediatric practice. Pediatrics 1995; 95:314–317.
Coverdale J, McCullough LB, Molinari V, Workman R. Ethically justified clinical strategies for promoting geriatric assent. Int J Geriatr Psychiatry 2006; 21:151–7.

253

Which of the following syndromes is the most common form of inherited mental retardation?

(A) Fragile X syndrome
(B) Williams syndrome
(C) Rett syndrome
(D) Prader-Willi syndrome
(E) Angelman syndrome

The correct response is option **A**: Fragile X syndrome

Fragile X syndrome is the most common cause of inherited mental retardation. It is reported to occur in 1 in 4000 males and 1 per 8000 females. Fragile X is caused by dysfunction of FMR1 gene at Xq27.3. It is characterized by large testicles, connective tissue disease, large head with prominent forehead and jaw, long face with large ears. Mental retardation is usually in the moderate to severe range.

The other entities listed are also genetic syndromes associated with mental retardation; their rates of occurrence are approximately:

Williams syndrome: 1 in 7,500;

Rett syndrome: 1 in 10,000;

Angelman syndrome: 1 in 10,000 to 20,000;

Prader-Willi syndrome: 1 in 30,000.

Smoller JW, Sheidley BR, Tsuang MT. Psychiatric Genetics: Applications in Clinical Practice. American Psychiatric Publishing, Inc.; 1st edition, 2008, p. 200–212

Dulcan MK (ed), Dulcan's Textbook of Child and Adolescent Psychiatry. American Psychiatric Publishing, Inc., Washington, DC. 2010, Chapter 12. Intellectual Disability (Mental Retardation), pp 157–159.

254

Hypertensive paroxysms associated with diaphoresis, tachycardia, flushing, nausea and significant apprehension suggests the presence of which of the following general medical conditions that mimics anxiety?

(A) Mitral valve problem
(B) Cocaine withdrawal
(C) Coronary insufficiency
(D) Hyperthyroidism
(E) Pheochromocytoma

The correct response is option **E**: Pheochromocytoma

The question describes the clinical features of pheochromocytoma, also known as chromaffin tumors. These are derived most often from the adrenal medulla, as well as the sympathetic ganglia. The clinical features of these tumors, most commonly hypertensive paroxysms, are predominantly due to the release of catecholamines.

Hales RE, Yudofsky SC, and Gabbard GO (eds): The American Psychiatric Publishing Textbook of Psychiatry, 5th ed. Arlington, VA, American Psychiatric Publishing, Inc., 2008. p 522.

Kay J, Tasman A. Essentials of Psychiatry. Hoboken, NJ, John Wiley and Sons, 2006. pp 399–401.

255

Behavioral therapy for a patient with OCD is most difficult when which of the following symptoms are present?

(A) Observable rituals
(B) Delusions
(C) Contamination fears
(D) Checking behaviors

The correct response is option **B**: Delusions

Preservation of insight is an OCD hallmark. While compelled to respond to inappropriate or bizarre rituals, good-prognosis OCD patients retain the awareness that their responses are unreasonable. Observable rituals, checking behaviors, and contamination fears lend themselves readily to behavioral manipulation, and severe symptoms may require extended therapy.

Greist JH, Baer L. Psychotherapy for obsessive-compulsive disorder. In: American Psychiatric Publishing Textbook of Anxiety Disorders. American Psychiatric Publishing, Washington DC 2002. Stein DJ, Hollander E (eds) p 228–229.

256

A psychiatrist is seeing a 35-year-old patient with schizophrenia who is accompanied by his mother. During a discussion about possible medication options, the psychiatrist turns to the patient and asks "What would you prefer to do?" This question is an example of which ethical principle?

(A) Altruism
(B) Respect for autonomy
(C) Beneficence
(D) Nonmaleficence

The correct response is option **B**: Respect for autonomy

Respect for autonomy is honoring the patient's right to make decisions for himself or herself. Altruism in health care delivery is the commitment of service to benefit others even at personal sacrifice. Beneficence is the obligation to try to help patients by relieving their suffering and enhancing their quality of life. Nonmaleficence is the duty to avoid harm.

Roberts LW. Ethical principles and skills in the care of mental illness. FOCUS: Forensic and Ethical Issues in Psychiatry. Fall 2003; 4:339–340.

257

Which of the following defines the virtue "veracity"?

(A) Saying only what is true, never misleading the patient, and pacing disclosure to the patient effectively.
(B) Practicing medicine consistent with the highest intellectual and moral standards, both professional and individual.
(C) Recognizing, preventing, and relieving pain, suffering, and distress and acting to prevent and relieve pain, suffering and distress.
(D) Not being excessively swayed by potential feared consequence.
(E) Taking reasonable risks to one's self-interest (in time, convenience, health and even life), to protect the interests of patients.

The correct response is option **A**: Saying only what is true, never misleading the patient, and pacing disclosure to the patient effectively.

Veracity refers to the physician's duty to tell the truth and not mislead through acts of commission or omission. The other options refer to integrity, compassion, courage and self-sacrifice, respectively.

Roberts LW, Dyer AR, Concise Guide to Ethics in Mental Health Care. American Psychiatric Publishing Inc., Washington D.C., 2004 p 8.
Roberts LW. Ethical principles and skills in the care of mental illness. FOCUS: Forensic and Ethical Issues, Fall 2003; 4:340.

258

A 25-year-old man has a history of facial and truncal tics since childhood. He presents to an outpatient clinic for evaluation of anxiety and is diagnosed as having OCD. Which of the following patterns of OCD symptoms is he most likely to exhibit?

(A) Obsessions and checking
(B) Cleanliness and washing
(C) Symmetry and ordering
(D) Hoarding

The correct response is option **C**: Symmetry and ordering

Factor analysis has determined that symptoms of OCD fall into several potentially meaningful subtypes. Chronic tic disorder has repeatedly been found to be associated with the subtype characterized by symmetry and ordering.

Eisen JL, Yip AG, Mancebo MC, Pinto A, Rasmussen SA. Phenomenology of Obsessive-Compulsive Disorder, in American Psychiatric Publishing Textbook of Anxiety Disorders, 2nd ed. Edited by Stein DJ, Hollander E, Rothbaum BO. Arlington, VA, American Psychiatric Publishing, 2010, pp 265–71.
Leckman JF, Grice DE, Boardman J, et al: Symptoms of obsessive-compulsive disorder. Am J Psychiatry 1997; 154:911–917.

259

The starting dose of lamotrigine should be reduced by half if a patient is taking which of the following medications?

(A) Carbamazepine
(B) Oral contraceptive
(C) Phenobarbital
(D) Divalproex
(E) Phenytoin

The correct response is option **D**: Divalproex

Divalproex will reduce the clearance of lamotrigine by about 50% resulting in a doubling of lamotrigine blood level. The risk of serious rash will be increased unless appropriate dose adjustments are made. Carbamazepine, oral contraceptives, phenytoin and phenobarbital are inducers of lamotrigine metabolism and will cause substantial reductions in lamotrigine blood levels.

Kanner AM, Frey M: Adding valproate to lamotrigine: a study of their pharmacokinetic interaction. Neurology 2000; 55:588–591.
Weintraub D, Buchsbaum R, Resor SR, Hirsch LJ: Effect of antiepileptic drug comedication on lamotrigine clearance. Arch Neurol 2005; 62:1432–1436.
Sidhu J, Job S, Singh S, Philipson R: The pharmacokinetic and pharmacodynamic consequences of the co-administration of lamotrigine and a combined oral contraceptive in healthy female subjects. Br J Clin Pharmacol 2006; 61:191–199.

A 75-year-old man with a history of mild Alzheimer's disease becomes increasingly aggressive at home. In addition, he is noted to have worsening memory and word-finding difficulty, inadequate self-care, and less interest in activities. Which of the patient's symptoms is most likely to be helped by risperidone?

    (A) Memory
    (B) Word finding
    (C) Independent functioning
    (D) Aggression
    (E) Interest in activities

The correct response is option **D**: Aggression

Aggression is a difficult acute symptom in dementia. Drugs should be used only when nonpharmacologic approaches have failed to adequately control behavioral disruption. There is concern regarding the potential for serious adverse outcomes.

The recently published CATIE-AD study reported that in usual care settings among patients continuing phase I treatment for 12 weeks in comparison to placebo, "antipsychotics may be more effective for particular symptoms, such as anger, aggression and paranoid ideation," but "they do not appear to improve cognition, functioning, care needs or quality of life." According to a June 2009 statement from the APA Council on Aging about the use of antipsychotics in Alzheimer patients, "their use should be preceded by a discussion of risks and benefits with the patient and/or other decision-makers. Clinicians should monitor patients closely, prescribe the lowest effective dosages, and discontinue the drugs as soon as possible."

Sultzer DL, Davis SM, Tariot PN, Dagerman KS, Lebowitz BD, Lyketsos CG, Rosenheck RA, Hsiao JK, Lieberman JA, Schneider LS; CATIE-AD Study Group. Clinical symptom responses to atypical antipsychotic medications in Alzheimer's disease: phase 1 outcomes from the CATIE-AD effectiveness trial. Am J Psychiatry. 2008; 165(7):844–854.

Salzman C, Jeste DV, Meyer RE, Cohen-Mansfield J, Cummings J, Grossberg GT, Jarvik L, Kraemer HC, Lebowitz BD, Maslow K, Pollock BG, Raskind M, Schultz SK, Wang P, Zito JM, Zubenko GS. Elderly patients with dementia-related symptoms of severe agitation and aggression: consensus statement on treatment options, clinical trials methodology, and policy. J Clin Psychiatry. 2008 Jun; 69(6):889–98.

Jeste DV, Blazer D, Casey D, Meeks T, Salzman C, Schneider L, Tariot P, Yaffe K. ACNP White Paper: update on use of antipsychotic drugs in elderly persons with dementia. Neuropsychopharmacology. 2008 Apr; 33(5):957–70.

Ballard C, Corbett A, Chitramohan R, Aarsland D. Management of agitation and aggression associated with Alzheimer's disease: controversies and possible solutions. Curr Opin Psychiatry. 2009 Aug 18.

Two teenagers randomly fire their guns at a 54-year-old man in their neighborhood. A week later the patient complains that he can't "get it out of my mind" and is having frequent nightmares about this incident. He is always "on the watch" when he drives down the road and avoids going out alone. The most likely diagnosis for this patient is:

    (A) generalized anxiety disorder.
    (B) obsessive-compulsive disorder.
    (C) acute stress disorder.
    (D) social phobia.
    (E) posttraumatic stress disorder.

The correct response is option **C**: Acute stress disorder

The essential feature of acute stress disorder is the development of characteristic anxiety, dissociative, and other symptoms that occur within 1 month after exposure to an extreme traumatic stressor (Criterion A). Either while experiencing the traumatic event or after the event, the individual has at least three of the following dissociative symptoms: a subjective sense of numbing, detachment, or absence of emotional responsiveness; a reduction in awareness of his or her surroundings; derealization; depersonalization; or dissociative amnesia (Criterion B). Following the trauma, the traumatic event is persistently re-experienced (Criterion C), and the individual displays marked avoidance of stimuli that may arouse recollections of the trauma (Criterion D) and has marked symptoms of anxiety or increased arousal (Criterion E). The symptoms must cause clinically significant distress, significantly interfere with normal functioning, or impair the individual's ability to pursue necessary tasks (Criterion F). The disturbance lasts for a minimum of 2 days and a maximum of 4 weeks after the traumatic event (Criterion G); if symptoms persist beyond 4 weeks, the diagnosis of posttraumatic stress disorder may be applied.

American Psychiatric Association: Diagnostic and Statistical Manual of Mental Disorders, 4th Edition, Text Revision (DSM-IV-TR). Washington DC, American Psychiatric Association. 2000. pp 471–472.

American Psychiatric Association Practice Guideline for the Treatment of Patients with Acute Stress Disorder and Posttraumatic Stress Disorder. 2004, p. 32, http://psychiatryonline.com/pracGuide/pracGuideHome.aspx

262

A 42-year-old patient complains of a fear of crowded places. This fear is present in any situation in which the patient perceives that escape may be difficult, including riding alone in elevators and cars. As a result of this fear, the patient rarely leaves home. Which of the following is the most likely diagnosis?

(A) Social phobia
(B) Agoraphobia
(C) Specific phobia
(D) Avoidant personality disorder
(E) Panic disorder

The correct response is option **B**: Agoraphobia

According to the DSM-IV, agoraphobia involves anxiety about being in a situation in which escape might be difficult or embarrassing and leads to avoidance of the situation or endurance of the situation with distress. Specific phobia should be considered only if the avoidance is limited to one or a few specific situations and social phobia should be considered if the avoidance is limited to social situations only. However, this patient avoids all situations in which escape is perceived to be difficult, including situations in which the patient is alone. While agoraphobia may be associated with panic disorder, the vignette does not include panic symptoms.

Diagnostic and Statistical Manual of Mental Disorders, Fourth Edition, Text Revision (DSM-IV-TR). Washington, DC, American Psychiatric Association, 2000, pp 433, 721.

263

Which of the following is an objective sleep disturbance that occurs in depression?

(A) Shortened sleep latency
(B) Decreased nighttime arousal
(C) Increased total sleep time
(D) Shortened REM latency
(E) Increased slow wave sleep

The correct response is option **D**: Shortened REM latency

The REM latency in depression is shortened. The sleep latency is prolonged, and there is increased nighttime arousal, decreased total sleep time and decreased slow wave sleep. There can be increased stage 1 sleep and a prolonged first REM period.

Schiffer RB, Rao SM, Fogel BS (eds): Neuropsychiatry, 2nd ed. Philadelphia, Lippincott, Williams & Wilkins, 2003. p 385.

264

The main factor of somatization disorder which differentiates it from factitious disorder or malingering is that in somatization disorder:

(A) patients seek to play the sick role.
(B) there are external incentives for the behavior.
(C) complaint of symptoms is exaggerated.
(D) patients often have had multiple hospitalizations.
(E) symptoms are not under voluntary control.

The correct response is option **E**: Symptoms are not under voluntary control.

Patients seek the sick role in factitious disorder, whereas external incentives are the motive in malingering. In both factitious disorder and malingering, symptoms are intentionally feigned or produced. Symptom complaint exaggeration and multiple hospitalizations can be present in all three.

In somatization, symptoms are not under conscious control of the patient.

American Psychiatric Association: Diagnostic and Statistical Manual of Mental Disorders, 4th Edition. Text Revision (DSM-IV-TR). Washington, DC, American Psychiatric Association, 2000. pp 486, 513–514, 739–740

265

A 38-year-old married woman presents to a psychiatrist complaining of difficulty in her sex life. She reports that, for much of her married life, she has had little interest in sexual intercourse with her husband. She has not had any affairs, and she denies any discord in her relationship with her husband aside from the lack of a satisfactory sex life. She does not masturbate and rarely has any sexual fantasies. On the few occasions that she does have intercourse with her husband, she is able to enjoy sex and achieve an orgasm. Which of the following diagnoses is most appropriate?

(A) Dyspareunia
(B) Sexual aversion disorder
(C) Hypoactive sexual desire disorder
(D) Female sexual arousal disorder
(E) Female orgasmic disorder

The correct response is option **C**: Hypoactive sexual desire disorder

Hypoactive sexual desire disorder is characterized by lack of or deficient sexual fantasies and sexual desire, as is present in this patient. Individuals with hypoactive sexual desire disorder often have no dysfunction once they are engaged in intercourse. Dyspareunia is characterized by pain with intercourse, sexual aversion disorder by an aversion to and avoidance of genital contact, female sexual arousal disorder by an inability to maintain physiological sexual excitement, and female orgasmic disorder by a delayed or absent orgasm.

Sadock BJ, Sadock VA, Ruiz P (eds): Kaplan & Sadock's Comprehensive Textbook of Psychiatry, 9th ed. Philadelphia, Lippincott Williams & Wilkins, 2009, pp 2040–43

266

The age at which a clinician should consider the possibility of the early onset subtype of dementia of the Alzheimer's type is:

(A) 35 years.
(B) 45 years or below.
(C) 55 years or below.
(D) 65 years or below.
(E) 75 years or below.

The correct response is option **D**: 65 years or below

According to the DSM-IV TR, the two subtypes of dementia of the Alzheimer's type include "late onset" and "early onset," with the latter more likely to be familial with autosomal dormant transmission. It may be more likely to be misdiagnosed because Alzheimer's dementia is more commonly associated with the elderly. Subtypes are specified for dementia of the Alzheimer's type: "with early onset" refers to cases "if onset is at age 65 years or below." "With late onset" is specified if onset is after age 65 years.

American Psychiatric Association: Diagnostic and Statistical Manual of Mental Disorders, 4th Edition. Text Revision (DSM-IV TR). Washington DC, American Psychiatric Association, 2000. pp 154–160
Meeks TW, Lanouette N, Vahia I, Dawes S, Jeste DV, Lebowitz B. Psychiatric assessment and diagnosis in older adults. FOCUS. 2009 winter; 7(1):3–13

267

A 22-year-old woman is driving her boyfriend home. The car hits a tree and he is killed. Six months after the accident she is still unable to drive, avoids going out, jumps when she hears loud noises and cannot feel any sadness or happiness. What is the most likely diagnosis for this patient?

(A) Adjustment disorder
(B) Agoraphobia
(C) Major depressive disorder
(D) Posttraumatic stress disorder
(E) Acute stress disorder

The correct response is option **D**: Posttraumatic stress disorder

The patient's symptoms are avoidance, numbing and increased arousal. These three symptom constellations comprise criteria B, C, and D for a DSM-IV-TR diagnosis of posttraumatic stress disorder

American Psychiatric Association: Diagnostic and Statistical Manual of Mental Disorders, 4th Edition. Text Revision (DSM-IV TR). Washington DC, American Psychiatric Association. 2000. pp 467–468

Which of the following actions is most likely to ease the fears of a dying patient and his family?

(A) Postponing the discussion of pain and pain management
(B) Giving the family and patient information on a need to know basis
(C) Telling the patient that only the family's input regarding care will be sought
(D) Educating the patient that he may have discomfort that cannot be alleviated
(E) Obtaining the patient's wishes regarding treatment decisions

The correct response is option **E**: Obtaining the patient's wishes regarding treatment decisions

Conveying a number of important messages to the dying patient and his family allows them to feel more confident and comfortable in dealing with end-of-life issues. These messages as described by Mitka include:

You will have the best medical treatment, aiming to prevent exacerbation, to improve function and survival, and to ensure comfort. You will never have to endure overwhelming pain, shortness of breath, or other symptoms. Your care will be continuous, comprehensive, and coordinated. You and your family will be prepared for everything that is likely to happen in the course of your illness.

Your wishes will be sought, respected, and followed whenever possible. We will help you consider your personal and financial resources, and we will respect your choices about their use. We will do all that we can to see that you and your family will have the opportunity to make the best of every day.

Sadock BJ, Sadock VA, Ruiz P (eds): Kaplan & Sadock's Comprehensive Textbook of Psychiatry, 9th ed. Philadelphia, Lippincott Williams & Wilkins, 2009, p 2355.
Mitka M: Suggestions for help when the end is near. JAMA 2000; 284:2441.

A 26-year-old bystander of a horrific motor vehicle accident is taken to the ED after reporting that suddenly she had gone blind. She does not appear to focus on anyone who is talking. However, her eyes are noted to track her reflection when a mirror is waved in front of her. After hospital admission, a complete medical and neurological workup is found to be normal. What should be the first intervention for her condition?

(A) Pointing out that she can see as a result of the mirror test
(B) Instituting a reward system for sight improvement
(C) Discussing the stress of the event under amobarbital
(D) Suggesting symptom improvement through hypnosis
(E) Reassuring her that her sight will soon return

The correct response is option **E**: Reassuring her that her sight will soon return

The patient is likely suffering from conversion disorder. Direct confrontation of symptom inconsistency is never recommended. While hypnosis, behavior therapy and amobarbital interviews can all be beneficial, they should only be tried if reassurance and relaxation are not effective.

Hales RE, Yudofsky SC, Gabbard GO (eds). The American Psychiatric Publishing Textbook of Psychiatry, 5th ed. Arlington, VA, American Psychiatric Publishing, Inc., 2008, pp 628-629

270

A 48-year-old obese man presents for an evaluation, at the prompting of his wife. The wife, who has accompanied the patient to the appointment, complains that the patient snores loudly and keeps her awake at night. She states he sometimes seems to be gasping for air. On questioning, the patient admits to falling asleep easily during the day, and even falling asleep while driving on occasion. He also complains of morning headaches and was recently diagnosed with hypertension. Which of the following is the best initial treatment for this patient's condition?

(A) Uvulopalatopharyngoplasty
(B) Temazepam
(C) Biofeedback
(D) Modafinil
(E) Nasal continuous positive airway pressure (CPAP)

The correct response is option **E**: Nasal continuous positive airway pressure (CPAP)

This patient most likely has moderate-severe obstructive sleep apnea. The best initial treatment is nasal CPAP. Uvulopalatopharyngoplasty is a treatment option, though it would not typically be considered first-line. Temazepam and biofeedback are not indicated for obstructive sleep apnea and temazepam may worsen daytime sleepiness, with its associated negative consequences. Although modafinil is used to treat daytime sleepiness, it does not address the underlying condition.

Hales RE, Yudofsky SC, Gabbard GO (eds): The American Psychiatric Publishing Textbook of Psychiatry. 5th ed. American Psychiatric Publishing, Inc., Washington, DC. 2008, pp 999–1000

271

A 55 year old patient with alcohol dependence treated with naltrexone 50mg daily has been abstinent from alcohol for the past 2 months. The patient has been advised to undergo surgical knee replacement. What is the minimum duration of time prior to the surgery for which naltrexone must be discontinued in order for opiate analgesia to be effective?

(A) 24 hours
(B) 72 hours
(C) 5 days
(D) 1 week
(E) 2 weeks

The correct response is option **B**: 72 hours

Naltrexone, which blocks μ-opioid receptors, must be discontinued 48-72 hours prior to receiving opiate analgesia.

Anton RF: Naltrexone for the management of alcohol dependence. NEJM 2008; 359:715–21

272

A 35-year-old patient worries obsessively that he will kill his mother. To alleviate the anxiety, he calls her repeatedly throughout the day to hear her voice and reassure himself that he has not harmed her. He has tried adequate trials of high doses of fluoxetine, paroxetine, lorazepam, and clonazepam, without improvement. Which of the following medications would be most appropriate to prescribe next?

(A) Citalopram
(B) Alprazolam
(C) Bupropion
(D) Lithium
(E) Clomipramine

The correct response is option **E**: Clomipramine

Clomipramine is the next best medication to prescribe. Clomipramine has substantial evidence to support its use in OCD, but due to its side effect profile, it is not typically prescribed until two SSRIs have failed (as in this patient). Citalopram would not be a good choice given that the patient has already failed therapeutic trials of two SSRIs. Benzodiazepines have not consistently shown efficacy. Bupropion and lithium are not typically prescribed for primary anxiety disorders.

Greist J, Jefferson J. Obsessive-compulsive disorder. FOCUS: OCD: Summer 2007, 3:283–298.

Schatzberg AF, Nemeroff CB (eds): Essentials of Clinical Psychopharmacology, 2nd ed, Washington, DC, American Psychiatric Publishing, 2006, pp 144, 185, 337–40.

Schruers K, Koning K, Leurmans J, et al. Obsessive-compulsive disorder: a critical review of therapeutic perspectives. Acta Psychiatr Scand 2005; 111:261–271.

American Psychiatric Association Practice Guideline for the Treatment of Patients with Obsessive-Compulsive Disorder 2007. http://psychiatryonline.com/pracGuide/pracGuideHome.aspx

A 60-year-old man with early Parkinson's disease presents to your office at the urging of his wife. She reports that the patient has begun "acting out" his dreams while asleep, and on at least one occasion this "acting out" led to his assaulting her. Polysomnogram is likely to demonstrate motor artifact and/or lack of complete hypotonia during which phase of sleep?

(A) Stage I
(B) Stage II
(C) Stage III
(D) Stage IV
(E) REM sleep

The correct response is option **E**: REM sleep

This patient likely has REM behavior disorder, which is characterized by lack of complete hypotonia during REM sleep. This results in patients displaying motor activity during sleep, often acting out their dreams. Older men with CNS disease, such as Parkinson's, are more likely to manifest this disorder.

Hales RE, Yudofsky SC, Gabbard GO (eds): The American Psychiatric Publishing Textbook of Psychiatry. 5th ed. American Psychiatric Publishing, Inc., Washington, DC. 2008. p 2040

Adding which one of the following medicines can increase the risk of toxicity in a patient stabilized on lamotrigine for bipolar maintenance therapy?

(A) Lithium
(B) Valproate
(C) Quetiapine
(D) Topiramate
(E) Olanzapine

The correct response is option **B**: Valproate

When administered with lamotrigine, valproate can result in a two-fold increase in lamotrigine levels. This is thought to be due to valproic acids inhibiting of CYPP450 microsomal function. It is the reason why the usual lamotrigine titration level should be decreased by 50% if a patient is on valproic acid.

Schatzberg AF, Cole JO, DeBattista C (eds): Manual of Clinical Psychopharmacology, 7th ed. Arlington VA, American Psychiatric Publishing Inc, 2010, p 340

A 52-year-old man presents with a rapidly progressive dementia, visual symptoms and cerebellar signs. Within a few weeks he is mute and has myoclonus. He dies four months later. Light microscopy of the brain reveals spongiform changes. This presentation is most consistent with which of the following diagnoses?

(A) Creutzfeldt-Jakob disease
(B) HIV infection
(C) Huntington's disease
(D) Progressive supranuclear palsy
(E) Wilson's disease

The correct response is option **A**: Creutzfeldt-Jakob disease

The transmissible spongiform encephalopathies are a group of rare dementias caused by an accumulation of abnormal prion protein within the brain. Creutzfeldt-Jakob disease is the most common human transmissible spongiform encephalopathy. It typically presents with a rapidly progressive dementia, and within weeks to months, marked cognitive impairment develops. The median duration of symptom onset to death is only 4 months. Spongiform changes are seen in the brain due to neuronal loss, gliosis, and deposition of "amyloid."

Levenson JL (ed): Essentials of Psychosomatic Medicine, American Psychiatric Publishing, Inc., Washington, DC, 2007, p 322

276

A family is seen in family therapy. During the process, the therapist attempts to increase differentiation, decrease triangulations, resolve cutoffs and improve the ability of the family to manage anxiety. This process is MOST consistent with which family therapeutic approach?

(A) Behavioral/cognitive-behavioral therapy
(B) Systemic family therapy
(C) Psychodynamic-psychoanalytic psychotherapy
(D) Strategic family therapy
(E) Transgenerational family therapy

The correct response is option **B**: Systemic family therapy

In Systemic Family Therapy, the core concepts are differentiation of the self, triangulation, emotional cutoffs, family emotional system and sibling position. The goals are to increase differentiation, de-triangulation, resolve cutoffs and improvement in the ability to manage anxiety. In Behavioral/Cognitive-Behavioral family therapy, the core concepts are based on social learning theory with the goal of enhancing communication and problem-solving skills. Psychodynamic-psychoanalytic approaches focus on object relations, projective identification, splitting and scapegoating. Strategic family therapy aims at resolving the presenting problem. The focus of transgenerational family therapy is the repair of ruptured relationships.

Sadock BJ, Sadock VA, Ruiz P (eds): Kaplan and Sadock's Comprehensive Textbook of Psychiatry, 9th ed. Philadelphia, Lippinicott Williams & Wilkins, 2009, pp 2845–2857
Textbook of Psychotherapeutic Treatments. Gabbard GO (ed). Arlington VA, American Psychiatric Publishing Inc, 2009, p 512

277

Which of the following is the most common male sexual disorder?

(A) Fetishism
(B) Male orgasmic disorder
(C) Male erectile disorder
(D) Premature ejaculation
(E) Sexual masochism

The correct response is option **D**: Premature ejaculation

The most prevalent male sexual disorder is premature ejaculation (27% prevalence estimate). It is frequently underestimated due to embarrassment issues as it is difficult for patients to discuss.

Hales RE, Yudofsky SC, Gabbard GO (eds): The American Psychiatric Publishing Textbook of Psychiatry. 5th ed. American Psychiatric Publishing, Inc., Washington, DC. 2008. pp 767–768
American Psychiatric Association: Diagnostic and Statistical Manual of Mental Disorders, 4th Edition, Text Revision (DSM-IV-TR). Washington DC, American Psychiatric Association. 2000, p 538

278

A 72 year old patient is admitted to the hospital with a fever of 101.8° F and a urinary tract infection. The patient believes that it is 1974 and that the hospital room is a kitchen. The nursing staff is concerned because the patient is agitated, trying to get out of bed, and trying to pull out the IV. Which of the following medications is the best choice for the patient's agitation?

(A) Lorazepam
(B) Haloperidol
(C) Diazepam
(D) Thioridazine
(E) Valproate

The correct response is option **B**: Haloperidol

The initial drug of choice for treatment of delirium is haloperidol, due to the low potential for anticholinergic or hypotensive effects, ability to be administered intravenously, and minimal cardiotoxicity. Benzodiazepines are only indicated in delirium due to substance withdrawal (primarily alcohol or sedative-hypnotic withdrawal). Valproate is not indicated for the treatment of delirium.

Wise MG, Rundell JR (eds): Clinical Manual of Psychosomatic Medicine: A Guide to Consultation-Liaison Psychiatry. Arlington VA, American Psychiatric Publishing Inc, 2005, pp 40–44
Sadock BJ, Sadock VA: Kaplan & Sadock's Comprehensive Textbook of Psychiatry, 9th ed. Philadelphia, Lippincott Williams & Wilkins, 2009, p 1165
Maldonado JR: Ask the Expert: Psychosomatic Medicine/Delirium. Focus 2009; 7(3):336–42

Which of the following stages has been identified by Kübler-Ross as a part of the process for dying patients?

(A) Anger
(B) Suicidal ideation
(C) Intellectualization
(D) Visual hallucinations
(E) Disorientation

The correct response is option **A**: Anger

Kübler-Ross postulated five stages that many dying patients pass through from the time they first become aware of their fatal prognosis to their actual death: Denial, Anger, Bargaining, Depression and Acceptance.

Sadock BJ, Sadock VA, Ruiz P (eds): Kaplan & Sadock's Comprehensive Textbook of Psychiatry, 9th ed. Philadelphia, Lippincott Williams & Wilkins, 2009, pp 2382–83.

In partial responders, which of the following classes of medications are effective adjuncts to SSRIs for the core symptoms of PTSD?

(A) Tricyclic antidepressants
(B) Lithium
(C) Anticonvulsants
(D) Benzodiazepines
(E) Atypical antipsychotics

The correct response is option **E**: Atypical antipsychotics

Atypical antipsychotics have been shown to be helpful with PTSD, anxiety, and psychotic spectrum positive symptoms. Because of concerns about toxicity, controlled trials of tricyclic antidepressants have not been done. Benzodiazepines are thought to disinhibit patients with PTSD and have been shown to be ineffective as monotherapy. There have been no controlled trials of lithium. Anticonvulsants have had mixed results as adjuvants in clinical trials.

Hales RE, Yudofsky SC, Gabbard GO (eds): The American Psychiatric Publishing Textbook of Psychiatry. 5th ed. American Psychiatric Publishing, Inc., Washington, DC. 2008. pp. 575–578
Benedek DM, Friedman MJ, Zatzick D, Ursano RJ. Guideline Watch (March 2009): Practice Guideline for the Treatment of Patients with Acute Stress Disorder and Posttraumatic Stress Disorder. FOCUS. 2009; 2:204–213 http://www.psychiatryonline.com/content.aspx?aid=156498

The treatment for body dysmorphic disorder that has been shown to be most effective includes which of the following psychotherapeutic techniques?

(A) Mindfulness training
(B) Exposure and response prevention
(C) Group psychotherapy
(D) Social skills training
(E) Biofeedback

The correct response is option **B**: Exposure and response prevention

The exposure and response prevention component of CBT has been found to be helpful in the treatment of body dysmorphic disorder. Part of the treatment includes exposing the patient to anxiety-provoking situations while not allowing the rituals to be performed. Group psychotherapy has not been demonstrated to be effective. Social skills training would be beneficial for social anxiety, which is often comorbid with body dysmorphic disorder. However, it would not address the core symptoms of BDD.

Phillips KA: Clinical features and treatment of body dysmorphic disorder. FOCUS. 2005; 3:179–183

A 69-year-old woman is hospitalized for pyelonephritis, which is successfully treated with antibiotics. Discharge to her home, where she lives alone, is planned. However, her daughter calls and informs the treatment team that she found several bottles of unused medications in the patient's home. The team wonders whether the patient can safely manage her medications at home, and asks psychiatry to evaluate her capacity. Which of the following potential reasons for medication noncompliance implies that the patient lacks capacity?

- (A) The patient was too delirious from her infection to remember to take her medications.
- (B) The patient's eyesight is too impaired to read the instructions on her pill bottles.
- (C) The patient is unable to understand the reasons the medications were prescribed.
- (D) The patient has a long history of noncompliance owing to a general mistrust of doctors.
- (E) The patient felt too hopeless and depressed to comply with her medication regimen.

The correct response is option **C**: The patient is unable to understand the reasons the medications were prescribed.

There are many potential reasons for medication noncompliance, and not all of them are reasons to consider a patient incapacitated. Physical reasons, such as arthritis or poor eyesight, can interfere, and these should be addressed with practical measures. Depression and delirium, although temporarily incapacitating a patient, are considered remediable conditions and should be treated before a capacity assessment is finalized. For some patients, noncompliance is consistent with their long-term personality and values. However, a patient's inability to understand the reasons a medication is prescribed during a psychiatric examination (which took place after her acute medical condition was resolved) suggests a more pervasive cognitive deficit affecting her ability to appreciate her condition. This inability to appreciate her illness and her need for medication is one of several generally accepted criteria for the capacity to make decisions.

Lai JM, Karlawish J. Assessing the capacity to make everyday decisions: a guide for clinicians and an agenda for future research. Am J Geriatr Psychiatry. 2007; 15(2):101–111

A 35-year-old man presents with memory deficits and emotional lability. Head CT reveals atrophy of the caudate. His father died from the same disorder when he was 38 years old. This presentation is most consistent with which of the following disorders?

- (A) Alzheimer's disease
- (B) Huntington's disease
- (C) Progressive multifocal leukodystrophy
- (D) Subacute sclerosing panencephalitis
- (E) Whipple's disease

The correct response is option **B**: Huntington's disease

The relationship between the onset of symptoms in the son and the same illness causing the death of his father at a very early age suggests that it is inherited. The only disease listed above which is inherited is Huntington's, which is transmitted autosomal dominant. Huntington's disease causes a combination of progressive motor, cognitive, psychiatric and behavioral dysfunction. The key pathological processes of Huntington's disease occur in the striatum, caudate, and putamen.

Levenson JL (ed): Essentials of Psychosomatic Medicine. American Psychiatric Publishing, Inc., Washington, DC, 2007. p 320

A 21-year-old patient has been diagnosed as having panic disorder. She reports that she frequently had difficulties with side effects in starting medications in the past. For this patient, which of the following would be the best beginning dose of sertraline?

- (A) 25 mg
- (B) 50 mg
- (C) 75 mg
- (D) 100 mg

The correct response is option **A**: 25 mg

Patients with panic disorder can be unusually sensitive to the side effects of the SSRIs, especially the activation. Adherence becomes a problem because restlessness, jitteriness, insomnia and agitation cannot be tolerated by the patient. It would be prudent to start this patient on a very low dose so side effects can be minimized as she adapts to the medication. Some psychiatrists initially give small amounts of a benzodiazepine like clonazepam to achieve symptom reduction while waiting the weeks for the SSRI to become effective. The benzodiazepine may treat panic while also reducing SSRI-induced activation symptoms.

Stein DJ, Hollander E, Rothbaum BO (eds): Textbook of Anxiety Disorders, 2nd ed. Arlington, VA, American Psychiatric Publishing, 2010, pp 399–401.

Paranoid personality disorder is marked by pervasive distrust and suspiciousness of others. For this diagnosis, distrust and suspiciousness can be manifested by which ONE of the following?

(A) Choosing solitary activities most of the time
(B) Experiencing social anxiety that persists even with familiarity
(C) Experiencing unusual perceptions such as bodily illusions
(D) Reading hidden, threatening meaning into benign events
(E) Showing emotional detachment

The correct response is option **D**: Reading hidden, threatening meaning into benign events

While a patient with paranoid personality disorder may display any one or more of the other features, they are not criteria for this diagnosis. Choosing solitary activities and showing emotional detachment are diagnostic criteria for schizoid personality disorder; experiencing social anxiety even in familiar contexts, and unusual bodily illusions are diagnostic criteria for schizotypal personality disorder.

Diagnostic and Statistical Manual of Mental Disorders, 4th ed, Text Revi (DSM-IV-TR). Washington, DC, American Psychiatric Association, 2000, pp 690–701

A 50-year-old man with a 20-year history of smoking 1–2 packs per day attempts to quit by using the nicotine patch. He relapses to smoking after four days of cessation. He comes for an appointment, saying he knew it was going to be harder than he thought and he's not sure he can go through the process again. The best response would be:

(A) "Most people need more than two tries before they successfully quit."
(B) "You will need to try harder next time."
(C) "With persistence about 75% of smokers successfully quit."
(D) "Let's try the same thing again."
(E) "Most smokers require more intensive treatment to quit."

The correct response is option **A**: "Most people need more than two tries before they successfully quit."

The psychiatrist should help maintain the patient's hope in the face of his demoralization. Most smokers who successfully quit have had 5–7 prior unsuccessful attempts. The 75% estimate is, however, too optimistic – about half of all smokers successfully quit. The next quit attempt should take advantage of lessons learned from this failed attempt, and not simply re-try the same interventions. Most smokers quit on their own or with minimal treatment.

American Psychiatric Association Practice Guideline for the Treatment of Patients with Substance Use Disorders, 2nd Edition, (2006), http://psychiatryonline.com/pracGuide/pracGuideHome.aspx.

In elderly patients, which of the following conditions is most important to address to prevent depressive symptoms after hip fracture surgery?

(A) Postoperative pain
(B) Requiring assistance with mobility
(C) Using benzodiazepines daily
(D) Using >4 medications

The correct response is option **A**: Postoperative pain

Depression after hip fracture surgery in the elderly is both common and a significant cause of morbidity. A number of investigators have looked for factors that might predict depression in an attempt to prevent it. Significant factors predicting postoperative depression in elderly individuals include postoperative anxiety and pain. The other variables listed have not been shown to have a significant effect (mobility problems reach some statistical significance when they are severe; however this significance is diminished when controlling for pain). These findings are important as pain and anxiety represent treatable problems that should be treated aggressively in elderly postsurgical patients.

Voshaar RC, Banerjee S, Horan M, Baldwin R, Pendleton N, Proctor R, Tarrier N, Woodward Y, Burns A. Predictors of incident depression after hip fracture surgery. Am J Geriatr Psychiatry. 2007; 15(9):807–814

A 36-year-old woman with breast cancer completed radiotherapy. However, three months later she continues to complain of disabling fatigue. In evaluating this patient, which of the following symptoms would suggest that the fatigue was directly due to her medical condition rather than depression?

(A) Late insomnia
(B) Impaired concentration
(C) Feelings of limb heaviness
(D) Decreased interest in activities
(E) Weight loss

The correct response is option **C**: Feelings of limb heaviness

Fatigue is a common problem with cancer patients, and it can be difficult to distinguish fatigue directly caused by comorbid illnesses such as depression. However, such a differentiation can be important for planning effective treatment. Many symptoms of cancer fatigue, such as insomnia, impaired concentration, lack of interest, poor appetite and associated weight loss are common to both disorders. However, certain physical symptoms, such as the subjective reports of weakness or limb heaviness, may be associated with cancer fatigue rather than depression.

Levy MR. Cancer fatigue: a neurobiological review for psychiatrists. Psychosomatics. 2008; 49(4):283–291

A 24-year-old woman is comatose with generalized myoclonic twitching and is found to have a serum lithium concentration of 4.2 mEq/L. The treatment of choice is:

(A) saline diuresis.
(B) hemodialysis.
(C) exchange transfusion.
(D) plasmapheresis.

The correct response is option **B**: Hemodialysis

In the presence of severe lithium poisoning which generally presents with neurotoxicity, hemodialysis is the treatment of choice because it most rapidly clears lithium from the body. Lithium is a simple structure (an element) that is water soluble and is neither protein bound nor metabolized; hence, it is readily dialyzable. Following dialysis, lithium redistribution from tissues may result in a rebound increase in blood level which, in turn, may necessitate further dialysis.

Jefferson JW, Greist JH: Lithium, in Kaplan & Sadock's Comprehensive Textbook of Psychiatry, 9th ed. Edited by Sadock BJ, Sadock VA, Ruiz P. Philadelphia, Lippincott Williams & Wilkins, 2009, pp 3132–45.

290

A 72-year-old man is referred by his primary care doctor to a geriatric psychiatrist for treatment of depression. Two weeks earlier the man had seen his primary care doctor who started citalopram 20 mg daily. The patient continues to report severe depressive symptoms. On interview, it becomes apparent that this is the man's first episode of depression, and he has no history of any prior psychiatric disorder. The psychiatrist should advise that the patient:

(A) discontinue citalopram and begin nortriptyline.
(B) discontinue citalopram and begin venlafaxine.
(C) continue citalopram, but add lithium.
(D) continue the current treatment as prescribed.
(E) increase the citalopram to 40 mg daily.

The correct response is option **D**: Continue the current treatment as prescribed.

Late onset depression is often thought to have a different course than early onset depression, and it is speculated that the approach should be different as well; however, there is little data to support this. The Sequenced Treatment Alternatives to Relieve Depression (STAR*D) study, when looking at late onset depression, did not find any difference in treatment response when compared with younger patients. Until new data suggests otherwise, the approach to late life depression should be similar to that for depression in younger individuals, which in this case would be to continue the citalopram as prescribed, as there remains a good possibility that the patient will respond in subsequent weeks without additional intervention. The addition of adjunctive medications as well as a premature dose increase would only increase the risk of side effects without increasing the chance of response.

Kozel FA, Trivedi MH, Wisniewski SR, Miyahara S, Husain MM, Fava M, Lebowitz B, Zisook S, Rush AJ. Treatment outcomes for older depressed patients with earlier versus late onset of first depressive episode: a Sequenced Treatment Alternatives to Relieve Depression (STAR*D) report. Am J Geriatr Psychiatry. 2008; 16(1):58–64

291

In addition to being effective in treating major depression, interpersonal psychotherapy has been shown to be highly effective in the treatment of which of the following disorders?

(A) Substance abuse
(B) Bulimia nervosa
(C) Obsessive-compulsive disorder
(D) Schizophrenia
(E) Dysthymia

The correct response is option **B**: Bulimia nervosa

The bulk of evidence for interpersonal psychotherapy (IPT) is for the treatment of major depression, however it has also been shown to be helpful in the treatment of bulimia, and IPT is included as an option in the American Psychiatric Association's Practice Guidelines for both disorders. Studies of IPT for substance abuse have not demonstrated efficacy. IPT experts have suggested that the treatment is less likely to be helpful for internally focused illnesses, such as schizophrenia and obsessive-compulsive disorder, however this opinion has not been systematically tested.

Markowitz JC: The clinical conduct of interpersonal psychotherapy. FOCUS 2006;4:179–184
Textbook of Psychotherapeutic Treatments. Gabbard GO (ed). Arlington VA, American Psychiatric Publishing Inc, 2009, p 342

292

A decrease of which neuropeptide has been linked most closely to narcolepsy?

(A) Neurotensin
(B) Oxytocin
(C) Somatostatin
(D) Hypocretin
(E) Melanocyte-stimulating hormone

The correct response is option **D**: Hypocretin

Patients with narcolepsy and cataplexy have low CSF concentrations of hypocretin, a peptide produced in the lateral hypothalamus. A narcolepsy-like condition has been produced in hypocretin receptor knockout mice.

Dauvilliers Y, Arnulf I, Mignot E. Narcolepsy with cataplexy. Lancet. 2007; 369:499–511
Moore DP. Textbook of Clinical Neuropsychiatry, 2nd ed. London, Hodder Arnold, 2008. pp 575–577.

293

Which of the following antidepressants could be pre-scribed for a depressed patient who has major concerns about the possible effects of medication on sexual functioning?

(A) Sertraline
(B) Venlafaxine
(C) Paroxetine
(D) Bupropion
(E) Trazodone

The correct response is option **D**: Bupropion

Bupropion has a favorable side-effect profile, in part because of its low affinity for muscarinic, adrenergic, and histaminic receptors. Sexual dysfunction and weight gain are rare side effects and are less frequent than with the other antidepressants listed. Bupropion has also been used in combined treatments with other antidepressants, particularly with SSRIs for treating patients with SSRI-induced sexual dysfunction.

Schatzberg AF, Nemeroff CB (eds): Essentials of Clinical Psychopharmacology, 2nd ed. Arlington, VA, American Psychiatric Publishing, Inc., 2006. pp 85–90

Hales RE, Yudofsky SC, Gabbard GO (eds): The American Psychiatric Publishing Textbook of Psychiatry, 5th ed. Washington, DC, American Psychiatric Publishing, 2008. pp 1060–1061

294

Which of the diagnostic criteria for PTSD is rarely fully-endorsed in preschool children?

(A) Disturbance of over one month
(B) Re-experiencing
(C) Avoidance/numbing
(D) Increased arousal
(E) Clinically significant impairment

The correct response is option **C**: Avoidance/numbing

Only 2% of highly traumatized preschool children endorsed at least three of the symptoms necessary to meet criteria for the avoidance/numbing cluster. However, once the number of required symptoms in the cluster is reduced to one, twenty-five percent of preschool children who have been highly traumatized meet criteria for PTSD.

Martin A, Volkmar FR (eds) Lewis's Comprehensive Textbook Child and Adolescent Psychiatry, 4th ed. Philadelphia, Lippincott Williams & Wilkins, 2007. p. 706

Sheeringa MS, Zeanah CH, Myers L, Putnam FW. New findings on alternative criteria for PTSD in preschool children. J Am Acad Child Adolesc Psychiatry. 2003; 42(5):564–565

295

When compared to individuals with Parkinson's disease dementia (PD-D), individuals with Alzheimer's disease dementia (AD-D) typically show more severe impairment in:

(A) apraxia.
(B) visual hallucinosis.
(C) depressive symptoms.
(D) visuospatial dysfunction.

The correct response is option **A**: Apraxia

While Alzheimer's disease dementia (AD-D) and Parkinson's disease dementia (PD-D) can occur simultaneously, *AD-D alone* has a neuropsychological profile distinct from PD-D. In early and moderate stages, AD-D findings are predominantly cortical, while PD-D findings are prefrontal and subcortical. All deficits except for apraxia are more likely to appear earlier and more severely in PD-D than AD-D, while apraxia, along with agitation, disinhibition, irritability, and euphoria, is more common in AD-D.

Emre M. What causes mental dysfunction in Parkinson's disease? Mov Disord. 2003; 18 Suppl 6: S63–S71

296

Generally, restraint and seclusion are considered appropriate treatment interventions when the patient is at imminent risk to harm himself or others AND:

(A) the patient is refusing medication.
(B) no less restrictive alternative is available.
(C) the hospital prefers physical to chemical restraint.
(D) the time period is expected to be brief.
(E) a physician is present to write the order.

The correct response is option **B**: no less restrictive alternative is available

Generally the courts have held that restraints and seclusion can be used only when the patient is at risk to harm himself or others and no less restrictive alternative exists. Most states have laws regulating the use of restraints, specifying the circumstances in which restraints can be used.

Simon RI. The law and psychiatry. FOCUS: Forensic and Ethical Issues in Psychiatry; Fall 2003; 4:365.

297

A bus carrying students from a local high school is swept down the side of the mountain following a mudslide. Despite rescue attempts, all the youth on the bus either die or are seriously wounded. Based on prevalence data, which of the following groups of individuals is most likely to develop PTSD symptoms after the disaster?

(A) Family members
(B) First responders
(C) Guidance counselors
(D) Classmates
(E) Teachers

The correct response is option **B**: First responders

In a systematic review of posttraumatic stress disorder following disasters, the highest prevalence of PTSD was found among survivors and first responders. The prevalence of PTSD among first responders assessed following involvement in rescue, recovery and cleaning efforts were especially high.

Neria Y, Nandi A, Galea S. Post-traumatic stress disorder following disasters: a systematic review. Psychol Med. 2008; 38(4):467–480

298

In association with research leading up to DSM-5, the core features of personality disorders are being re-examined. Investigators are assessing which characteristics are stable, trait-like and "attitudinal", and which tend to vary with life-stresses over time. For which one of the following personality disorder diagnoses were rigidity and problems delegating found to be the least changeable criteria?

(A) Schizotypal personality disorder
(B) Narcissistic personality disorder
(C) Borderline personality disorder
(D) Avoidant personality disorder
(E) Obsessive-compulsive personality disorder

Answer **E**. Obsessive-compulsive personality disorder

As research into personality disorders proceeds in the direction of DSM-5, investigators are re-examining core features of diagnoses. Investigators tracked the course of individual diagnostic criteria of four DSM-IV diagnoses, borderline (BPD), schizotypal, avoidant and obsessive compulsive (OCPD) personality disorders in 474 patients who completed 24 months of a longitudinal study. The least changeable criteria for BPD were affective instability, impulsivity and anger; for schizotypal PD, paranoid ideation and unusual thinking; for avoidant PD, feelings of inadequacy and social ineptness; and for OCPD, rigidity and problems delegating. Each diagnosis was found to be comprised of both stable personality trait-like and "attitudinal criteria," and criteria that vary with life-stresses over time.

McGlashan TH, Grilo CM, Sanislow CA, Ralevski E, Morey LC, Gunderson JG, Skodol AE, Shea MT, Zanarini MC, Bender D, Stout RL, Yen S, Pagano M. Two-year prevalence and stability of individual DSM-IV criteria for schizotypal, borderline, avoidant, and obsessive-compulsive personality disorders: toward a hybrid model of axis II disorders. Am J Psychiatry, 2005; 162:883–889.

299

Which of the following antiepileptic drugs has been shown to be effective in treating binge eating disorder associated with obesity in short-term, placebo-controlled studies?

(A) Topiramate
(B) Lamotrigine
(C) Oxcarbazepine
(D) Valproate
(E) Tiagabine

The correct response is option **A**: Topiramate

The anticonvulsant medication topiramate is effective for binge reduction and weight loss, although adverse effects may limit its clinical utility for some individuals. In short-term trials, topiramate has been shown to significantly reduce binge frequency. In one study, 58% of patients on topiramate reached remission versus 29% on placebo.

McElroy SL, Hudson JI, Capece JA, Beyers K, Fisher AC, Rosenthal NR; Topiramate Binge Eating Disorder Research Group. Topiramate for the treatment of binge eating disorder associated with obesity: a placebo-controlled study. Biol Psychiatry. 2007; 61(9): 1039–1048

McElroy SL, Shapira NA, Arnold LM, Keck PE, Rosenthal NR, Wu SC, Capece JA, Fazzio L, Hudson JI. Topiramate in the long-term treatment of binge-eating disorder associated with obesity. J Clin Psychiatry. 2004; 65(11):1463–1469

300

A 32-year-old man is admitted to the hospital with a severe episode of bipolar disorder, mixed. Which of the following would be the best first-line pharmacologic treatment for him?

(A) Lithium alone
(B) Lithium plus a benzodiazepine
(C) Lithium plus an antidepressant
(D) Lithium plus an antipsychotic
(E) Lithium plus valproate

The correct response is option **D**: Lithium plus an antipsychotic

The first-line pharmacological treatment for more severe manic or mixed episodes is the initiation of lithium plus an antipsychotic or valproate plus an antipsychotic. For less ill patients, monotherapy with lithium, valproate, or an antipsychotic such as olanzapine may be sufficient. Short-term adjunctive treatment with a benzodiazepine may also be helpful.

American Psychiatric Association Practice Guideline for the Treatment of Patients with Bipolar Disorder, 2nd ed (2002), Reprinted in FOCUS: Bipolar Disorder, Winter 2003, 1:64.

301

Which of the following medications has the strongest body of evidence for the treatment of bulimia nervosa?

(A) Bupropion
(B) Fluoxetine
(C) Duloxetine
(D) Paroxetine
(E) Venlafaxine

The correct response is option **B**: Fluoxetine

In November 1996, the FDA approved fluoxetine for the treatment of moderate to severe bulimia nervosa based on the results of two 8-week and one 16-week placebo-controlled trials.

American Psychiatric Association Practice Guideline for Treatment of Patients with Eating Disorders, 3rd ed. Am J Psychiatry. 2006; http://psychiatryonline.com/pracGuide/pracGuideHome.aspx

Hales RE, Yudofsky SC, Gabbard GO (eds): The American Psychiatric Publishing Textbook of Psychiatry, 5th ed. American Psychiatric Publishing, Inc., 2008. p 989

302

Which of the following patterns is most likely to be seen on an EEG of a delirious patient?

(A) Generalized slowing
(B) Increased alpha
(C) Decreased theta
(D) Triphasic sharp waves
(E) Focal high frequency spikes

The correct response is option **A**: Generalized slowing

Delirious patients have progressive disorganization of rhythms and generalized slowing. There is slowing of the peak and average frequencies in addition to increased theta and delta but decreased alpha rhythms.

Hales RE, Yudofsky SC, Gabbard GO (eds): The American Psychiatric Publishing Textbook of Psychiatry, 5th ed. Washington, DC, American Psychiatric Publishing, Inc., 2008. p 864

Fearing MA, Inouye SK. Delirium. American Psychiatric Publishing Textbook of Geriatric Psychiatry. 2009. Blazer DG, Steffens DC (eds). Reprinted in FOCUS. 2009; 1:53–63

303

Which of the following types of psychotherapy focuses on a patient's current social functioning within one of four problem areas (reaction, interpersonal disputes, role transition, or interpersonal deficits)?

(A) Supportive psychotherapy
(B) Interpersonal psychotherapy
(C) Cognitive therapy
(D) Psychodynamic psychotherapy
(E) Psychoanalytic psychotherapy

The correct response is option **B**: Interpersonal psychotherapy

Interpersonal psychotherapy was developed out of the work of Henry Stack Sullivan by Klerman and colleagues to focus on interpersonal functioning in four common problem areas. The focus tends to be on current relationships and can include the teaching of new behavioral skills.

Hales RE, Yudofsky SC (eds): The American Psychiatric Publishing Textbook of Psychiatry. 4th ed. American Psychiatric Publishing, Inc., Washington, DC. 2008, pp 1186–1188
Markowitz JC: The clinical conduct of interpersonal psychotherapy. Focus 2006; 4(2): 179–84

304

A patient with a long history of successful treatment with 20 mg of fluoxetine has been found to be HIV+ and has initiated antiretroviral therapy. The patient sees you because of a return of symptoms of depression. Which of the following is the most likely pharmacologic cause?

(A) As the patient gained weight from an increased appetite, more of the imipramine became bound to fat cells.
(B) The protease inhibitor caused lipodystrophy which decreased fluoxetine levels.
(C) The protease inhibitor began to compete with fluoxetine for protein-binding sites.
(D) The protease inhibitor induced the activity of an enzyme that enhanced the metabolism of fluoxetine and norfluoxetine.
(E) The protease inhibitor has a direct interaction on the fluoxetine, causing it to lose efficacy.

The correct response is option **D**: The protease inhibitor induced the activity of an enzyme which enhanced metabolism of fluoxetine or norfluoxetine.

Some protease inhibitors induce the activity of cytochrome P450 2D6, which increases the metabolism of many medications like fluoxetine and TCAs. Induction of this enzyme would decrease the plasma concentration of fluoxetine and norfluoxetine. Lipodystrophy is a complication of antiretroviral therapy but would not occur immediately after initiating treatment. Disreplacement of fluoxetine from protein would increase, not decrease, fluoxetine levels. Current HAART treatment is not believed to cause direct drug interactions that would decrease fluoxetine's effectiveness.

Hales RE, Yudofsky SC, Gabbard GO (eds): The American Psychiatric Publishing Textbook of Psychiatry, 5th ed. Arlington VA, American Psychiatric Publishing Inc, 2008, pp 1055–1057

305

A 24-year-old man is arrested after repeated episodes of rubbing his genitals against women's buttocks while riding on the subway. The most likely paraphilic diagnosis is which of the following?

(A) Fetishism
(B) Frotteurism
(C) Exhibitionism
(D) Voyeurism
(E) Sexual masochism

The correct response is option **B**: Frotteurism

According to DSM-IV-TR, "The paraphilic focus of Frotteurism involves touching or rubbing against a nonconsenting person." The behavior typically takes place in crowded locations from which escape is more likely. Fetishism involves "recurrent, sexually arousing fantasies, sexual urges, or behaviors involving the use of nonliving objects."

American Psychiatric Association: Diagnostic and Statistical Manual of Mental Disorders, 4th Edition, Text Revision (DSM-IV-TR). Washington DC, American Psychiatric Association, 2000, p 570

306

Which ONE of the following is the most consistently agreed upon characteristic of supportive psychotherapy?

(A) It is a form of psychodynamic psychotherapy.
(B) It is based on the use of transference or other interpretation.
(C) It is best for patients with axis- II disorders.
(D) Its practice requires only common sense, interpersonal skills, and a capacity for empathy.
(E) It serves primarily to strengthen patient's self-esteem.

The correct response is option **E**: It serves primarily to strengthens patient's self-esteem.

A number of texts on supportive psychotherapy are available, but no universally agreed upon definitions of supportive psychotherapy and its methods exist. Agreed upon elements of supportive psychotherapy include 1) that it strengthens the patient's self-esteem and 2) it enhances the therapeutic alliance.

Douglas CJ: Teaching supportive psychotherapy to psychiatric residents. Am J Psychiatry 2008; 165:445–452
Hellerstein DJ, Markowitz JC: Developing supportive psychotherapy as evidence-based treatment. Am J Psychiatry 2008; 165: 1355-–1356

307

Which of the following treatments has the greatest body of evidence demonstrating efficacy for treatment of specific phobia?

(A) Eye movement desensitization and reprocessing (EMDR)
(B) In vivo exposure therapy
(C) Hypnotherapy
(D) Pharmacotherapy
(E) Imaginal exposure therapy

The correct response is option **B**: In vivo exposure therapy

The best data supports exposure therapy as the most reliable treatment. "Imaginal exposure" therapy uses an imagined picture of the feared object. It has not proved to be as effective as in vivo treatment. EMDR uses an imagined phobic object as well, but with horizontal eye movements stimulated by hand movements of the therapist. It has not been successful. Studies of pharmacotherapy and hypnotherapy are inconclusive.

Stein DJ, Hollander E, Rothbaum BO (eds): Textbook of Anxiety Disorders, 2nd ed. Arlington, VA, American Psychiatric Publishing, 2010, pp 533–35.

308

A 23-year-old man is the sole survivor of a fire aboard a crowded plane. In the immediate aftermath of exposure to the trauma, which of the following interventions is most likely to be successful in preventing psychological sequelae?

(A) Encourage him to imagine positive emotions.
(B) Have the man ventilate about how he is feeling.
(C) Normalize the stress reaction.
(D) Prescribe a short-acting benzodiazepine.
(E) Use critical incident debriefing.

The correct response is option **C**: Normalize the stress reaction.

For both those who develop more severe stress reactions and the general population of exposed individuals, normalization of stress reactions is a key intervention principle to enhance calming. A major reason why ventilation and psychological debriefing have been criticized is that they serve to enhance arousal in the immediate aftermath of trauma exposure. Benzodiazepines are effective for acute symptom relief and immediate calming, but have been shown to increase the likelihood of PTSD among symptomatic trauma survivors when used as monotherapy. Exposure therapy is only effective when the event can be paired with freedom from anxiety.

Hobfoll SE, Watson P, Bell CC, Bryant RA, Brymer MJ, Friedman MJ, Friedman M, Gersons BP, de Jong JT, Layne CM, Maguen S, Neria Y, Norwood AE, Pynoos RS, Reissman D, Ruzek JI, Shalev AY, Solomon Z, Steinberg AM, Ursano RJ: Five essential elements of immediate and mid-term mass trauma intervention: empirical evidence. Psychiatry. 2007; 70(4):283–315. Reprinted in FOCUS. 2009; 2:221–242

American Psychiatric Association Practice Guideline for the Treatment of Patients with Acute Stress Disorder and Posttraumatic Stress Disorder. Am J Psychiatry. 2004; 161(11): 1013 http://www.psychiatryonline.com/pracGuide/ pracGuideTopic_11.aspx

309

Following survival from a tornado that killed 38 people in a local community, a woman is provided with education and training of coping skills that includes deep muscle relaxation, breathing control, assertiveness, role playing, covert modeling, thought stopping, positive thinking, and self-talks. The intervention described is:

(A) aversion therapy.
(B) insight-oriented psychotherapy.
(C) interpersonal therapy.
(D) stress inoculation training.

The correct response is option **D**: Stress inoculation training.

Stress inoculation training (SIT) is a type of cognitive behavioral therapy that can be thought of as a toolbox, or set of skills, for managing anxiety and stress. A number of studies have found SIT to be effective with rape victims, accident survivors and soldiers experiencing combat stress reactions.

Hobfoll SE, Watson P, Bell CC, Bryant RA, Brymer MJ, Friedman MJ, Friedman M, Gersons BP, de Jong JT, Layne CM, Maguen S, Neria Y, Norwood AE, Pynoos RS, Reissman D, Ruzek JI, Shalev AY, Solomon Z, Steinberg AM, Ursano RJ: Five essential elements of immediate and mid-term mass trauma intervention: empirical evidence. Psychiatry. 2007; 70(4):283–315. Reprinted in FOCUS. 2009; 2:221–242

310

Which of the following symptoms is most consistent with a medication side effect rather than progression of Huntington's disease?

(A) Flowing movements
(B) Postural instability
(C) Effects on swallowing
(D) Akathisia
(E) Facial apraxia

The correct response is option **D**: Akathisia

Characteristics specific to side effects of anti-psychotic medications, but not Huntington's disease, are akathisia and marching in place. Characteristics specific to Huntington's disease include forehead chorea, flowing movements, facial apraxia, oculomotor defects, gait disorder, postural instability, and effects on swallowing.

Gabbard GO (ed): Treatments of Psychiatric Disorders 4th ed. American Psychiatric Publishing, Inc., Washington, DC. 2007. p 486

Scott B. Movement Disorders. American Psychiatric Publishing Textbook of Geriatric Psychiatry. 2009. Blazer DG, Steffens DC (eds).

311

The hormone that masculinizes the human brain during uterine life is:

(A) testosterone.
(B) dihydrotestosterone.
(C) estrone.
(D) estradiol.
(E) progesterone.

The correct response is option **D**: Estradiol

While the fetal testis is required to produce the testosterone that serves as precursor, the actual hormone of masculinization is estradiol, produced from testosterone by the enzyme aromatase. The developing female brain is ordinarily exposed neither to testosterone nor to estrogen derivatives. A second breakdown product of testosterone – dihydrotestosterone – is responsible for the development of male genitalia – testes, scrotum, and penis – from female anlagen initially found in all embryos. In the absence of dihydrotestosterone, the female habitus is the default option.

Schwarz JM, McCarthy MM: Steroid-induced sexual differentiation of the developing brain: multiple pathways, one goal. J Neurochem. 2008; 105:1561–1572

Bostwick JM, Martin KA: A man's brain in an ambiguous body: a case of mistaken gender identity. Am J Psychiatry. 2007; 164: 1499–1505

312

Which of the following cognitive abilities is preserved in normal aging?

(A) Working memory
(B) Perceptual-motor skills
(C) Vocabulary
(D) Fluency
(E) Logical problem solving

The correct response is option **C**: Vocabulary

While perceptual-motor skills, working memory, fluency and logical problem solving all decline with increasing age, vocabulary may stay stable or even increase with age.

Spar JE, La Rue A. Normal aging. In Spar JE, La Rue A (eds). Clinical Manual of Geriatric Psychiatry, 1st ed. Arlington, VA: American Psychiatric Publishing Inc; 2006. pp 213–214

Meeks TW, Lanouette N, Vahia I, Dawes S, Jeste DV, Lebowitz B. Psychiatric assessment and diagnosis in older adults. FOCUS. 2009; 7:3–16

313

Explicit feelings of shame, shame proneness, and self-stigma associated with higher ratings of anger and hostility have been empirically demonstrated to be increased in patients with which of the following disorders?

(A) Social phobia
(B) Borderline personality disorder
(C) Histrionic personality disorder
(D) Dysthymia
(E) Paranoid personality disorder

The correct response is option **B**: Borderline personality disorder

Shame proneness is common in patients with borderline personality disorder, and is related to anger-hostility, lower quality of life, and low self-esteem. Clinicians have long recognized that shame is an important characteristic of patients with borderline personality disorder (BPD) often associated with suicidality, self-harm, rage, and impulsivity, and some have even suggested that borderline personality disorder is largely a chronic shame response. A recent study compared women with BPD, social phobia, and normal controls, using self-report measures to assess "explicit shame" (i.e. consciously accessible self-cognitions) and "implicit shame"or shame proneness (i.e. measures of implicit or automatic self concepts and attitudes based on speed and closeness of word and phrase associations evoked in response to vignettes of potentially embarrassing and anxiety-provoking situations). In general, measures of explicit and implicit shame were not highly correlated. In comparison to the other groups, women with BPD scored higher in measures of shame and shame-proneness, and in contrast to the other groups were more prone to associate with shame than anxiety in response to the vignettes. After controlling for depression, shame proneness was associated with lower quality of life and lower self-esteem, and positively correlated with measures of anger-hostility. Empirical studies of these constructs in patients with other personality disorders have not yet been conducted or published.

Rüsch N, Lieb K, Göttler I, Hermann C, Schramm E, Richter H, Jacob GA, Corrigan PW, Bohus M. Shame and Implicit Self-Concept in Women With Borderline Personality Disorder. Am J Psychiatry, September 2007 164:500–508.

Rüsch N, Hölzer A, Hermann C, Schramm E, Jacob GA, Bohus M, Lieb K, Corrigan PW. Self-stigma in women with borderline personality disorder and women with social phobia. J Nerv Ment Dis. 2006 Oct;194(10):766–73

314

Following a massive hurricane, the occupants of a city are placed in a temporary refugee camp until other housing can be obtained. Which of the following ways of organizing the refugee camp is likely to be most successful in preventing PTSD?

(A) Bring in citizen leaders from nearby cities to run the camp.
(B) Develop the camp into a village with a village council.
(C) Have the military oversee operation of the camp.
(D) Organize the camp along racial, religious, and ethnic divisions.
(E) Provide individuals with their own tents.

The correct response is option **B**: Develop the camp into a village with a village council

Large-scale interventions in the majority of countries consistently find that efforts to promote social support networks in temporary refugee camps are effective in preventing PTSD symptoms. This is related to self- and collective efficacy. This is best embodied in the idea of developing the camp into a village with village councils, welcoming committees, places of worship, places to for services, etc. Further, citizens of the village, rather than outsiders, fill the social roles and do so within their natural cultural traditions and practices. If people spend most of their time alone in their own tents, they are not as likely to be as connected to others.

Hobfoll SE, Watson P, Bell CC, Bryant RA, Brymer MJ, Friedman MJ, Friedman M, Gersons BP, de Jong JT, Layne CM, Maguen S, Neria Y, Norwood AE, Pynoos RS, Reissman D, Ruzek JI, Shalev AY, Solomon Z, Steinberg AM, Ursano RJ: Five essential elements of immediate and mid-term mass trauma intervention: empirical evidence. Psychiatry. 2007; 70(4):283–315. Reprinted in FOCUS. 2009; 2:221–242

315

Which of the following signs and symptoms is most reliable in distinguishing between delirium and dementia?

(A) Orientation
(B) Short-term memory
(C) Long-term memory
(D) Sleep pattern
(E) Level of consciousness

The correct response is option **E**: Level of consciousness

Memory impairment, sleep disruption, and other cognitive disturbances may be present in both dementia and delirium. The characteristic feature of delirium is a disturbance of arousal or level of consciousness; this is typically not present in dementia. Other features that characterize delirium are disorientation, development of perceptual disturbance, attention deficits, disordered sleep wake, fluctuation in presentation (waxing and waning), and changes in psychomotor activity depending on the type of delirium.

Maldonado JR. Ask the Expert: Delirium. FOCUS. 2009; 3:336–342
Sadock BJ, Sadock VA, Ruiz P (eds): Kaplan & Sadock's Comprehensive Textbook of Psychiatry, 9th ed. Philadelphia, Lippincott Williams & Wilkins, 2009, pp 4069–70

316

A 64-year-old patient is hospitalized for an injury that occurred while he was inebriated. Three days after admission the patient is disoriented, hallucinating, and has a grand mal seizure. His blood pressure is 160/100, with a pulse of 105. Which of the following medications is most appropriate for managing this patient's condition?

- (A) Haloperidol
- (B) Sertraline
- (C) Quetiapine
- (D) Lorazepam
- (E) Propranolol

The correct response is option **D**: Lorazepam

This patient has developed delirium secondary to alcohol withdrawal (i.e., delirium tremens). The most appropriate initial treatment for alcohol withdrawal delirium is a benzodiazepine. Antipsychotic medications may be appropriate in combination with benzodiazepines, but caution must be used as antipsychotic agents can lower the seizure threshold. The patient's age and history of alcohol use suggest that a drug with a shorter half-life and renal clearance would be of greatest benefit. Antidepressants are not indicated in alcohol withdrawal.

American Society of Addiction Medicine (ASAM). Principles of Addiction Medicine, 3rd ed. ASAM, 2003; pp 626, 630

Hales RE, Yudofsky SC, Gabbard GO (eds): The American Psychiatric Publishing Textbook of Psychiatry, 5th ed. Washington, DC, American Psychiatric Publishing, 2008, p 571

317

Which of the following chromosomal abnormalities is associated with an increased risk of early onset Alzheimer's dementia?

- (A) Angelman syndrome (Deletion of the 15q11-q13 region of chromosome 15)
- (B) Down syndrome (trisomy 21)
- (C) Turner syndrome (monosomy X)
- (D) Klinefelter syndrome (46, xy/47, xxy mosaicism)

The correct response is option **B**: Down syndrome (trisomy 21)

Down syndrome (trisomy 21) has been associated with an increased risk for dementia. Such a risk has not been identified with chromosome 15 deletions (Angelman syndrome), monosomy X (Turner syndrome), 46, xy/47, xxy mosaicism (Klinefelter syndrome).

Coppus AM, Evenhuis HM, Verberne GJ, Visser FE, Arias-Vasquez A, Sayed-Tabatabaei FA, Vergeer-Drop J, Eikelenboom P, van Gool WA, van Duijn CM. The impact of apolipoprotein E on dementia in persons with Down's syndrome. Neurobiol Aging. 2008; 29(6): 828–835

National Institutes of Health, US Department of Health & Human Services: Your Guide to Understanding Genetic Conditions Handbook. http://ghr.nlm.nih.gov/handbook/genetics

318

Which of the following is the most common psychiatric diagnosis among patients with cancer who have no prior psychiatric history?

- (A) Posttraumatic stress disorder
- (B) Major depressive disorder
- (C) Acute stress disorder
- (D) Adjustment disorder
- (E) Generalized anxiety disorder

The correct response is option **D**: Adjustment disorder

While the other disorders listed may occur in patients with cancer, the largest group of psychiatric disorders present in cancer patients are the adjustment disorders (with depressed mood, anxious mood, and/or mixed features).

Sadock BJ, Sadock VA, Ruiz P (eds): Kaplan & Sadock's Comprehensive Textbook of Psychiatry, 9th ed. Philadelphia, Lippincott Williams & Wilkins, 2009, p 2322

319

A 40-year-old woman with bipolar I disorder complains of a lengthy, paralyzing period of depression following an episode of mania that led to hospitalization. Her symptoms have not responded to treatment with lamotrigine alone. Which of the following medications has the best evidence for efficacy as monotherapy to treat this patient's depression?

(A) Aripiprazole
(B) Haloperidol
(C) Quetiapine
(D) Valproic acid

The correct response is option **C**: Quetiapine

Quetiapine monotherapy has been shown in a large randomized, double-blind placebocontrolled trial to be effective in treatment of bipolar I or II depression. Although valproic acid would be an appropriate choice for maintenance therapy in a patient with bipolar I disorder, it would be expected to have limited utility in acutely treating bipolar depression. Aripiprazole monotherapy has evidence for efficacy in the acute treatment of manic or mixed episodes but has not been sufficiently studied to recommend its use in the acute treatment of bipolar depression. Haloperidol also does not have evidence for efficacy and extrapyramidal side effects could be associated with an apparent worsening of depressive symptoms.

Hirschfeld RMA: "Guideline Watch: Practice Guideline for the Treatment of Patients with Bipolar Disorder, 2nd Edition" *APA Practice Guidelines* pp 3–4, November 2005. Reprinted in FOCUS, Winter 2007,1:36.

American Psychiatric Association Practice Guideline for the Treatment of Patients with Bipolar Disorder, 2nd ed (2002) Reprinted in FOCUS: Bipolar Disorder, Winter 2003; 1:64–110.

American Psychiatric Association Practice Guideline for the Treatment of Patients with Schizophrenia, 2nd ed (2004). http://psychiatryonline.com/pracGuide/pracGuideHome.aspx

320

A 28-year-old man presents with the chief complaint of excessive daytime sleepiness. He reports the sudden onset of brief periods of daytime sleep that are very restful. On a few occasions, he has experienced brief muscle paralysis after laughter. Recently, he has had two episodes of temporary paralysis when he awakens during the morning accompanied by vivid visual hallucinations. A polysomnogram is most likely to show which of the following?

(A) Episodes of decreased blood oxygen saturation in spite of ventilatory effort
(B) Sleep-onset REM periods within 15 minutes of falling asleep
(C) Increased sleep spindles and K-complexes in stage 2 non-REM sleep
(D) Multiple awakenings during stage 3 and 4 of non-REM sleep
(E) Prolonged episodes of REM sleep in the first half of the night

The correct response is option **B**: Sleep-onset REM periods within 15 minutes of falling asleep

The patient presents with classic symptoms of narcolepsy including excessive daytime somnolence; cataplexy; sleep paralysis; hypnagogic and hypnopompic hallucinations; and sleep-onset REM periods (SOREMPS). On polysomnogram, the most common finding is SOREMPS within 15 minutes of falling asleep (normal is 90 minutes).

Saddock BJ, Saddock VA. Pocket Handbook of Clinical Psychiatry. 4th ed. Philadelphia, PA. Lippincott Williams and Wilkins, 2005. pp 238–239

Which of the following is most likely to be predictive of a good prognosis in schizophrenia?

    (A) Early age at onset of symptoms
    (B) Presence of predominantly negative symptoms
    (C) Acute onset with underlying precipitating factors
    (D) Presence of neurological signs and symptoms
    (E) Low IQ

The correct response option **C**: Acute onset with underlying precipitating factors

Factors that may indicate a good prognosis for schizophrenia include good premorbid functioning, older age at the time of first symptoms, acute onset with precipitating factors, female gender, being married, good support system, higher IQ, family history of affective disorder, absence of obvious negative symptoms and no significant history of drug or alcohol use.

Lauriello J, Bustillo JR, Shingler KC: The first interview of a patient with psychosis: symptoms, safety, and stabilization. FOCUS: Schizophrenia. Winter 2004; 2(1):7–12.

Hales RE, Yudofsky SC, Gabbard GO (eds): The American Psychiatric Textbook of Psychiatry, 5th ed. Arlington, VA, American Psychiatric Publishing, Inc., 2008, pp 424–426.

Which of the following medications is considered to be a first-line pharmacological treatment for delirium?

    (A) Lorazepam
    (B) Haloperidol
    (C) Quetiapine
    (D) Trazodone
    (E) Hydroxyzine

The correct response is option **B**: Haloperidol

Nonpharmacological treatments should be implemented as the first line of treatment of delirium. Pharmacological management should only be used in patients with severe agitation that interferes with medical treatment or in patients who pose a danger to themselves, other patients or staff. When such pharmacological treatment becomes necessary, neuroleptics are the first-line treatment. Among them, haloperidol is the most widely used and studied. Atypical antipsychotics such as quetiapine may be helpful but have only been tested in small, uncontrolled studies, and may be associated with higher mortality. Benzodiazepines typically lead to over-sedation and confusion. Antidepressants generally have not been shown to be useful, and the heterocyclic antidepressants may worsen delirium. Similarly, antihistamines such as diphenhydramine and hydroxyzine can cause or worsen delirium.

Hales RE, Yudofsky SC, Gabbard, GO (eds): The American Psychiatric Publishing Textbook of Psychiatry, 5th ed. Washington, DC, American Psychiatric Publishing, 2008. pp. 1462

Fearing MA, Inouye SK: Delirium, in The American Psychiatric Publishing Textbook of Geriatric Psychiatry. Edited by Blazer DG, Steffens DC. Washington, DC, American Psychiatric Publishing, 2009, pp 229–241. Reprinted in FOCUS. 2009; 7:53–63

A 67-year-old woman presents with visual hallucinations, memory loss, apathy and extrapyramidal symptoms. The patient's extrapyramidal symptoms increase markedly when given olanzapine 2.5 mg. This presentation is most consistent with:

(A) vascular dementia.
(B) dementia of the Alzheimer's type.
(C) Lewy body dementia.
(D) dementia due to HIV.
(E) dementia due to Huntington's disease.

The correct response is option **C**: Lewy body dementia

Lewy body dementia presents with well-formed visual hallucinations, delusions, depression, apathy, anxiety, and extrapyramidal symptoms. Patients with Lewy body dementia are extremely sensitive to the extrapyramidal effects of antipsychotic medication.

Hales RE, Yudofsky SC, Gabbard GO (eds): The American Psychiatric Publishing Textbook of Psychiatry, 5th ed, Washington, DC, American Psychiatric Publishing, Inc., 2008. pp 330–331

A 70-year-old woman presents with a history of a fixed belief that her arms and legs are infested with bugs that are crawling and biting her. She has no known associated medical condition and is physically healthy. Which of the following is best supported as a treatment of her condition?

(A) Methylphenidate
(B) Imipramine
(C) Pimozide
(D) Selegiline
(E) Fluoxetine

The correct response is option **C**: Pimozide

The patient appears to be suffering from delusional parasitosis which is a fixed belief of being infested with living organisms despite a lack of medical evidence of such infestation. It is often associated with various medical conditions such as tuberculosis, syphilis, polycyathemia vera, congestive heart failure, diabetes mellitus, vitamin B12 deficiency, renal and hepatic disorders, dementia and Huntington's disease. It can also be caused by use of amphetamines, cocaine, etc. Delusional parasitosis can present as a monosymptomatic hypochondriacal psychosis and labeled as delusional disorder, somatic type. Patients with this condition respond to the potent antipsychotic pimozide, which also serves as an opiate antagonist and possibly decreases pruritis and pain by that mechanism. Other antipsychotics, such as haloperidol and risperidone, have also been used in such trials. Methylphenidate may worsen the symptoms, while there are no positive studies reported with imipramine, selegiline and psychotherapy.

Gupta AK. Psychocutaneous disorders, in Kaplan & Sadock's Comprehensive Textbook of Psychiatry, 9th ed. Edited by Sadock BJ, Sadock VA, Ruiz P. Philadelphia, Lippincott Williams & Wilkins, 2009, pp 2435–36.

325

For the treatment of vaginismus, which of the following interventions in combination with education and counseling would be most effective?

(A) A short-acting benzodiazepine prior to intercourse
(B) Guided imagery during intercourse
(C) Limiting intercourse to the female superior position
(D) Use of a vibrator applied to the clitoris to induce orgasm
(E) Vaginal dilation exercises using plastic dilators

The correct response is option **E**: Vaginal dilation exercises using plastic dilators

Vaginismus is an involuntary muscle constriction of the outer third of the vagina that interferes with penile insertion and intercourse. This dysfunction most frequently afflicts women following sexual trauma. For treatment, women are advised to dilate their vaginal opening with their fingers or dilators.

Saddock BJ, Saddock VA. Pocket Handbook of Clinical Psychiatry. 4th ed. Philadelphia, PA. Lippincott Williams and Wilkins, 2005. pp 214, 218

326

Which antidepressant group is most likely to induce significant anticholinergic side effects that should be considered when treating late-life depression?

(A) Serotonin norepinephrine reuptake inhibitors
(B) Monoamine oxidase inhibitors
(C) Selective serotonin reuptake inhibitors
(D) Reversible monoamine oxidase inhibitors
(E) Tricyclic antidepressants

The correct response is option **E**: Tricyclic antidepressants

The geriatric population is particularly susceptible to anticholinergic-induced urinary retention and confusional states. Tricyclics have significant anticholinergic effects which can also result in dry mouth, constipation, and blurred vision.

Schatzberg AF, Nemeroff CB (eds): Essentials of Clinical Psychopharmacology, 2nd ed., Washington, DC, American Psychiatric Publishing, Inc., 2006. pp 64
Schatzberg AF, Cole JO, DeBattista C (eds): Manual of Clinical Psychopharmacology, 6th ed. Washington, DC. American Psychiatric Publishing Inc., 2007. pp 112–115

327

A 69-year old man with chronic obstructive pulmonary disease, cirrhosis of the liver, benign prostatic hypertrophy and alcohol dependence is prescribed acamprosate as part of his comprehensive treatment plan for his alcoholism. Which of the following laboratory tests would be most appropriate to obtain in order to determine the best starting dose of acamprosate?

(A) Alanine aminotransferase
(B) Electrolytes
(C) Creatinine clearance
(D) Serum osmolality
(E) Serum total protein

The correct response is option **C**: Creatinine clearance

The dose of acamprosate will need to be adjusted for patients with renal impairment as determined by creatinine clearance. Acamprosate absorption across the gastrointestinal tract is moderate, slow and sustained. Acamprosate is not protein bound. An extensive portion of the drug is eliminated via the gastrointestinal tract with the feces. The portion of the drug that is absorbed does not undergo metabolism. Acamprosate is excreted in the urine as acamprosate. There is a linear relationship between renal clearance and plasma half-life of the drug.

Sadock BJ, Sadock VA (eds): Kaplan and Sadock's Comprehensive Textbook of Psychiatry, 9th ed. Philadelphia, Lippincott Williams & Wilkins, 2009, pp. 3102–3104

328

Social rhythm therapy for bipolar disorder is based on which of the following types of psychotherapy?

    (A) Cognitive-behavioral therapy
    (B) Family therapy
    (C) Group therapy
    (D) Interpersonal therapy
    (E) Psychodynamic psychotherapy

The correct response is option **D**: Interpersonal therapy

Social rhythm therapy is an adaptation of Klerman and Weissman's interpersonal psychotherapy as an individual psychotherapy for the treatment for bipolar disorder. It proposes that sleep-wake cycle abnormalities found in bipolar disorder may be responsible for some of the symptomatic manifestations of the illness. Both positive and negative life events may cause disruptions in patients' social rhythms that, in turn, alter sleep-wake cycles and lead to the development of bipolar symptoms. Features of the therapy include having the patient regularize their daily routines, diminish interpersonal problems, and adhere to medication regimens.

Frank E, Kupfer DJ, Thase ME, Mallinger AG, Swartz HA, Fagiolini AM, Grochocinski V, Houck P, Scott J, Thompson W, Monk T: Two-year outcomes for interpersonal and social rhythm therapy in individuals with bipolar I disorder. Archives of General Psychiatry. 2005; 62:996–1004.

Frank E, Swartz HA, Kupfer DJ: Interpersonal and social rhythm therapy: managing the chaos of bipolar disorder. Biological Psychiatry 2000; 48:593–604.

American Psychiatric Association Practice Guideline for the Treatment of Patients with Bipolar Disorder, 2nd Edition (2002). Reprinted in FOCUS: Bipolar Disorder 2003; 1:99.

329

A 15-year-old girl is diagnosed with anorexia nervosa. She has had symptoms for 18 months. Her medical status is stable and she maintains an acceptable weight. The treatment that would be most beneficial for ongoing care is:

    (A) behavioral management.
    (B) psychodynamic psychotherapy.
    (C) cognitive-behavioral therapy.
    (D) family therapy.
    (E) dialectical behavior therapy.

The correct response is option **D**: Family therapy

Understanding the current evidence supporting psychotherapeutic interventions for anorexia nervosa is important for clinical practice. In controlled trials, anorexics who were younger than 16 years old, with symptoms less than 3 years benefited more from family therapy than individual therapy.

American Psychiatric Association Practice Guideline for the Treatment of Patients with Eating Disorders. Am J Psychiatry. 2006; 163(7):27 http://www.psychiatryonline.com/pracGuide/pracGuideTopic_12.aspx

330

Which one of the following medications is associated with causing Ebstein's anomaly in the newborn if taken regularly by pregnant women?

    (A) Lithium
    (B) Valproic acid
    (C) Carbamazepine
    (D) Lamotrigine
    (E) Aripiprazole

The correct response is option **A**: Lithium

Lithium use in the first trimester of pregnancy is associated with Ebstein's anomaly, a serious defect in the formation of the tricuspid valve of the heart. Valproic acid and carbamazepine in the first trimester are associated with and increased risk of neural tube defects. Lamotrigine use in pregnancy is of concern because of the theoretical risk the fetus could get Stephens-Johnson syndrome but the mother would not get it, and so not be aware of the need to stop the lamotrigine. There is not much data on the use of atypical antipsychotics as mood stabilizers during pregnancy.

Hales RE, Yudofsky SC, Gabbard GO (eds): The American Psychiatric Publishing Textbook of Psychiatry, 5th ed. Arlington VA, American Psychiatric Publishing, Inc, 2008, p 1500

A 42-year-old woman receiving chemotherapy for non-Hodgkin's lymphoma develops anorexia-cachexia syndrome. She is started on a medication to address her symptoms. A few weeks later she returns with reports of an increase in her sense of well-being, and decreased pain and nausea. However, she has gained no weight and has new onset muscle weakness. Which of the following agents is most likely responsible?

(A) Corticosteroids
(B) Cyproheptadine
(C) Medroxyprogesterone acetate
(D) Metoclopramide
(E) Ondansetron

The correct response is option **A**: Corticosteroids

Anorexia-cachexia syndrome occurs frequently in patients with cancer. There are a number of agents available for treatment. Corticosteroids increase the sense of well-being and often decrease pain and nausea. However, they are associated with osteoporosis, muscle weakness, immunosupression, delirium and have no demonstrated effects on body weight. Cyproheptadine increases appetite, but does not prevent weight loss. Medroxyprogesterone acetate increases appetite and body weight, but does not impact the overall sense of well being or reduction in pain. Metoclopramide only addresses emesis. Ondansetron does not prevent weight loss.

Levenson JL (ed): Essentials of Psychosomatic Medicine. American Psychiatric Publishing, Inc., Washington, DC, 2007. pp 114–115

A 42-year man is being treated with cognitive-behavior therapy (CBT) for depression. He describes several mistakes he made at work, and voices the belief that "no matter what I try, I always fail." This is an example of:

(A) automatic thought.
(B) maladaptive schema.
(C) full consciousness.
(D) modified cognition.
(E) unconscious conflict.

The correct response is option **B**: Maladaptive schema.

Schemas are defined as "fundamental rules or templates for information processing that are shaped by developmental influences and other life experiences." They are the deepest level of cognition as defined by CBT, and are an important target for the therapy. The other two levels are full consciousnessm, the state of full awareness in which decisions are made, and automatic thoughts, rapid, automatic thoughts that occur in one's stream of consciousness which are not generally evaluated carefully by the thinker. Identifying cognitive errors and modifying cognition are among the goals of CBT.

Jesse H. Wright. Cognitive behavior therapy: basic principles and recent advances. FOCUS 2006;4:173–178
Textbook of Psychotherapeutic Treatments. Gabbard GO (ed). Arlington VA, American Psychiatric Publishing Inc, 2009, pp 170–72

Which of the following mood stabilizers is FDA-approved for acute mania in children older than 12 years?

(A) Lithium
(B) Sodium valproate
(C) Carbamazepine
(D) Lamotrigine
(E) Topiramate

The correct response is option **A**: Lithium

Lithium is approved for acute mania and maintenance therapy for children older than 12 years. While all mood stabilizers and antipsychotic agents are commonly used for early-onset bipolar disorder in clinical settings, none of these agents has been well studied in the pediatric population. The few double-blind placebo-controlled studies of lithium in this population are generally positive, but are limited by very small sample sizes and diagnostic variability. The FDA approval of lithium for use in children older than 12 years was largely based on the response in adult studies.

McClellan J, Kowatch R, Findling RL; Work Group on Quality Issues. Practice parameter for the assessment and treatment of children and adolescents with bipolar disorder. J Am Acad Child Adolesc Psychiatry. 2007; 46(1):107–25.

A 66-year-old man being treated for bipolar disorder is noted to have asymptomatic hypercalcemia and elevated levels of parathyroid hormone. Which of the following medications is the most likely cause?

(A) Divalproex
(B) Lamotrigine
(C) Lithium
(D) Topiramate
(E) Olanzapine

The correct response is option **C**: Lithium

Lithium is the only psychiatric medication for which there is well-documented evidence for causing hypercalcemia and hyperparathyroidism. While quite uncommon, this side effect has, on occasion, led to surgical intervention to remove hyperplastic or adenomatous parathyroid glands.

Jefferson JW, Greist JH: Lithium, in Kaplan & Sadock's Comprehensive Textbook of Psychiatry, 9th ed. Edited by Sadock BJ, Sadock VA, Ruiz P. Philadelphia, Lippincott Williams & Wilkins, 2009, pp 3132–45.

Abdullah H, Bliss R, Guinea AI, Delbridge L: Pathology and outcome of surgical treatment for lithium-associated hyperparathyroidism. Br J Surgery 1999; 86:91–93.

McHenry CR, Lee K: Lithium therapy and disorders of the parathyroid glands. Endocrine Practice 1996; 2:103–109.

335

A 28-year-old hospitalized patient is started on an antipsychotic medication for schizophrenia. Within 3 weeks, the patient complains of chest pain, shortness of breath, and swelling of the lower extremities. Which medication is the patient most likely taking?

(A) Fluphenazine
(B) Quetiapine
(C) Risperidone
(D) Aripiprazole
(E) Clozapine

The correct response is option **E**: Clozapine

The patient's symptoms are suggestive of cardiac dysfunction. Of the choices listed, only clozapine has been associated with myocarditis and cardiomyopathy, typically in the early stages of treatment. A study of 213 cases of myocarditis indicated that 85% of these occurred at the recommended dosage of clozapine in the first two months of therapy. The presence of eosinophilia in many of the reported cases indicates that an immunoglobulin E medicated hypersensitivity reaction may have been involved.

Clozaril® package insert, Novartis Pharmaceuticals Corporation, East Hanover, NJ, 2005. http://www.pharma.us.novartis.com/product/pi/pdf/Clozaril.pdf.
Hales RE, Yudofsky SC and Gabbard GO (eds): The American Psychiatric Publishing Textbook of Psychiatry, 5th ed. Arlington, VA, American Psychiatric Publishing, Inc., 2008. pp 1097–1098.
Schatzberg AF, Nemeroff CB (eds): Textbook of Psychopharmacology, 3rd ed. Arlington, VA, American Psychiatric Publishing, Inc., 2006. p 449.

336

A requirement for initiating hospice care is that the patient must have:

(A) a cognitive-impairing terminal illness.
(B) a health care power-of-attorney.
(C) a prognosis of ≤ 6 months to live.
(D) no family members able to provide care.
(E) Medicare and/or Medicaid benefits.

The correct response is option **C**: A prognosis of ≤ 6 months to live

Although a Medicare hospice benefit is available, Medicare or Medicaid is not a requirement, nor are the other incorrect answers. The prognosis requirement is a barrier for those with uncertain prognoses, such as with Alzheimer's disease.

Blazer DG, Steffens DC (eds): The American Psychiatric Publishing Textbook of Geriatric Psychiatry, 4th ed. Arlington, VA, American Psychiatric Publishing, 2009, p 610.

337

A 38-year-old patient with schizophrenia is observed holding her arms in bizarre positions for hours at a time. On interview, the patient does not answer any questions, but rather repeats everything the psychiatrist says. Which of the following is the most appropriate initial treatment?

(A) Lorazepam
(B) Propranolol
(C) Diphenhydramine
(D) Phenobarbital
(E) Botulinum toxin

The correct response is option **A**: Lorazepam

This patient is experiencing catatonia, with posturing and echolalia. Benzodiazepines are recommended for the initial treatment of catatonic reactions.

American Psychiatric Association Practice Guideline for the Treatment of Patients with Schizophrenia, 2nd ed (2004), pp 659–60 http://www.psychiatryonline.com/pracGuide/pracGuideHome.aspx

338

Procedural justice in the process of civil commitment refers to:

(A) physician decision-making that supports a beneficial outcome for patients.
(B) a style of communication that alleviates patients' experience of coercion.
(C) the inclusion of a patient's family in commitment decisions.
(D) judicial decision-making that takes into account patients' therapeutic options.
(E) choosing the least restrictive alternative for patients.

The correct response is option **B**: A style of communication that alleviates patients' experience of coercion

Procedural justice is a style of communication that is intended to limit patients' experience of coercion during the processes of civil commitment. Relevant components include listening to patients and validating their concerns, informing patients about the issues at stake and treating them with dignity and respect. The style of communication that is most important to avoid when committing patients, because it is most closely associated with their experience of coercion, is the use of threats and force. Therapeutic jurisprudence applies to judges choosing options that are "therapeutic" for the patient. Including a patient's family in commitment decisions might be helpful, with the patient's agreement, but is not relevant to the concept. Similarly, the remaining options do not directly relate to patients' experience of coercion.

McKenna BG, Simpson AIF, Laidlaw TM. Patient perception of coercion on admission to acute psychiatric services: the New Zealand experience. International Journal of Law and Psychiatry. 1999; 22:143–153.

Simon RI, Shuman DW. Clinical Manual of Psychiatry and Law. Arlington, VA, American Psychiatric Publishing, 2007, p 127.

339

A review of the current evidence suggests that the BEST explanation for an increase in the rate of autism spectrum disorders is:

(A) exposure to childhood vaccines.
(B) rates of genetic mutations.
(C) exposure to environmental toxins.
(D) screening and diagnosis.
(E) survival of premature infants.

The correct response is option **D**: Screening and diagnosis

Based on the current evidence, the best explanation for the increased rate of autism spectrum disorders is broader diagnosis, improved screening and diagnosis and identification at an earlier age. The current evidence does not support the other options.

Westphal A, Volkmar F. An update on autism. FOCUS: Child and Adolescent Psychiatry. Summer 2008; 6(3):286:288–291.

Wazana A, Bresnahan M, Kline J. The autism epidemic: fact or artifact? J Am Acad Child Adolesc Psychiatry. 2007;46:723–30.

Naqvi S. Review of Child and Adolescent Psychiatry. FOCUS: Child and Adolescent Psychiatry. Fall 2004; 2(4):536.

340

A 22-year-old male college student has a positive HIV test. History reveals he had unprotected sex with multiple partners. His CBC is consistent with anemia. Which of the following factors places him at highest risk for eventually developing an HIV dementia?

(A) Age
(B) Anemia
(C) Educational level
(D) Gender
(E) Multiple sexual partners

The correct response is option **B**: Anemia

HIV-associated dementias are reported in up to two-thirds of AIDS patients. Risk factors associated with eventual development of HIV dementia include lower educational level, older age, anemia, illicit drug use, and female gender.

Levenson JL (ed): Essentials of Psychosomatic Medicine, American Psychiatric Publishing, Inc., Washington, DC, 2007, p 209

341

The symptom that is most suggestive that an individual has generalized anxiety disorder is worrying about:

(A) specific behaviors.
(B) physical symptoms.
(C) embarrassment.
(D) all experiences.
(E) past events.

The correct response is option **D**: All experiences

Worry is a relatively generic feature of anxiety disorders. The primary distinction between generalized anxiety disorder and other anxiety disorders is the focus of the patient's concern. Worrying about physical symptoms occurs in panic disorder. Concern about being embarrassed is usually the focus of individuals with social phobia. Patients with GAD experience uncontrollable worry about a number of different areas and often worry about their worrying (meta-worrying). Ruminating about past events tends to be associated with depression.

Huppert JD, Rynn M. Generalized anxiety disorder in Clinical Manual of Anxiety Disorders. Edited by Stein DJ. American Psychiatric Publishing Inc, Washington DC, 2004; pp 150–151.
Hoge EA, Oppenheimer JE, Simon NM: Generalized anxiety disorder. FOCUS: Anxiety Disorders, Summer 2004; 3:346–347.

342

A 7-year-old boy with an anxiety disorder is in cognitive behavior therapy. The parents ask how they should approach getting the child to do activities that he is fearful about, such as socializing with peers and participating in competitive situations. Which of the following is the MOST appropriate response?

(A) Wait until the anxiety and fearfulness have been resolved.
(B) Start when the child understands his anxieties.
(C) Gradually approach with reinforcement for trying.
(D) Find appropriate non-anxiety-producing substitutes.
(E) Make fun activities contingent on doing anxiety-provoking things.

The correct response is option **C**: Gradually approach with reinforcement for trying.

Cognitive and behavioral therapies for anxiety have demonstrated effectiveness for a variety of anxiety disorders. While there is some variation in approaches, the focus is on helping children and adolescents identify and manage their anxiety as well as reinforcing ongoing attempts to deal with anxiety-provoking situations successfully.

Naqvi S. Review of Child and Adolescent Psychiatry. FOCUS: Child and Adolescent Psychiatry. Fall 2004; 2(4):536–7.
AACAP practice parameter for the assessment and treatment of children and adolescents with anxiety disorders. J Am Acad Child Adolesc Psychiatry. 2007; 46:273–274.

343

A patient presents with a well-defined history of recurrent hypomanic episodes but denies ever having had depressive symptoms or full manic episodes. According to DSM-IV-TR criteria, the most appropriate diagnosis would be:

(A) cyclothymic disorder.
(B) schizoaffective disorder.
(C) bipolar I disorder.
(D) bipolar II disorder.
(E) bipolar disorder, not otherwise specified.

The correct response is option **E**: Bipolar disorder, not otherwise specified

According to DSM-IV-TR, a diagnosis of bipolar I disorder requires at least one manic or mixed episode; a diagnosis of bipolar II disorder is defined by one or more major depressive episodes accompanied by at least one hypomanic episode; cyclothymic disorder is characterized by numerous periods with hypomanic symptoms and numerous periods with depressive symptoms; and criteria for schizoaffective disorder include at least one manic, mixed or major depressive episode. Unless additional history is obtained to the contrary, the patient's diagnosis would be bipolar disorder, not otherwise specified.

Diagnostic and Statistical Manual of Mental Disorders, Fourth Edition, Text Revision (DSM-IV-TR). Washington, DC, American Psychiatric Association, 2000, pp 319–323, 382–401.

344

Which of the following is a required criterion for the diagnosis of depression with melancholic features?

(A) Mood worse in the late afternoon
(B) Middle or late insomnia
(C) Significant hyperphagia or weight gain
(D) Mood changes similar to those found in bereavement
(E) Loss of pleasure in all, or almost all, activities

The correct response is option **E**: Loss of pleasure in all, or almost all, activities

To diagnose depression with melancholic features, a person must have either a loss of pleasure in all or almost all activities OR a lack of reactivity to usually pleasurable stimuli (criteria A). They also must have three of six additional criteria, including: depression worse in the morning, early morning awakening, significant anorexia or weight loss, a distinct quality of depressed mood that is different than that found in normal bereavement.

American Psychiatric Association: Diagnostic and Statistical Manual of Mental Disorders, 4th Edition. Text Revision (DSM-IVTR). Washington, DC, American Psychiatric Association, 2000. pp 419–20.

345

A 10-year-old boy is referred for psychiatric assessment after setting his family's home on fire. His mother smoked cigarettes during the pregnancy. The patient grew up in an extremely impoverished neighborhood with his mother as his sole caregiver. His mother describes the boy as being extremely oppositional and defiant as a preschooler. She has primarily used corporal punishment including beating him with a belt and electric cords. Since starting school he has had multiple suspensions for fighting with peers and teachers. Intelligence testing is consistent with borderline intellectual functioning. Which of these factors from the patient's history is MOST predictive of a poor outcome in this patient's conduct disorder?

(A) Early age at onset of symptoms.
(B) Exposure to toxins in utero.
(C) Lack of a father figure in his life.
(D) Impaired intellectual functioning.

The correct response is option **A**: Early age at onset of symptoms

Early age at onset is the factor most consistently found to be associated with poor outcome in conduct disorder. A combination of demographic, individual, school, and family variables predicts age at onset. However, each variable individually does not predict the persistence of symptoms as well as the development of symptoms at an early age.

AACAP practice parameter for the assessment and treatment of children and adolescents with depressive disorders. J Am Acad Child Adolesc Psychiatry. 2007. FOCUS. 2008; 6(3):380–381.

Dulcan MK, Weiner JM. Essentials of Child and Adolescent Psychiatry. Arlington (VA): American Psychiatric Publishing, Inc., 2006, p374.

Hales RE, Yudofsky SC, Gabbard GO (eds): The American Psychiatric Publishing Textbook of Psychiatry, 5th ed. Arlington, VA, American Psychiatric Publishing, Inc., 2008. p 895

346

During the assessment of a $3\frac{1}{2}$-year-old boy who has been referred for biting other children at preschool, the mother discloses that the boy's stepfather has been physically abusive towards her. The child may have witnessed some of the abusive episodes. Which of the following MUST be done prior to the end of the session?

(A) Explain that the child is at risk for PTSD.
(B) Refer the mother for her own treatment.
(C) Find contact information for shelters.
(D) Explore whether the child has been abused.
(E) Explore mother's reasons for staying with the stepfather.

The correct response is option **D**: Explore whether the child has been abused.

In terms of safety, it is essential to determine if the child is being abused. A significant risk factor for child maltreatment is living in a household with domestic violence. The other options are important but not necessarily immediate.

Kaufman J. Child abuse and neglect, in Martin A, Volkmar FR (eds) Lewis' Comprehensive Textbook of Child and Adolescent Psychiatry 4th ed. Philadelphia, Lippincott Williams & Wilkins; 2007, pp 692–701.

347

Which of the following signs differentiate patients with pseudodementia from patients who are severely demented?

(A) Less attention to self care
(B) Cognitive impairment
(C) Complaints of memory loss
(D) Less attention to environment
(E) Memory storage and retrieval

The correct response is option **C**: Complaints of memory loss

Unlike patients with pseudodementia, demented patients with impaired insight are not aware of their cognitive losses and therefore do not complain about them. In addition, depressed patients lack signs of cortical dysfunction such as apraxia, aphasia, and agnosia. Diagnosing patients who have pseudodementia is critical so they can be treated. Distinguishing dementia from depression-related cognitive dysfunction can be difficult, particularly as the two may coexist.

American Psychiatric Association Practice Guideline for the Treatment of Patients with Major Depressive Disorder, 3rd ed. (2010), http://psychiatryonline.com/pracGuide/pracGuideHome.aspx.

348

A 32-year-old woman who does not want to take medication complains about shortness of breath, chest pain and diaphoresis. She has had multiple attacks in the past 3 weeks. Her medical work-up is negative. Which of the following treatments has the strongest evidence supporting it as first choice for this patient?

(A) Dialectical behavioral therapy
(B) Family therapy
(C) Group therapy
(D) Patient support groups
(E) Cognitive-behavioral therapy

The correct response is option **E**: Cognitive-behavioral therapy

Cognitive-behavioral therapy has the most robust evidence of all the psychosocial treatments listed. Family therapy, group therapy, and patient support groups may be useful as supplementary approaches depending on the patient's profile and needs. Dialectical behavioral therapy is currently used as a treatment for borderline personality disorder.

American Psychiatric Association Practice Guideline for the Treatment of Patients With Panic Disorder, 2nd ed (2008). http://www.psychiatryonline.com/pracGuide/pracGuideHome.aspx.

A 74-year-old man with known dementia is admitted to the hospital for workup and treatment of a presumed delirium. He scores a 21 on the Mini Mental State Exam (MMSE) on admission, and a 15 two days later. Nursing notes from his hospitalization indicate that there are times when he is completely alert and other times when he is nearly stuporous. Without appearing bothered, he has occasionally described seeing brightly colored birds perching on the windowsill of his room. A thorough delirium workup reveals no cause for his waxing and waning mental status findings. This description is most consistent with which dementing process?

(A) Vascular dementia
(B) Alzheimer dementia
(C) Frontotemporal dementia
(D) Lewy body dementia
(E) Korsakoff dementia

The correct response is option **D**: Lewy body dementia

Lewy body dementia is distinguished from other common dementias by marked day-to-day fluctuations in cognitive performance, and it must be differentiated from delirium. Spontaneous vivid visual hallucinations, with detailed evocations of humans and animals, are common. Also characteristic are relatively preserved memory function, prominent attentional and visuospatial dysfunction, and extrapyramidal motor signs. Systematic clinical evaluations, such as the National Institute of Neurological and Communicative Disorders and Stroke – AD and Related Disorders Association criteria, are remarkably accurate for diagnosing Alzheimer's disease, with a positive predictive value of as much as 88% when compared with neuropathological diagnosis. Although the criteria are accurate at distinguishing Alzheimer's disease from most other forms of dementia, clinical diagnosis appears to have the most difficulty differentiating Lewy body disease from Alzheimer's disease. This is likely because, at least early on, patients often do not develop the extrapyramidal symptoms and hallucinations that help to distinguish this disorder from Alzheimer's disease.

Ranginwala NA, Hynan LS, Weiner MF, White CL, III Clinical criteria for the diagnosis of Alzheimer disease: still good after all these years. Am J Geriatr Psychiatry. 2008; 16(5):384–388
Geser F, Wenning GK, Poewe W, McKeith I. How to diagnose dementia with Lewy bodies: state of the art. Mov Disord. 2005; 20 Suppl 12: S11–S20

Which of the following features differentiates autism from Asperger's syndrome?

(A) Obsessive and compulsive behaviors
(B) Failure to develop peer relationships appropriate to the developmental level
(C) Inflexible adherence to specific non functional routines
(D) Single words used by age 2, phrases by age 3
(E) Stereotyped and repetitive motor mannerisms

The correct response is option **D**: Single words used by age 2, phrases by age 3

In contrast to autistic disorder, in Asperger's syndrome there are no clinically significant delays in language. The essential features of Asperger's syndrome are severe and sustained impairment in social interaction and the development of restricted repetitive patterns of behavior, interests and activities. In autism, impairment in communication is marked and sustained and affects verbal and non verbal skills along with the essential features of impaired development in social interaction. The pervasive developmental disorders (autism spectrum disorders) must be distinguished from one another, and from disorders such as selective mutism, child onset schizophrenia, and some degenerative CNS disorders.

Volmar F, Westphal A. An update on autism. FOCUS: Child and Adolescent Psychiatry. Summer 2008; 6(3):289.
American Psychiatric Association: Diagnostic and Statistical Manual of Mental Disorders, 4th Edition. Text Revision (DSM-IVTR). Washington DC, American Psychiatric Association, 2000. p 75.

Which of the following psychosocial treatments for depression has the most robust data supporting its use?

(A) Cognitive-behavioral therapy
(B) Dialectical behavioral therapy
(C) Group therapy
(D) Psychodynamic psychotherapy
(E) Supportive therapy

The correct response is option **A**: Cognitive-behavioral therapy

Cognitive-behavioral therapy, interpersonal psychotherapy (IPT), and behavioral psychotherapies (e.g., behavioral activation) have demonstrated acute efficacy in treating major depressive disorder. There is less evidence for other psychotherapies.

American Psychiatric Association: Practice Guideline for the Treatment of Patients with Major Depressive Disorder, 3rd ed (2010), p 47 http://www.psychiatryonline.com/pracGuide/pracGuideHome.aspx.

A 25-year-old patient with schizophrenia is admitted to the hospital with auditory hallucinations and persecutory delusions. The psychiatrist initiates haloperidol 5mg orally twice per day. After 48 hours of receiving medication, the patient becomes increasingly irritable, agitated, and is noted to be restless and pacing. The patient's blood pressure is 130/85 with a pulse of 88. The next step in management of this patient's symptoms should be to:

(A) increase the haloperidol to 10mg orally twice per day.
(B) administer benztropine 1mg orally twice per day.
(C) administer a one-time dose of haloperidol 5mg intramuscularly.
(D) administer a one-time dose of diphenydramine 25mg intramuscularly.
(E) initiate propranolol 20mg orally three times per day.

The correct response is option **E**: Initiate propranolol 20mg orally three times per day.

Akathisia is a common reaction to treatment with typical neuroleptic agents. Because akathisia may be mistaken for an increase in psychosis or anxiety, it is sometimes inappropriately addressed by increasing the antipsychotic dosage, which results in a worsening of symptoms. The treatment of choice is either to change to an atypical neuroleptic agent or to add a β blocking agent, such as propranolol. Anticholinergic agents have not been found to be effective.

Haddad PM, Dursun SM. Neurological complications of psychiatric drugs: clinical features and management. Hum Psychopharmacol. 2008 Jan: 23 Suppl 1:15–26.

Rathbone J, Soares-Weiser K. Anticholinergics for neuroleptic-induced acute akathisia. Cochrane Database Syst Rev. 2006 Oct 18; (4): D003727.

American Psychiatric Association: Diagnostic and Statistical Manual of Mental Disorders, 4th Edition. Text Revision (DSM-IVTR). Washington DC, American Psychiatric Association, 2000. pp 800–802

Hales RE, Yudofsky SC, and Gabbard GO (eds): The American Psychiatric Publishing Textbook of Psychiatry, 5th ed. Arlington, VA, American Psychiatric Publishing, Inc., 2008. pp 1089–1090.

Which of the following doses of haloperidol decanoate has been shown to have the lowest rate of symptomatic exacerbation, yet minimal increased risk of adverse effect or subjective discomfort?

(A) 25 mg/month
(B) 50 mg/month
(C) 100 mg/month
(D) 200 mg/month

The correct response is option **D**: 200 mg/month

In a multidose study of haloperidol decanoate in the maintenance treatment of schizophrenia, 200 mg/month was associated with the lowest rate of symptomatic exacerbation combined with a minimal increased risk of adverse effect of subjective discomfort when compared to doses of 25, 50 and 100 mg/month.

Kane JM, Davis JM, Schooler N, Marder S, Casey D, Brauzer B, Mintz J, Conley R A multidose study of haloperidol decanoate in the maintenance treatment of schizophrenia. Am J Psychiatry. 2002; 159:554–60

Which of the following medications has the potential for a significantly increased risk of hemorrhagic pancreatitis?

(A) Clozapine
(B) Divalproex
(C) Nefazodone
(D) Pemoline
(E) Thioridazine

The correct response is option **B**: Divalproex

Divalproex is associated with hemorrhagic pancreatitis and hepatic failure. All of the above medications have the potential for serious side effects: clozapine for agranulocytosis and myocarditis; nefazodone for acute liver failure; pemoline for acute liver failure; and thioridazine for torsades de pointes or QT and QTc prolongation.

Sadock BJ, Sadock VA (eds): Kaplan and Sadock's Comprehensive Textbook of Psychiatry, 9th ed. Philadelphia, Lippincott Williams & Wilkins, 2009, p. 2972

Which of the following situations is the individual with social phobia likely to avoid?

(A) Crossing bridges
(B) Eating in public
(C) Being in closed spaces
(D) Proximity to spiders
(E) Sitting in movie theatres

The correct response is option **B**: Eating in public

Anxiety that characterizes social phobia occurs when the individual is expected to perform or interact in social situations in which he/she could be embarrassed, especially with strangers or people he feels might judge him. Eating in public for some patients becomes impossible because of the fear that others are judging the way she consumes food. Others with this disorder may not be able to write in public, use public urinals or speak in public – the latter is the most common phobia. Avoidance of crossing bridges and movie theatres can be a feature of panic disorder or agoraphobia. Avoidance of closed spaces or spiders is associated with specific phobia.

American Psychiatric Association: Diagnostic and Statistical Manual of Mental Disorders, 4th Edition. Text Revision (DSM-IVTR). Washington DC, American Psychiatric Association, 2000. pp 450–3

A 32-year-old woman with a history of early childhood abuse and abandonment begins dynamic psychotherapy. Although the initial stages of treatment proceed well, after three months her psychiatrist notices that she is becoming more critical of the therapy and frequently questions the value of it. In addition, she is dismissive of the psychiatrist and begins to question whether the psychiatrist is adequately trained. As a result, the psychiatrist begins to dread the sessions, and occasionally begins the sessions late. This mode of interaction is best described as a type of:

(A) Projective identification
(B) Displacement
(C) Sublimation
(D) Paranoid-schizoid position
(E) Ambivalent/resistant pattern

The correct response is option **A**: Projective identification

A core psychoanalytic concept derived from object relations theory is that patients reenact early internalized relationship patterns through the externalization of these patterns. The recapitulating of old relationships into the present is called "projective identification," in which the patient exerts pressure on the therapist to conform to the pattern of interaction that he or she is generating. In this case, the patient, fearful of attachment (with its risk of subsequent abandonment) resorts to earlier modes of interaction in which she behaves in a way that irritates the psychiatrist to the point where the professional begins to behave in a way reminiscent of earlier abusive figures in the patient's life.

Displacement refers to the shifting of uncomfortable impulses to a more acceptable or less threatening target (for example, yelling at one's spouse when angry at an employer). Sublimation is the transformation of negative impulses into positive or productive actions or emotions (for example, frustrated by a failing relationship, one turns to painting). The paranoid-schizoid position is another concept from object relations theory in which one can only form partial object relationships. The result is the defense mechanism referred to as "splitting." The ambivalent/resistant pattern is a reference to attachment theory and refers to a child's reaction to a neglectful or inconsistent caregiver by both seeking closeness with the person, but then resisting it when offered.

Gabbard GO: Psychodynamic approaches to personality disorders. FOCUS 2005; 3:363–367

The parents of a 16-year-old year old boy ask if he can be treated to prevent the development of schizophrenia. For the last year, the boy has been more irritable, staying in his room most of the time playing music. His grades have declined. His uncle was diagnosed with schizophrenia at the age of 17. Which of the following statements BEST describes the current knowledge about the early identification and treatment of individuals who will become schizophrenic?

(A) Many adolescents with these symptoms will not become schizophrenic.
(B) Treatment with low dose atypical antipsychotics will prevent schizophrenia.
(C) Long term use of atypical antipsychotics does not have major adverse effects.
(D) Psychosocial interventions are more effective than medication treatment.

The correct response is option **A**: Many adolescents with these symptoms will not become schizophrenic.

There is increased interest in early identification of adolescents who are at high risk to become schizophrenic and in early interventions to either prevent the development of the disorder or ameliorate its course. Current problems include: many adolescents have prodromal symptoms but do not develop schizophrenia, the adverse effects of long term use of atypical antipsychotics, unnecessary treatment of individuals and the unclear benefits of early treatment with atypical antipsychotics. There have been no identified psychosocial treatments that prevent the onset of schizophrenia. At this point, further evaluation would be helpful to determine what is going on and whether the adolescent has a condition that would warrant treatment (e.g., psychosis, depression, substance abuse).

AACAP practice parameters for the assessment and treatment of children and adolescents with schizophrenia. J Am Acad Child Adolesc Psychiatry. 2001; 40(7) Supplement:4S–23S

Which of the following is a common adverse effect of monoamine oxidase inhibitors therapy?

(A) Serotonin syndrome
(B) Hypertensive crisis
(C) Priapism
(D) Orthostatic hypotension
(E) Weight loss

The correct response is option **D**: Orthostatic hypotension

Hypotension is a frequent adverse effect of MAOIs. Other common side effects include: insomnia, dry mouth, weight gain, edema, sexual dysfunction, headache, and afternoon somnolence. Orthostatic hypotension can lead to dizziness and falls. Therefore, cautious upward titration of MAOI dosage should be used. Treatment for orthostatic hypotension includes avoidance of caffeine, intake of 2 L of fluid per day, addition of dietary salt, adjustment of antihypertensive drugs, support stockings, and in severe cases, treatment with fludrocortisones. Hypertensive crises and serotonin syndrome are rare but life-threatening events.

Sadock BJ, Sadock VA (eds): Kaplan and Sadock's Synopsis of Psychiatry: Behavioral Sciences/Clinical Psychiatry. Philadelphia, Lippincott Williams & Wilkins, 10th edition, 2007, p.1067

Yudofsky SC, Hales RE (eds): The American Psychiatric Publishing Textbook of Neuropsychiatry and Behavioral Sciences, 5th ed. Arlington VA, American Psychiatric Publishing Inc, 2008, pp. 1061, 1071–1074

A patient who was recently diagnosed with panic disorder complains 2 days after starting citalopram that she continues to be very anxious about having another panic attack. Even her sleep has been disrupted. Which of the following would treat her anxiety best?

    (A) Increase the citalopram.
    (B) Add lithium.
    (C) Lower citalopram.
    (D) Add clonazepam.
    (E) Add trazodone.

The correct response is option **D**: Add clonazepam.

The patient's complaint is likely due to anticipatory anxiety. Clonazepam or another benzodiazepine would lower her anxiety until the citalopram can both treat anxiety and reassure her that a panic attack is unlikely in the future. If she complained about jitteriness in general, lowering the citalopram dose would be indicated. The addition of trazodone would address the sleep problem, but that is not her primary problem. Currently there is no indication for increasing the citalopram or adding lithium.

American Psychiatric Association Practice Guideline for the Treatment of Patients With Panic Disorder, 2nd ed (2008). http://www.psychiatryonline.com/pracGuide/pracGuide Home.aspx

A 32-year-old woman presents to the emergency department after being raped. She appears confused and extremely frightened. She mentions a history of prior rapes. Which of the following psychotherapies, if administered soon after the event, has the best body of evidence in preventing the patient from progressing to a posttraumatic stress disorder?

    (A) Supportive psychotherapy
    (B) Psychological debriefing
    (C) Hypnosis
    (D) Cognitive-behavioral therapy
    (E) Single session exposure therapy

The correct response is option **D**: Cognitive-behavioral therapy

Victims of multiple traumas are at particular risk for developing PTSD. A number of psychotherapeutic techniques have been attempted to prevent the onset of PTSD. By desensitizing individuals to trauma-related triggers, cognitive behavioral therapies have been shown to speed recovery and prevent PTSD in rape and accident victims. In patients who have experienced multiple recurrent traumas there is little evidence that supportive therapy or psychoeducation will, in and of themselves, result in lasting reductions in symptoms, although they are unlikely to do harm. In contrast, single session techniques such as psychological debriefing and single session exposure therapies may exacerbate symptoms in some patients. Hypnosis has been used for PTSD patients, generally not as a preventive treatment, nor has it been used in the acute setting.

American Psychiatric Association Practice Guideline for the Treatment of Patients with Acute Stress Disorder and Posttraumatic Stress Disorder. 2004. p. 13 http://www.psychiatryonline.com/pracGuide/pracGuideTopic_11.aspx

361

A 28-year-old patient with schizophrenia is prescribed an atypical antipsychotic medication. A baseline fasting plasma glucose level is obtained and is within normal limits. After what period of time should this test be repeated?

(A) 2 weeks, and then quarterly
(B) 3 months, and then annually
(C) 6 months, and then annually
(D) Every 6 months
(E) Annually

The correct response is option **B**: 3 months, and then annually

According to the Consensus Development Conference on Antipsychotic Drugs and Obesity and Diabetes, individuals prescribed an antipsychotic medication should have a fasting plasma glucose level performed at baseline, then again in 3 months, and then annually thereafter. The APA Guidelines on Schizophrenia (2004) mention "Fasting blood glucose or hemoglobin A1c at 4 months after initiating a new treatment and annually thereafter."

American Psychiatric Association Practice Guideline for the Treatment of Patients with Schizophrenia, 2nd ed (2004) pp. 272–273. http://www.psychiatryonline.com/pracGuide/pracGuideHome.aspx
Consensus Development Conference on Antipsychotic Drugs and Obesity and Diabetes. (Reviews/Commentaries/Position Statements). Diabetes Care. 2004; 27:596–601

362

Which of the following reflects the APA's position on psychiatrists' participation in legally authorized executions?

(A) Sanctioning of participation is determined by state associations.
(B) Psychiatrists should not participate in executions.
(C) Participation is left up to the discretion of the psychiatrist.
(D) Psychiatrists may only perform a mental status exam prior to execution.
(E) Psychiatrists may participate if they are only in a supervisory role.

The correct response is option **B**: Psychiatrists should not participate in executions.

APA ethical guidelines state that psychiatrists should not participate in executions.

American Psychiatric Association. The Principles of Medical Ethics with Annotations Especially Applicable to Psychiatry, 2006 edition, p 4.

363

A 20-year-old college student presents to the mental health clinic because he is worried about an exam that he must take in two days. He has chronic problems with concentration and sleep, and complains that he is easily fatigued. He states that he is tired of the pressure he always feels. He adds that he has been to the medical clinic as well because he feared that his frequent muscle tension and headaches meant he had a neurological disease. Which of the following is the most likely diagnosis?

(A) Major depression
(B) Hypochondriasis
(C) Generalized anxiety disorder
(D) Adjustment disorder
(E) Somatization disorder

The correct response is option **C**: Generalized anxiety disorder

The patient's history includes virtually all the criteria for GAD. The disorder can be comorbid with depression but this history doesn't provide much evidence for that diagnosis. Choices B and E refer to disorders where the chief complaints are focused on the body. Adjustment disorder requires a known precipitant and would have less extensive and intensive symptomatology.

Diagnostic and Statistical Manual of Mental Disorders, Fourth Edition, Text Revision (DSM-IV-TR). Washington, DC, American Psychiatric Association, 2000, pp 472–476.

Which medication has the most evidence supporting its use as an augmenting agent for treatment of a major depression?

(A) Divalproex sodium
(B) Lamotrigine
(C) Lithium
(D) Lorazepam
(E) Phenelzine

The correct response is option **C**: Lithium

Augmentation of antidepressant medications can utilize another non-MAOI antidepressant, generally from a different pharmcological class, or a non-antidepressant medication such as lithium. Lithium carbonate has been found to be effective in augmenting antidepressants when treating depressive disorders and has the most evidence for its use. Lorazepam can be used to reduce associated anxiety which may indirectly relieve depressive symptoms. Several anticonvulsants have been studied as augmentation agents, but the evidence for agents like lamotrigine or divalproex sodium is not as strong as it is for lithium. Phenelzine is a monoamine oxidase inhibitor (MAOI) which should not be given with a selective serotonin reuptake inhibitor (SSRI, e.g. fluoxetine) because it can result in serious life-threatening reactions.

Crossley NA, Bauer M. Acceleration and augmentation of antidepressants with lithium for depressive disorders: two metaanalyses of randomized, placebo-controlled trials. J Clin Psychiatry. 2007 Jun; 68(6):935–40.

Nierenberg AA, Katz J, Fava M. A critical overview of the pharmacologic management of treatment-resistant depression. Psychiatr Clin North Am 2007 Mar; 30(1):13–29.

American Psychiatric Association Practice Guideline for the Treatment of Patients with Major Depressive Disorder, 3rd ed. (2010). http://psychiatryonline.com/pracGuide/pracGuideHome.aspx.

EMDR (eye movement desensitization and reprocessing) has several features that distinguish it from the other cognitive behavioral treatments for PTSD. In addition to the directed eye movements, which of the following also distinguishes EMDR?

(A) Having patients think about the trauma rather than verbalize it
(B) Encouraging patients to learn to identify cognitive distortions
(C) Utilizing and emphasizing exposures to the traumatic material
(D) Teaching relaxation and imaging techniques to manage anxiety
(E) Employing homework assignments to reinforce session work

The correct response is option **A**: Having patients think about the trauma rather than verbalize it

EMDR is a form of psychotherapy that includes an exposure-based therapy (with multiple brief, interrupted exposures to traumatic material), eye movement, and recall of traumatic memories of an event or events. It combines multiple perspectives and techniques, including cognitive behavior therapy. The use of directed eye movements as a feature distinguishes this form of therapy from other cognitive behavior approaches additionally, The traumatic material need not be verbalized; instead, patients are directed to think about their traumatic experiences without having to discuss them.

American Psychiatric Association Practice Guideline for the Treatment of Patients with Acute Stress Disorder and Posttraumatic Stress Disorder. Am J Psychiatry. 2004; 161(11):18 http://www.psychiatry online.com/pracGuide/pracGuideTopic_11.aspx

A 28-year-old woman with bipolar II disorder has been using an oral contraceptive for birth control. She currently presents with a hypomanic episode. Which of the following medications would be best to treat her hypomania without impairing the efficacy of the oral contraceptive?

(A) Carbamazepine
(B) Lithium
(C) Oxcarbamazepine
(D) Topirimate

The correct response is option **B**: Lithium

Carbamazepine, oxcarbamazepine, and topiramate increase the metabolism of oral contraceptives. As a result, women taking these medications should not rely on oral contraceptives for birth control. This effect does not occur with other medications used to treat bipolar disorder.

American Psychiatric Association Practice Guideline for the Treatment of Patients with Bipolar Disorder, 2nd Edition (2002). Reprinted in FOCUS: Bipolar Disorder 2003; 1:74.

Altshuler LL, Hendrick V, Cohen LS: Course of mood and anxiety disorders during pregnancy and the postpartum period. J Clin Psychiatry 1998; 59(suppl 2):29–33 87.

Spina E, Pisani F, Perucca E: Clinically significant pharmacokinetic drug interactions with carbamazepine: an update. Clin Pharmacokinet 1996; 31:198–214.

Which psychotherapeutic modality involves teaching patients to tolerate distress, regulate their emotions, reduce vulnerability to cues, and avoid or distract without problem behavior, while concomitantly reducing reinforcement of maladaptive behavior?

(A) Psychoanalytic psychotherapy
(B) Cognitive behavioral therapy
(C) Interpersonal psychotherapy
(D) Dialectical behavior therapy
(E) Supportive therapy

The correct response is option **D**: Dialectical behavior therapy

Dialectical behavior therapy (DBT) focuses on expanding the patient's repertoire of coping skills, reducing reinforcement of maladaptive behavior and increasing reinforcement of adaptive behaviors, generalizing new behaviors from the therapeutic environment to the natural environment, and supporting the motivation and capability of the therapist.

Sadock BJ, Sadock VA: Kaplan and Sadock's Synopsis of Psychiatry, 10th ed. Philadelphia, Lippincott Williams & Wilkins, 2007, pp 944–5

Textbook of Psychotherapeutic Treatments. Gabbard GO (ed). Arlington VA, American Psychiatric Publishing Inc, 2009, pp 727–731

Which of the following drug classes is the preferred initial pharmacotherapy for social anxiety disorder (generalized)?

(A) Tricyclic antidepressant (TCA)
(B) Monoamine oxidase inhibitor (MAOI)
(C) Benzodiazepine (BDZ)
(D) Selective serotonin reuptake inhibitor (SSRI)
(E) Beta-blockers

The correct response is option **D**: Selective serotonin reuptake inhibitor (SSRI)

Both paroxetine and sertraline are SSRIs that are FDA-approved for treating social phobia. Research studies have also supported the efficacy of other SSRIs. Venlafaxine XR (serotonin/norepinephrine reuptake inhibitor SNRI) is also FDA-approved for anxiety disorders (SNRI). Research evidence does support efficacy for both MAOIs and benzodiazepines, although neither is FDA-approved, and they have disadvantages that prevent them from being first-line medications for social phobia. Beta-blockers may have some value for treatment performance anxiety, but their effectiveness for generalized social phobia is marginal. There is little evidence that TCAs are useful for treating generalized social phobia.

Delong H, Pollack M. Update on the assessment, diagnosis, and treatment of individuals with social anxiety disorder. FOCUS: Panic and Social Phobia. Fall 2008; (6)4

Davidson JRT. Pharmacotherapy of social anxiety disorder: what does the evidence tell us? J Clin Psychiatry. 2006; 67(suppl 12):20–26

Muller JE, Koen L, Seedat S, Stein DJ. Social anxiety disorder: current treatment recommendations. CNS Drugs 2005; 19:377–391

Hales RE, Yudofsky SC and Gabbard GO (eds): The American Psychiatric Publishing Textbook of Psychiatry, 5th ed. Arlington, VA, American Psychiatric Publishing, Inc., 2008. p542

Which of the following factors is most likely to be associated with bacterial softtissue infections in drug users?

(A) Cleaning the skin before injection
(B) Being HIV negative
(C) Being an experienced injector
(D) Intravenous injection
(E) Subcutaneous injection

The correct response is option **E**: Subcutaneous injection

Subcutaneous injection or intramuscular injection ("skin popping"), repeatedly flushing and pulling back during an injection ("booting"), being human immunodeficiency virus positive, and failing to clean the skin before injection all increase the risk of bacterial sot-tissue infections. Intravenous injection, particularly by an experienced injector with a single drug does not increase the risk as much as these other factors. Being an inexperienced injector and combining heroin and cocaine ("speed balls") may increase the risk of infection. Staphylococcus aureus and streptococcus species are the most common sources of infection.

Gordon RJ, Lowy FD: Bacterial infections in drug users. N Engl J Med 2005; 353:1945–54.

A 40-year-old patient complains of episodes of intense fear with associated somatic symptoms that have a sudden onset and peak within minutes. Which of the following is the essential feature required for a diagnosis of panic *disorder*?

(A) Anticipatory anxiety and avoidance of public speaking
(B) Unexpected, "out-of-the-blue" nature of the episodes
(C) Presence of 4 or more characteristic symptoms during episodes
(D) Episodes precipitated by memories of a past trauma
(E) Episodes triggered by contact with "contaminated" objects

The correct response is option **B**: Unexpected, "out-of-the-blue" nature of the episodes

According to DSM-IV-TR, the occurrence of unexpected, uncued, "out-of-the-blue" panic attacks is required for a diagnosis of panic disorder. Panic attacks can also occur in association with many other conditions such as social phobia (e.g., public speaking), posttraumatic stress disorder (e.g., when recalling the stressor), and obsessive-compulsive disorder. While at least 4 of 13 listed symptoms are necessary to diagnose a panic attack, this criterion applies to panic attacks occurring under any circumstance.

Diagnostic and Statistical Manual of Mental Disorders DSM-IV-TR. Fourth Edition (Text Revision). American Psychiatric Association, Inc., 2000. pp 430–441

A 53-year-old man with a history of alcohol dependence has been abstinent from alcohol for three months. Although he continues to attend peer support groups, he reports that he has recently begun drinking one to two drinks approximately every other day, and is fearful that his relapse will worsen. Which of the following medications would be the most appropriate first-line pharmacological intervention for this patient?

(A) Naltrexone
(B) Acamprosate
(C) Bupropion
(D) Fluoxetine
(E) Disulfiram

The correct response is option **B**: Acamprosate

Of medications used for the treatment or prevention of alcohol abuse and dependence, naltrexone and acamprosate have the best support in the literature. Naltrexone, an opioid antagonist, appears to be most effective at reducing heavy drinking. Acamprosate, which is thought to work through an effect on NMDA-mediated glutamatergic transmission, appears to have a unique role in supporting abstinence in individuals who are abstinent or only recently relapsed. Disulfiram, which has had mixed results, should not be used in patients who are actively drinking even small amounts, and antidepressants have only equivocal results for treating alcohol dependence.

Mason BJ: Acamprosate for alcohol dependence: An update for the clinician. FOCUS 2006;4:505–511

Yudofsky SC, Hales RE (eds): The American Psychiatric Publishing Textbook of Neuropsychiatry and Behavioral Sciences, 5th ed. Arlington VA, American Psychiatric Publishing Inc, 2008, p. 380

372

A 20-year-old patient with schizophrenia receiving antipsychotic treatment complains of breast tenderness, galactorrhea, and amenorrhea. Which of the following medications is the patient most likely taking?

(A) Aripiprazole
(B) Risperidone
(C) Quetiapine
(D) Clozapine
(E) Ziprasidone

The correct response is option **B**: Risperidone

This patient is experiencing the effects of hyperprolactinemia. Of all of the atypical antipsychotic agents, risperidone is most likely to cause increased prolactin levels.

Schatzberg AF, Nemeroff CB (eds): Essentials of Clinical Psychopharmacology, 2nd ed. Washington, DC, American Psychiatric Publishing, Inc., 2006, p 291–2

373

Which of the following statements most accurately reflects the position of the *APA's Principles of Medical Ethics* on faculty psychiatrists having sex with trainees?

(A) There is no established APA position on sexual relationships with trainees.
(B) Sexual relationships with trainees are absolutely unethical.
(C) Sexual relationships are permissible when both parties are consenting adults.
(D) Sexual behavior in faculty/trainee relationships may negatively impact patient care.

The correct response is option **D**: Sexual behavior in faculty/trainee relationships may negatively impact patient care.

APA ethical guidelines state that sexual involvement between supervisors and trainees may be unethical because the patient whose treatment is being supervised may be negatively impacted, trust between the student and teacher may be damaged and teachers are important role models for trainees and affect their trainees' future professional behavior.

American Psychiatric Association. The Principles of Medical Ethics with Annotations Especially Applicable to Psychiatry, 2006 edition, p 7.

374

In which of the following situations would a high potency benzodiazepine be the preferred initial pharmacotherapy for panic disorder?

(A) Co-morbid major depression
(B) Need for rapid onset of action
(C) Anticipation of long-term treatment
(D) Associated agoraphobia
(E) Co-morbid cardiovascular disease

The correct response is option **B**: Need for rapid onset of action

While SSRIs are usually the preferred treatment for panic disorder, their onset of action is slow compared to that of benzodiazepines. On the other hand, benzodiazepines are not effective antidepressants, and they carry risks of dependence and abuse with long term treatment. Both classes of drugs can benefit associated agoraphobia and are well tolerated in the presence of cardiovascular disease.

Bakker A, van Balkom AJ, Stein DJ. Evidence-based pharmacotherapy of panic disorder. Int J Neuropsychopharmacol 2005; 8:473–482

Pollack MH, Allgulander C, Bandelow B, Cassano GB, Greist JH, Hollander E, Nutt DJ, Okasha A, Swinson RP. WCA recommendations for the long-term treatment of panic disorder. CNS Spectrums 2003; 8(suppl 1):17–30

Roy-Byrne PP, Craske MG, Stein MG. Panic disorder. Lancet 2006; 368:1023–1032

American Psychiatric Association Practice Guideline for the Treatment of Patients With Panic Disorder, 2nd ed (2008). (suppl; in press)

375

Which of the following substance abuse therapist attributes has the greatest and most consistent impact on patient retention and reduced substance use?

(A) Therapists skilled at limit setting
(B) Therapists who were successfully treated for substance dependence
(C) Therapists who have a first degree relative who was substance dependent
(D) Therapists with strong interpersonal skills
(E) Therapists who are knowledgeable about both biological and psychosocial interventions

The correct response is option **D**: Therapists with strong interpersonal skills

Limit setting has an important role in treatment of substance use disorders and may be particularly important for individuals with co-occurring personality disorders. However, a review of the literature on effective characteristics of therapists concluded that the characteristic most associated with patient retention and reduced substance use was strong interpersonal skills.

American Psychiatric Association Practice Guideline for the Treatment of Patients with Substance Use Disorders, Second Edition, 2nd Edition (2006), p 316–317, http://psychiatryonline.com/pracGuide/pracGuideHome.aspx

376

The daughter of an 89-year-old man with severe dementia requests that her father be deemed incompetent. The ultimate decision to determine competence is made by the:

(A) daughter.
(B) court.
(C) psychiatrist.
(D) treating physician.
(E) health care power-of-attorney.

The correct response is option **B**: Court

Although anyone can offer an opinion as to whether or not someone should be deemed incompetent, the final decision is made by the court.

Blazer DG, Steffens DC (eds): The American Psychiatric Publishing Textbook of Geriatric Psychiatry, 4th ed. Arlington, VA, American Psychiatric Publishing, 2009, pp 612–13.

377

Anger is most closely associated with which of the following temperament traits?

(A) Harm Avoidance
(B) Novelty Seeking
(C) Reward Dependence
(D) Persistence

The correct response is option **B**: Novelty Seeking

Temperament, a heritable factor in personality development, has been divided into four dimensions: Harm Avoidance, Novelty Seeking, Reward Dependence, and Persistence. These are associated with the four basic emotions of fear, anger, attachment, and ambition, respectively.

Sadock BJ, Sadock VA: Kaplan & Sadock's Comprehensive Textbook of Psychiatry. 9th Ed, 2009 pp 2199–2204.
Angres DH. The Temperament and Character Inventory in addiction treatment. Focus 2010 8: 192

378

An 80-year-old man is brought to the emergency room after suffering a grand mal seizure. His serum sodium concentration is 107 mmol/L. Which of the following medications is most likely to have caused the hyponatremia?

(A) Topiramate
(B) Lamotrigine
(C) Gabapentin
(D) Oxcarbazepine
(E) Valproate

The correct response is option **D**: Oxcarbazepine

Of the options given, only oxcarbazepine use has been associated with hyponatremia. The mechanism has not been resolved fully, but considerations include increased antidiuretic hormone (ADH) release, increased renal vasopressin receptor sensitivity, and vasopressinase inhibition. Risk factors include increased age, low baseline sodium concentration, smoking and diuretic use.

Dong X, Leppik IE, White J, Rarick J: Hyponatremia from oxcarbazepine and carbamazepine. Neurology 2005; 65:1976–1978
Van Amelsvoort T, Bakshi R., Devaux CB, Schwabe S: Hyponatremia associated with carbamazepine and oxcarbazepine therapy: a review. Epilepsia 1994; 35:181–188

379

In children with major depressive disorder, which of the following is MORE likely to occur in boys than girls?

(A) Feelings of anxiety
(B) Acting-out behaviors
(C) Poorer self-esteem
(D) Severe symptoms of depression
(E) Shorter period of recovery

The correct response is option **B**: Acting-out behaviors

Epidemiological students have demonstrated gender differences in children and adolescents with depressive disorders. Gender is not believed to affect recovery from depression. Girls tend to report higher levels of depressive symptoms than boys and have more inwardly directed symptoms related to feeling anxious. Girls have lower self-worth and poorer self-esteem than boys. Boys have higher rates of irritability and acting-out behaviors such as running away, theft, or substance abuse.

Dulcan MK, Weiner JM. Essentials of Child and Adolescent Psychiatry. Arlington (VA); 2006, p. 270

380

A 21-year-old patient dropped out of college and has been unable to attend social gatherings as a result of extreme fear of embarrassing herself. She has failed to respond to therapeutic trials of paroxetine, fluvoxamine, sertraline, clonazepam, and buspirone. Which of the following medications would be most appropriate to prescribe next?

(A) Fluoxetine
(B) Propranolol
(C) Phenelzine
(D) Lithium
(E) Risperidone

The correct response is option **C**: Phenelzine

MAOIs such as phenelzine are very effective in the treatment of social phobia, but due to side effects and the requirement of extensive medication and dietary restrictions, they are not first-line treatments. However, in individuals who have failed to respond to therapeutic trials of several other agents with better side effect profiles, such as the patient described in this case, MAOIs are another option. Fluoxetine would not be a good choice, given failed trials of more than two other SSRI's. Propranolol is typically useful on an as-needed basis for performance anxiety, and is not likely to be helpful in treatment-refractory social phobia. Lithium and risperidone have not been proven to be effective in the treatment of social phobia.

Hales RE, Yudofsky SC, Gabbard GO (eds): The American Psychiatric Publishing Textbook of Psychiatry, 5th ed. Arlington, VA, American Psychiatric Publishing, 2008, pp 542–44.

Blanco C, Raza MS, Schneier FR, et al. The evidence-based pharmacological treatment of social anxiety disorder. Int J Neuropsychopharmacol 2003; 6:427–442.

381

Which of the following psychotropic medications has been associated with polycystic ovarian syndrome?

    (A) Lithium
    (B) Divalproex
    (C) Methylphenidate
    (D) Citalopram
    (E) Aripiprazole

The correct response is option **B**: Divalproex

Divalproex has been associated with the polycystic ovarian syndrome. Patients taking valproic acid medications should be counseled to avoid weight gain. If they have oligomenorrhea or hirsutism, then a referral may be appropriate for initiation of treatment with either a combination oral contraceptive or progestin and treatments for hirsutism. The mood stabilizers (e.g., lithium, lamotrigine) do not appear to be associated with PCOS and may be substituted for divalproex, if needed.

Correll CU, Carlson HE: Endocrine and metabolic adverse effects of psychotropic medications in children and adolescents. J Am Acad Child & Adolescent Psychiatry. 2006; 45:771–91

382

A 58-year-old patient with diabetic peripheral neuropathic pain presents with major depressive disorder. Which of the following antidepressants is most likely to have beneficial effects on both conditions?

    (A) Bupropion
    (B) Duloxetine
    (C) Escitalopram
    (D) Nefazodone
    (E) Mirtazapine

The correct response is option **B**: Duloxetine

While all of the options are FDA-approved for the treatment of major depressive disorder, only duloxetine is also approved for the treatment of diabetic peripheral neuropathic pain.

Smith TR. Duloxetine in diabetic neuropathy. Expert Opin Pharmacother 2006; 7:215–223

383

When initiating treatment with risperidone long-acting injection, oral risperidone should be concomitantly prescribed for what length of time?

    (A) 1 week
    (B) 3 weeks
    (C) 6 weeks
    (D) 8 weeks
    (E) 12 weeks

The correct response is option **B**: 3 weeks

According to the package insert, oral risperidone (or another oral antipsychotic medication) should be prescribed for 3 weeks following the first injection (and then discontinued) to maintain therapeutic plasma concentrations.

Lasser RA, Bossie CA, Zhu Y, Locklear JC, Kane JM. Long-acting risperidone in young adults with early schizophrenia or schizoaffective illness. Ann Clin Psychiatry. 2007 Apr-Jun; 19(2):65–71.
Risperdal® Consta® package insert, Janssen LP, Titusville, NJ, 2007

384

Which of the following personality disorders most closely resembles social phobia?

    (A) Schizoid
    (B) Borderline
    (C) Avoidant
    (D) Dependent
    (E) Histrionic

The correct response is option **C**: Avoidant

According to DSM-IV-TR, avoidant personality disorder may be a more severe variant of social phobia that is not qualitatively distinct. Schizoid personality is characterized by odd behavior and beliefs. Borderline personality disorder is characterized by problems with boundaries and others. Histrionic individuals tend to call attention to themselves by their actions, while dependent individuals are seeking means to cling to others.

Diagnostic and Statistical Manual of Mental Disorders, 4th ed. Text Revision (DSM-IV-TR). Washington, DC, American Psychiatric Association, 2000, pp 455

Which antidepressant has been shown to be most efficacious in the treatment of depression in patients with HIV/AIDS with chronic diarrhea?

- (A) Fluoxetine
- (B) Mirtazapine
- (C) Paroxetine
- (D) Sertraline
- (E) Venlafaxine

The correct response is option **B**: Mirtazapine

Several studies reported efficacy of various antidepressants in HIV-infected patients, but no single antidepressant has been found superior in treating HIV-infected patients as a group. The side effects of certain antidepressants can render them advantageous or disadvantageous in particular patients with HIV. For example, SSRIs are best avoided in patients with chronic diarrhea. SNRIs should also be avoided in patients with chronic diarrhea.

Levenson JL (editor): Essentials of Psychosomatic Medicine. Arlington, VA, American Psychiatric Publishing, Inc., 2007, pp 213–14.

386

Which of the following is the best predictor of a recurrence of depression in someone with major depressive disorder?

- (A) Family history of depression
- (B) Prior episodes of depression
- (C) Prior suicidal attempt
- (D) Co-morbid Axis I disorder
- (E) Co-morbid medical condition

The correct response is option **B**: Prior episodes of depression

The number of lifetime major depressive episodes is significantly associated with the probability of recurrence, such that the risk of recurrence increases by 16% with each successive episode.

Diagnostic and Statistical Manual of Mental Disorders, 4th ed, Text Revision (DSM-IV-TR). Washington, DC, American Psychiatric Association, 2000, pp 372–373

American Psychiatric Association Practice Guideline for the Treatment of Patients with Major Depressive Disorder, 3rd ed (2010), p 57 http://www.psychiatryonline.com/pracGuide/pracGuideHome. aspx

387

A patient has been successfully treated with an SSRI for acute panic episodes. What is the minimum length of time recommended for maintenance pharmacotherapy for this patient?

- (A) 2–4 months
- (B) 6–12 months
- (C) 18 months
- (D) Over 24 months

The correct response is option **B**: 6–12 months

The American Psychiatric Association Practice Guideline Watch for the Treatment of Patients with Panic Disorder recommends maintenance pharmacotherapy for at least 6–12 months following acute treatment. Studies of fluoxetine, paroxetine, sertraline, imipramine and clomipramine have demonstrated a benefit of continuing medication for 6–12 months. Maintenance pharmacotherapy should be considered for most patients as a means of preventing recurrence of panic disorder symptoms and promoting continued symptom relief and better functioning.

American Psychiatric Association Practice Guideline for the Treatment of Patients with Panic Disorder (2009). http://psychiatryonline. com/pracGuide/pracGuideHome.aspx

388

Which of the following is a required gateway symptom for a major depressive disorder?

- (A) Insomnia or hypersomnia
- (B) Recurrent thoughts of death
- (C) Feelings of worthlessness
- (D) Psychomotor agitation or retardation
- (E) Loss of interest or pleasure

The correct response is option **E**: Loss of interest or pleasure

According to DSM-IV-TR, the diagnosis of a major depressive episode requires the presence of either a depressed mood or a loss of interest or pleasure as 1 of 9 symptoms listed. For the diagnosis to be made, at least 4 of other symptoms must be present. In addition, symptoms must have been evident for at least 2 weeks and "represent a change from previous functioning."

Diagnostic and Statistical Manual of Mental Disorders, 4th ed, Text Revision (DSM-IV-TR). Washington, DC, American Psychiatric Association, 2000, pp 356

389

In contrast to delusional disorders, schizophrenia is characterized by:

(A) disorganized speech.
(B) grandiosity.
(C) mood episodes.
(D) paranoid beliefs.
(E) physiological effects of a general medical condition.

The correct response is option **A**: Disorganized speech

The differential diagnosis between schizophrenia and delusional disorder rests on the nature of the delusion (bizarre in schizophrenia), versus non-bizarre in delusional disorder and the presence of other characteristic symptoms of schizophrenia (hallucinations, disorganized speech or behavior, prominent negative symptoms). Both paranoid beliefs and grandiosity may be common to schizophrenia and delusional disorder. General medical conditions must be ruled out prior to making a diagnosis of schizophrenia.

Diagnostic and Statistical Manual of Mental Disorders, 4th ed, Text Revision (DSM-IV-TR). Washington, DC, American Psychiatric Association, 2000, pp 298–317, 323–329

390

Which of the following symptoms of PTSD is classified as an avoidance symptom?

(A) Difficulty falling asleep
(B) Recurrent nightmares
(C) Exaggerated startle response
(D) Sense of foreshortened future
(E) Difficulty concentrating

The correct response is option **D**: Sense of foreshortened future

Only option D is an avoidance symptom. Some other avoidance symptoms include efforts to avoid thoughts, feelings, conversations, activities, places, or people that arouse recollection of the event, inability to recall important aspects of the trauma, and a restricted range of affect. Options A, C and E are symptoms of increased arousal, while B is a symptom of re-experiencing.

Diagnostic and Statistical Manual of Mental Disorders, 4th ed, Text Revision (DSM-IV-TR). Washington, DC, American Psychiatric Association, 2000, pp 468

391

The personality disorder most closely associated with social anxiety disorder is which of the following?

(A) Schizoid
(B) Obsessive-compulsive
(C) Histrionic
(D) Avoidant
(E) Borderline

The correct response is option **D**: Avoidant

DSM-IV-TR lists the essential features of avoidant personality disorder (APD) as "a pervasive pattern of social inhibition, feelings of inadequacy, and hypersensitivity to negative evaluation that begins by early adulthood. . .". There is considerable overlap between the features of generalized social anxiety disorder and those of APD and there is a stronger association with social anxiety disorder and APD than with other personality disorders. Avoidant personality disorder is sometimes viewed as occupying the most severe end of the social anxiety disorder continuum.

Diagnostic and Statistical Manual of Mental disorders, Fourth Edition, Text Revision (DSM-IV-TR). Washington, DC, American Psychiatric Association, 2000, pp 450–456, 718–721

Hummelen B, Wilberg T, Pedersen G, Karterud S: The relationship between avoidant personality disorder and social phobia. Compr Psychiatry 2007; 48:348–356

Stein MB, Stein DJ: Social anxiety disorder. Lancet 2008; 371:1115–1125

392

In order to make a diagnosis of bulimia nervosa, the symptoms must have duration of at least:

(A) 1 month.
(B) 3 months.
(C) 6 months.
(D) 9 months.
(E) 12 months.

The correct response is option **B**: 3 months

According to the DSM-IV-TR, symptoms of bulimia nervosa must be present for at least 3 months. Prior to three months the patient would be diagnosed with eating disorder, not otherwise specified.

American Psychiatric Association: Diagnostic and Statistical Manual of Mental Disorders, 4th Edition, Text Revision (DSM-IV-TR). Washington DC, American Psychiatric Association. 2000. pp 589, 594

A 65-year-old man whose wife died 3 months ago presents to the clinic, accompanied by his daughter. The daughter states that the couple had been married for 40 years, and that he now feels utterly worthless without his wife. Since her death, he has stayed in the house, letting the newspapers pile up, and he doesn't answer the phone. He stopped his weekly fishing trips with his neighbor, a pastime of his for 20 years. He denies suicidal ideation, but states that he wishes to join his wife. He has had a weight loss of 30 pounds over the past 3 months and has stopped taking his hypertension medications. What is the most likely diagnosis?

(A) Bereavement
(B) Adjustment disorder with depressed mood
(C) Major depressive disorder
(D) Depressive disorder, NOS
(E) Dysthymic disorder

The correct response is option **C**: Major depressive disorder

While the death of his spouse clearly precipitated his current symptoms, their severity places his diagnosis past the point of simple bereavement or an adjustment disorder, which, by definition, cannot be represented by bereavement. Moreover, the time frame for making a diagnosis of depression after bereavement is two months. He has enough symptoms to meet criteria for major depressive disorder.

Diagnostic and Statistical Manual of Mental Disorders, 4th ed, Text Revision (DSM-IV-TR). Washington, DC, American Psychiatric Association, 2000, pp 355

In dialectical behavior therapy (DBT), the term "dialectical" refers to which of the following therapeutic principles?

(A) Psychic integration of good and bad objects
(B) A simultaneous emphasis on validation and change
(C) Efforts to treat both the manic and depressed phases of bipolar disorder
(D) A simultaneous focus on both thoughts and behaviors
(E) A dual focus on one's feelings and their impact on others

The correct response is option **B**: A simultaneous emphasis on validation and change

Dialectical behavior therapy (DBT) was developed by Linehan, in part based on the observation that patients with borderline personality disorder often find an emphasis on behavioral change to feel as though it invalidates their painful inner experiences. The "dialectic" of this new therapy would be a dual emphasis on both validation of these painful feelings, alongside change strategies, which are also necessary for providing hope and improving functioning. The first choice refers to the psychodynamic concept of integrating split objects, most attributable to Melanie Klein but also further developed within object relations theory. Dialectical behavior therapy does not target bipolar disorder. Option D describes cognitive behavioral therapy (CBT), and option E does not refer to any specific type of psychotherapy formally, though may be a target of many therapeutic treatments.

Shearin EN, Linehan MM: Dialectical behavior therapy for borderline personality disorder: theoretical and empirical foundations. Acta Psychiatr Scand Suppl, 1994; 379:61−8

Textbook of Psychotherapeutic Treatments. Gabbard GO (ed) Arlington VA, American Psychiatric Publishing Inc, 2009, p 731−732

Which of the following approaches to neurotransmitter modulation would be most appropriate in treating a patient with Tourette's disorder?

(A) Dopaminergic modulation at the striatum and serotonergic modulation at the orbitofrontal cortex
(B) Dopaminergic modulation at the striatum
(C) Serotonergic modulation at the orbitofrontal cortex
(D) Noradrenergic modulation

The correct response is option **B**: Dopaminergic modulation at the striatum

Body dysmorphic disorder and non-tic-related OCD respond best to serotonergic modulation. Tic related OCD responds best to a combination of serotonergic and dopaminergic modulation. Tourette's disorder responds to dopaminergic modulation at the level of the striatum but not to serotonergic modulation at the orbitofrontal cortex. Noradrenegeric modulation does not seem to be active in the treatment of Tourette's disorder.

Fineberg NA, Gale TM, Sivakumaran T. A review of antipsychotics in the treatment of obsessive compulsive disorder. J Psychopharmacology 2006; 20:97–103. Reprinted in FOCUS: OCD summer 2007; 3:354–360.
Dougherty DD, Rauch SL, Greenberg BD. Pathophysiology of Obsessive-Compulsive Disorders, in American Psychiatric Publishing Textbook of Anxiety Disorders. Edited by Stein DJ, Hollander E, Rothbaum BO. Arlington, VA, American Psychiatric Publishing, 2010, pp 291–92.

Features that support the diagnosis of somatization disorder include involvement of multiple organ systems, early onset, absence of expected lab abnormalities, and:

(A) chronic course without development of physical signs.
(B) distinct, clearly delineated symptoms of limited duration.
(C) symptoms that are different from those of organic disorders.
(D) symptoms that do not cause functional impairment.
(E) signs not acknowledged or recognized by the patient.

The correct response is option **A**: Chronic course without development of physical signs

Individuals with somatization disorder tend to have ongoing symptoms without physical signs or structural abnormalities. Often the symptoms are vague, multiple, confusing and persistent and similar to the symptoms of organically based disorders.

Sadock BJ, Sadock VA, Ruiz P (eds): Kaplan & Sadock's Comprehensive Textbook of Psychiatry, 9th ed. Philadelphia, Lippincott Williams & Wilkins, 2009, pp 1928–35

Demographic and clinical factors associated with suicide in patients with schizophrenia include:

(A) older age.
(B) female gender.
(C) higher cognitive function.
(D) lower socioeconomic status.
(E) good social support.

The correct response is option **C**: Higher cognitive function

About 20–50% patients with schizophrenia attempt suicide while up to 10% eventually commit suicide. Demographic and clinical factors associated with suicide include young age, male gender, single marital status, depressive symptoms and hopelessness, more severe illness, frequent relapses, recent hospitalization, good insight, higher cognitive functions, higher socioeconomic background, poor social functioning and lack of social support.

American Psychiatric Association Practice Guideline for the Treatment of Patients with Schizophrenia, 2nd ed (2004), pp 577–78, 607–608 http://www.psychiatryonline.com/pracGuide/pracGuideHome.aspx.
Kirkpatrick B and Tek C. Schizophrenia: Clinical Features and Psychopathology Concepts, in: Sadock BJ, Sadock VA (eds): Kaplan and Sadock's Comprehensive Textbook of Psychiatry, 8th ed. Philadelphia, Lippincott Williams & Wilkins, 2005, pp 1416–36.
VanOs J and Allardyce J. The Clinical Epidemiology of Schizophrenia, in Sadock BJ, Sadock VA, Ruiz P (eds): Kaplan & Sadock's Comprehensive Textbook of Psychiatry, 9th ed. Philadelphia, Lippincott Williams & Wilkins, 2009, pp 1475–87.

Which of the following therapeutic strategies for OCD maintains treatment success for the longest period of time after active therapy is discontinued?

(A) Psychoeducation
(B) Record keeping
(C) A selective serotonin reuptake inhibitor
(D) Exposure and response prevention
(E) Supportive psychotherapy

The correct response is option **D**: Exposure and response prevention

Exposure and response prevention (ERP) has the strongest research supporting effectiveness in maintaining long-term gains after active treatment. SSRIs and other agents are as effective while the patient is on the drugs but relapse may occur when patients discontinue pharmacotherapy. Supportive therapy has not been shown to be efficacious. Psychoeducation and record keeping are useful adjuncts to treatment.

American Psychiatric Association Practice Guideline for the Treatment of Patients with Obsessive-Compulsive Disorder 2007, http://psychiatryonline.com/pracGuide/pracGuideHome. aspx.
Greist J, Jefferson J. Obsessive-compulsive disorder. FOCUS: OCD: Summer 2007; 3:283–298.

The highest level of decision making capacity is required for which of the following actions?

(A) Making a will
(B) Appointing a substitute decision maker
(C) Agreeing to participate in a research study
(D) Making a decision about treatment
(E) Consenting to phlebotomy

The correct response is option **C**: Agreeing to participate in a research study

Drane proposed a sliding scale for capacity: the more serious the issue at stake, the higher the threshold for decisional capacity. Agreement to participate in clinical research requires the highest standard because the patient must be able to understand that she will not necessarily be in an active treatment arm.

Rosenstein DL, Miller FG. Ethical issues. in: American Psychiatric Publishing Textbook of Psychosomatic Medicine, edited by Levenson JL. Arlington VA, American Psychiatric Publishing, 2005, pp 58.
Drane JF. Competency to give an informed consent. A model for making clinical assessments. JAMA. 1984 Aug 17; 252(7):925–7.

Which of the following agents has been shown to be effective in the treatment of trauma-related nightmares and sleep disruption?

(A) Phenelzine
(B) Prazosin
(C) Bupropion
(D) Cyproheptadine
(E) Diphenhydramine

The correct response is option **B**: Prazosin

A series of controlled studies have shown that the alpha-adrenergic antagonist prazosin is effective in increasing total sleep time and REM sleep, and in reducing nightmares and PTSD symptoms and improving the total Clinical Global Impression—Improvement Scale (CGI-I).

Raskind MA, Peskind ER, Hoff DJ, Hart KL, Holmes HA, Warren D, et al. A parallel group placebo controlled study of prazosin for trauma nightmares and sleep disturbance in combat veterans with post-traumatic stress disorder. Biol Psychiatry. 2007; 61: 928–934
Taylor FB, Martin P, Thompson C, Williams J, Mellman TA, Gross C et al. Prazosin effects on objective sleep measures and clinical symptoms in civilian trauma posttraumatic stress disorder: a placebo-controlled study. Biol Psychiatry 2008; 63:629–632
Maher MJ, Rego SA, Asnis GM. Sleep disturbances in patients with post-traumatic stress disorder: epidemiology, impact and approaches to management. CNS Drugs. 20(7):567–590
Benedek DM, Friedman MJ, Zatzick D, Ursano RJ. Guideline Watch (March 2009): Practice Guideline for the Treatment of Patients with Acute Stress Disorder and Posttraumatic Stress Disorder. FOCUS. 2009; 2:204–213 http://www. psychiatryonline.com/content.aspx?aid=156498

FOCUS Psychiatry Review (Volume 2): Answer Sheet

1. A	51. D	101. D	151. A	201. A	251. C	301. B	351. A
2. B	52. E	102. E	152. E	202. B	252. B	302. A	352. E
3. D	53. D	103. E	153. D	203. A	253. A	303. B	353. D
4. C	54. C	104. C	154. A	204. B	254. E	304. D	354. B
5. B	55. B	105. E	155. C	205. C	255. B	305. B	355. B
6. B	56. C	106. D	156. A	206. C	256. B	306. E	356. A
7. A	57. A	107. A	157. C	207. E	257. A	307. B	357. A
8. C	58. C	108. C	158. C	208. E	258. C	308. C	358. D
9. E	59. A	109. D	159. A	209. C	259. D	309. D	359. D
10. C	60. B	110. D	160. A	210. A	260. D	310. D	360. D
11. B	61. B	111. C	161. E	211. A	261. C	311. D	361. B
12. B	62. C	112. C	162. C	212. A	262. B	312. C	362. B
13. C	63. B	113. D	163. D	213. A	263. D	313. B	363. C
14. E	64. D	114. B	164. E	214. D	264. E	314. B	364. C
15. B	65. D	115. A	165. B	215. D	265. C	315. E	365. A
16. A	66. B	116. C	166. C	216. A	266. D	316. D	366. B
17. C	67. A	117. A	167. A	217. C	267. D	317. B	367. D
18. A	68. A	118. E	168. B	218. A	268. E	318. D	368. D
19. C	69. B	119. C	169. D	219. D	269. E	319. C	369. E
20. B	70. C	120. D	170. C	220. A	270. E	320. B	370. B
21. B	71. B	121. D	171. D	221. C	271. B	321. C	371. B
22. D	72. B	122. E	172. C	222. B	272. E	322. B	372. B
23. A	73. D	123. C	173. A	223. D	273. E	323. C	373. D
24. D	74. C	124. B	174. A	224. C	274. B	324. C	374. B
25. B	75. B	125. B	175. B	225. D	275. A	325. E	375. D
26. E	76. C	126. A	176. C	226. A	276. B	326. E	376. B
27. E	77. C	127. E	177. D	227. D	277. D	327. C	377. B
28. A	78. A	128. B	178. A	228. A	278. B	328. D	378. D
29. E	79. C	129. B	179. E	229. E	279. A	329. D	379. B
30. A	80. A	130. B	180. B	230. D	280. E	330. A	380. C
31. C	81. B	131. A	181. E	231. A	281. B	331. A	381. B
32. D	82. C	132. C	182. E	232. C	282. C	332. B	382. B
33. A	83. A	133. D	183. C	233. E	283. B	333. A	383. B
34. B	84. C	134. B	184. C	234. A	284. A	334. C	384. C
35. D	85. A	135. C	185. C	235. A	285. D	335. E	385. B
36. C	86. B	136. D	186. C	236. D	286. A	336. C	386. B
37. A	87. B	137. C	187. E	237. A	287. A	337. A	387. B
38. C	88. C	138. C	188. B	238. D	288. C	338. B	388. E
39. D	89. E	139. C	189. B	239. A	289. B	339. D	389. A
40. D	90. A	140. B	190. D	240. E	290. D	340. B	390. D
41. A	91. B	141. B	191. B	241. E	291. B	341. D	391. D
42. E	92. B	142. B	192. D	242. B	292. D	342. C	392. B
43. A	93. B	143. D	193. D	243. E	293. D	343. E	393. C
44. B	94. C	144. B	194. A	244. A	294. C	344. E	394. B
45. E	95. D	145. B	195. B	245. C	295. A	345. A	395. B
46. E	96. C	146. D	196. A	246. C	296. B	346. D	396. A
47. D	97. C	147. C	197. B	247. D	297. B	347. C	397. C
48. A	98. E	148. E	198. B	248. E	298. E	348. E	398. D
49. C	99. C	149. B	199. B	249. C	299. A	349. D	399. C
50. E	100. E	150. C	200. D	250. D	300. D	350. D	400. B

FOCUS Psychiatry Review (Volume 2): Blank Answer Sheet

1. ____	51. ____	101. ____	151. ____	201. ____	251. ____	301. ____	351. ____
2. ____	52. ____	102. ____	152. ____	202. ____	252. ____	302. ____	352. ____
3. ____	53. ____	103. ____	153. ____	203. ____	253. ____	303. ____	353. ____
4. ____	54. ____	104. ____	154. ____	204. ____	254. ____	304. ____	354. ____
5. ____	55. ____	105. ____	155. ____	205. ____	255. ____	305. ____	355. ____
6. ____	56. ____	106. ____	156. ____	206. ____	256. ____	306. ____	356. ____
7. ____	57. ____	107. ____	157. ____	207. ____	257. ____	307. ____	357. ____
8. ____	58. ____	108. ____	158. ____	208. ____	258. ____	308. ____	358. ____
9. ____	59. ____	109. ____	159. ____	209. ____	259. ____	309. ____	359. ____
10. ____	60. ____	110. ____	160. ____	210. ____	260. ____	310. ____	360. ____
11. ____	61. ____	111. ____	161. ____	211. ____	261. ____	311. ____	361. ____
12. ____	62. ____	112. ____	162. ____	212. ____	262. ____	312. ____	362. ____
13. ____	63. ____	113. ____	163. ____	213. ____	263. ____	313. ____	363. ____
14. ____	64. ____	114. ____	164. ____	214. ____	264. ____	314. ____	364. ____
15. ____	65. ____	115. ____	165. ____	215. ____	265. ____	315. ____	365. ____
16. ____	66. ____	116. ____	166. ____	216. ____	266. ____	316. ____	366. ____
17. ____	67. ____	117. ____	167. ____	217. ____	267. ____	317. ____	367. ____
18. ____	68. ____	118. ____	168. ____	218. ____	268. ____	318. ____	368. ____
19. ____	69. ____	119. ____	169. ____	219. ____	269. ____	319. ____	369. ____
20. ____	70. ____	120. ____	170. ____	220. ____	270. ____	320. ____	370. ____
21. ____	71. ____	121. ____	171. ____	221. ____	271. ____	321. ____	371. ____
22. ____	72. ____	122. ____	172. ____	222. ____	272. ____	322. ____	372. ____
23. ____	73. ____	123. ____	173. ____	223. ____	273. ____	323. ____	373. ____
24. ____	74. ____	124. ____	174. ____	224. ____	274. ____	324. ____	374. ____
25. ____	75. ____	125. ____	175. ____	225. ____	275. ____	325. ____	375. ____
26. ____	76. ____	126. ____	176. ____	226. ____	276. ____	326. ____	376. ____
27. ____	77. ____	127. ____	177. ____	227. ____	277. ____	327. ____	377. ____
28. ____	78. ____	128. ____	178. ____	228. ____	278. ____	328. ____	378. ____
29. ____	79. ____	129. ____	179. ____	229. ____	279. ____	329. ____	379. ____
30. ____	80. ____	130. ____	180. ____	230. ____	280. ____	330. ____	380. ____
31. ____	81. ____	131. ____	181. ____	231. ____	281. ____	331. ____	381. ____
32. ____	82. ____	132. ____	182. ____	232. ____	282. ____	332. ____	382. ____
33. ____	83. ____	133. ____	183. ____	233. ____	283. ____	333. ____	383. ____
34. ____	84. ____	134. ____	184. ____	234. ____	284. ____	334. ____	384. ____
35. ____	85. ____	135. ____	185. ____	235. ____	285. ____	335. ____	385. ____
36. ____	86. ____	136. ____	186. ____	236. ____	286. ____	336. ____	386. ____
37. ____	87. ____	137. ____	187. ____	237. ____	287. ____	337. ____	387. ____
38. ____	88. ____	138. ____	188. ____	238. ____	288. ____	338. ____	388. ____
39. ____	89. ____	139. ____	189. ____	239. ____	289. ____	339. ____	389. ____
40. ____	90. ____	140. ____	190. ____	240. ____	290. ____	340. ____	390. ____
41. ____	91. ____	141. ____	191. ____	241. ____	291. ____	341. ____	391. ____
42. ____	92. ____	142. ____	192. ____	242. ____	292. ____	342. ____	392. ____
43. ____	93. ____	143. ____	193. ____	243. ____	293. ____	343. ____	393. ____
44. ____	94. ____	144. ____	194. ____	244. ____	294. ____	344. ____	394. ____
45. ____	95. ____	145. ____	195. ____	245. ____	295. ____	345. ____	395. ____
46. ____	96. ____	146. ____	196. ____	246. ____	296. ____	346. ____	396. ____
47. ____	97. ____	147. ____	197. ____	247. ____	297. ____	347. ____	397. ____
48. ____	98. ____	148. ____	198. ____	248. ____	298. ____	348. ____	398. ____
49. ____	99. ____	149. ____	199. ____	249. ____	299. ____	349. ____	399. ____
50. ____	100. ____	150. ____	200. ____	250. ____	300. ____	350. ____	400. ____

Index of Questions by Topic

This index provides a guide for review of questions by topic area. Many questions apply to more than one topic area but are indexed by a single topic.